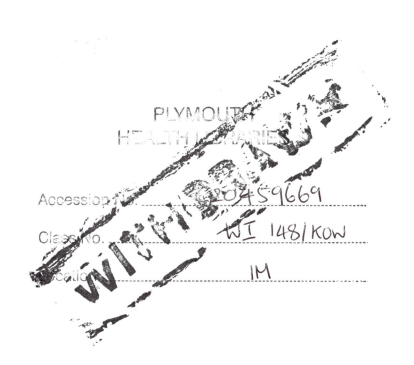

ATLAS OF COMPLICATED ABDOMINAL EMERGENCIES

**Tips on Laparoscopic and
Open Surgery, Therapeutic Endoscopy
and Interventional Radiology**

ATLAS OF COMPLICATED ABDOMINAL EMERGENCIES

Tips on Laparoscopic and Open Surgery, Therapeutic Endoscopy and Interventional Radiology

Edited by

Ti Thiow Kong
Davide Lomanto

National University Hospital, Singapore & National University of Singapore, Singapore

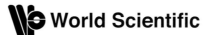

World Scientific

NEW JERSEY · LONDON · SINGAPORE · BEIJING · SHANGHAI · HONG KONG · TAIPEI · CHENNAI

Published by

World Scientific Publishing Co. Pte. Ltd.

5 Toh Tuck Link, Singapore 596224

USA office: 27 Warren Street, Suite 401-402, Hackensack, NJ 07601

UK office: 57 Shelton Street, Covent Garden, London WC2H 9HE

Library of Congress Control Number: 2014934356

British Library Cataloguing-in-Publication Data
A catalogue record for this book is available from the British Library.

ATLAS OF COMPLICATED ABDOMINAL EMERGENCIES
Tips on Laparoscopic and Open Surgery, Therapeutic Endoscopy and Interventional Radiology
With DVD-ROM

ISBN 978-981-4412-14-8

Typeset by Stallion Press
Email: enquiries@stallionpress.com

Printed by FuIsland Offset Printing (S) Pte Ltd Singapore

Dedication

To our teachers, students and colleagues everywhere who strive to provide best care
for patients with abdominal emergencies.

Acknowledgements

Grateful thanks to Aslam Bashir for the artwork, Lilian Ng-Quek, Cecilia Chao, Hasbalela bte Hassan, Ann Paul and June Terng for secretarial assistance.

Foreword

by

Professor Lee Chuen Neng
Chair, University Surgical Cluster
National University Health System
Head, Department of Surgery,
National University of Singapore

Associate Professor Benjamin Ong
Chief Executive
National University Health System, Singapore
Senior Vice President (Health Affairs)
National University of Singapore

Professor Sydney Chung Sheung Chee
Yeoh Ghim Seng Visiting Professor
National University of Singapore

Sir Roy Calne
Emeritus Professor of Surgery
University of Cambridge Fellow of Trinity Hall
University of Cambridge Yeoh Ghim Seng
Professor of Surgery
National University of Singapore
18 Trumpington Road
Cambridge, CB2 2AS UK

Lee Chuen Neng

A key role of an academic Department of Surgery is to teach. Recent and continued advances in technology have greatly impacted the therapeutic options in patient care. This ever changing standard of care requires guidance from experienced clinician–teachers.

Publication of this book is a milestone of our Academic Medical Center: The National University Health System, Singapore.

It is a multi-disciplinary work of surgeons, radiologists, gynecologists, gastroenterologists and Accident and Emergency specialists. It is a work that reflects the evolution of therapeutic avenues now available to our patients.

The authors, ably led by Professors Ti Thiow Kong and Davide Lomanto have presented an excellent resource of reference standards for all involved in the care of patients with abdominal emergencies.

This succinct update of the current multi-modality approach is excellent reading.

It will become a definitive work in the field and will certainly help save lives and improve patient outcomes.

By writing a book, we also focus our mind on the subject and learn in the process.

The desire to continue to learn is essential for us to be a world leader in patient care.

I encourage everyone to publish and examine our processes of care and the impact of new technology on choice of therapeutic options.

When we teach, or make the effort to write a book on treatment, we multiply our personal capability beyond treating one patient at a time.

Benjamin Ong

I am pleased to pen a few thoughts on what I personally feel is a timely publication drawing from the talent and vast experience of the Department of Surgery of the Yong Loo Lin School of Medicine at the National University of Singapore.

Less invasive techniques have increasingly become default and mainstream procedures and open surgery utilised less even in emergent settings. Hence I believe there is a particular need for this insightful book which covers the indications and techniques in the multi-modality approach that is vital when doctors confronted with complicated abdominal emergencies. Perusing the chapters, the book is organised in an intuitive manner centred around clinical presentations — an emphasis that is apt.

I am confident that this book will not only become a valued guide to residents and surgical trainees in the 21st century, but will be counted as a reference text for surgical consultants and practitioners in their care of patients with complicated abdominal emergencies.

The editors have assembled these book contributors not only from the NUHS University Surgical Cluster but also NUHS gastroenterologists as well as an interventional radiologist and a gynecologist. The combined experience of these experts has been integrated in a well organised and high quality reference book.

Sydney Chung Sheung Chee

The last few decades have seen many important advances that radically changed the management of patients with the acute abdomen. Notable examples include endoscopic therapy for patients with biliary sepsis and stones, intravascular embolisation for bleeding and laparoscopic surgery for cholecystitis and appendicitis. Computed tomography is now routine and exploratory laparotomy has become a thing of the past. Even patients with appendicitis, the veritable test of surgical acumen of yesteryear, will have their diagnosis confirmed on CT before going to the operating theatre.

With increasing sub-specialisation the surgical consultant on-call is unlikely to personally have all the skills needed to treat the patients admitted under his care. His role is no longer "the port of last call" for his patients, but rather a triage point where he has to decide whether to summon help, and if so which one of his multi-disciplinary colleagues to call in. To make this decision wisely he needs to be honest about his own ability, know what surgical specialists in other fields can offer, and understand the capabilities and limitations of therapeutic endoscopy and interventional radiology.

This book, written by the multi-disciplinary team at the National University Hospital in Singapore, describes the current practice in 2012. It is a useful reference of the possible diagnostic and therapeutic options available for patients with abdominal emergencies, and reflects the high standard of clinical care at that hospital.

Multi-disciplinary care does not mean management by a committee. The surgeon, under whose care the patient is admitted, must maintain overall authority and responsibility. The results of surgery, just like those of therapeutic endoscopy and interventional radiology, are highly dependent on the skill of the operator. Clinical guidelines are based on published data, which tend to be produced by expert exponents of that particular technique in centers of excellence. The surgeon with an ill patient in the emergency room must take into account the availability of facilities and expertise locally, and exercise common sense in deciding whether published guidelines are relevant in his particular case. For patients with acute abdominal emergencies, time is often of essence. One must not let sophisticated technology delay life saving surgery. To have a precise diagnosis prior to going to theatre is all very well, but remember the CT scanner can be the "tunnel of death" for a rapidly exsanguinating patient.

Roy Calne

I congratulate the editors and contributors of this book which will be of aid on many occasions to young doctors working in the emergency centres of the future.

As specialisation increases so emergency medicine and surgery has become the "Cinderella" of medical care which is especially apparent at weekends. A recent UK study showed that the chances of a fatal outcome after presentation at hospital were considerably higher at weekends than during the week. The super-specialist does not wish to be on call and is often not competent to cope with the wide spectrum of conditions that may require urgent resuscitation.

In my surgical teaching round on a Saturday morning, I would take the students to two or three patients and each student was expected to have an individual responsibility for his or her personal patients. The student would then present, in a formal manner, the case history and demonstrate the physical signs of the patient. On one occasion, we considered a man in his 50s with abdominal pain who had come into hospital for observation. On admission, he was tender in the mid-abdomen, but other findings were negative. The patient being admitted on Friday, the surgical team looking after him changed for the weekend and the new surgical registrar saw the patient on his rounds and noted that the abdominal pain seemed to be worse, but since an abdominal scan had been ordered by the previous team, he felt that this was reasonable management as the vital signs had not deteriorated. In the course of my teaching round it was clear that the patient was in considerable pain and distress, his abdominal pain was much worse and he had muscular rigidity and a silent abdomen. I asked the student looking after him what he felt should be done and he reminded me that the scan had been ordered and presumably would be performed on Monday morning. I suggested that this was now an inappropriate course to take, especially since the scanning department would be reluctant to scan a corpse. I arranged for the patient to have an immediate laparotomy, which I performed myself as no-one else with competence in abdominal surgery was around, and found and dealt with a perforated duodenal ulcer. On the next round, I did try and explain to the students that the "dimension of time" is extremely important in disease and an acute abdominal emergency can change from mild symptoms to a life-threatening condition in a matter of hours. Since that ward-round, the British surgical training system has been sabotaged by regulations from Europe, which do not permit one of the most important duties of doctors, namely to look after patients in continuity, instead of according to the clock. The other transformation that has been extremely rapid is ever-increasing specialisation. In the dim and distant past when I trained in surgery, I was trained to be able to handle abdominal emergencies, aneurisms, acutely ischaemic legs and abscesses in most parts of the body, based on the careful history and the eliciting of physical signs. Above all we were repeatedly reminded that we should never neglect careful and attentive listening to the patient and only to use the laboratory and the X-ray department as a back-up.

No doubt covering such a wide field of surgery, with hindsight our competence in each area could be questioned. We now have narrow and exclusive specialisation so that for instance a professional life devoted to surgery of the knee is common and accepted. This requires extreme detailed knowledge of the anatomy and physiology of the knee and how to use the latest endoscopic instruments to effect appropriate management with minimal trauma. A surgeon trained for the knee will seldom stray from this territory. Even orthopaedic conditions occurring in other parts of the body or in children may be "off limits".

A good case can be made for a complete reorganisation of the medical curriculum to enable early specialisation and avoid time spent to studies irrelevant to the speciality in question. So how can we give the patient the best care for serious trauma and abdominal emergencies? To have appropriate staff available in every general hospital is extremely expensive and probably unnecessary. The "bullet has to be bitten" that the patient and the patient's relatives may need to travel longer distances to get the best care, available in a few fully staffed emergency units. In these centres, there would be on 24 hour duty an abdominal, vascular and trauma surgeon, a physician to handle medical emergencies, an experienced anaesthetist, a conventional and interventional radiologist and a team that can provide appropriate scanning. Also needed are sufficient available fully-staffed operating theatres and intensive-care beds. None of this comes cheaply and a great many patients who present at an emergency centre have only trivial disorders. We need to provide safe care for the patient who may appear reasonably healthy but is nevertheless at the beginning of a severe and dangerous condition, where the gravity of the illness can accelerate with alarming speed. For example, a child with a fever and headache, who starts to develop rose spots. Every year we hear of such cases where the patient has been sent home by an inexperienced doctor, without the benefits of the opinion of a practitioner, who realises that the patient is seriously ill and administers penicillin in sufficient doses immediately. To manage this problem a form of triage is essential with a senior nurse on duty who can deal with minor trauma, upset stomachs, drunks and other conditions not requiring admission, but can direct patients with obvious serious emergency conditions to the appropriate specialist in the emergency unit, who is capable of managing the patient or, if indicated, rapidly contacting a specialist colleague "on call". For patients causing concern, without a diagnosis, there should be observation beds so the patients can be under careful surveillance with repeated recording of vital statistics and any changes in the patient's complaints until the natural history of the case is revealed.

This may all sound too idealistic, but if sufficient resources are devoted to a few high quality centres, such facilities could be made available in most developed countries. The training of staff suitable for the emergency facility needs to be carefully worked out and available to young doctors, some of whom will find this kind of work challenging, exciting and rewarding, providing a chance for a wide medical and surgical education. Just as a postscript, the surgical and anaesthetic team at the emergency unit should be capable of removing organs for transplantation, in accordance with the law, from patients who were bought in dead or who die soon after admission.

This book is timely and should be available and will be of great practical value to those working in emergency centres.

Preface

During the past decades, the management of "abdominal emergencies" is no longer the prerogative of surgeons. With advancing technological innovations and skills, the "surgical abdomen" is now increasingly managed by endoscopists and interventional radiologists. Minimally invasive surgery has further reduced the role of open surgery.

Thus, progress made in the pathogenesis and therapeutics of peptic ulcer disease and endoscopic arrest of ulcer haemorrhage has minimized the need for gastric surgery. ERCP extraction of ductal biliary calculi has made surgical exploration of the bile duct rarely necessary. Interventional radiology has achieved equally impressive progress, especially with TIPSS in the control of variceal haemorrhage, vascular emergencies and in the drainage of purulent abdominal collections.

Nevertheless, prompt surgery continues to be the only life-saving option in patients suffering from bowel perforation, gangrenous viscera, and severe traumatic injuries.

Additionally, surgery has a salvage role when endoscopic or radiological intervention fails. Realistically, a successful outcome would only be achievable if referral to the attending surgeon is timely and not delayed until the patient is moribund!

The attending surgeon has to be well trained. This is becoming problematical in the present era of sub-specialisation. It has been helpful that Sir Roy Calne, in our book's "Foreword," has thoughtfully alluded to how this dilemma could be solved.

At the National University Hospital, emergencies are initially managed at the Accident and Emergency Department. The attending surgeon on call has the option of referring patients to surgeons in other specialties who all participate in emergency care. A common roster of gastroenterologists and surgeons provide emergency endoscopic skills, while an emergency interventional radiological service is also available.

Our experience has been that the best interest of the patient is served by conversation and close collaboration amongst members of the care giver team. This necessitates that each team member (trainee or consultant) is not only proficient in his/her specialty but also keeps abreast of the best practice in allied disciplines.

This book has been written to promote such a holistic approach. Emergency physicians, gastroenterologists, interventional radiologists and surgeons of all specialties in the National University Health System share their experience in the present book. Through a step-by-step narrative and an abundance of medical illustrations, the contributors impart to the reader how best to perform and overcome difficulties encountered in the management of complicated abdominal emergencies.

It is hoped that this single volume would serve as a convenient companion manual for all emergency care-givers. To enhance learning, a CD-ROM showing snippets from a number of procedures is provided with each book.

We are indeed happy that the publication of this book in 2013 coincides with the centennial celebration of our National University of Singapore Department of Surgery.

Editors

Ti Thiow Kong, MBBS, MD, FRCS, FRACS, FRCSE ad hominen
Emeritus Consultant, National University Hospital
Professorial Fellow (formerly Professor of Surgery)
National University of Singapore

Davide Lomanto, MD, PhD, FAMS (Surgery)
Associate Professor, National University of Singapore
Director, Khoo Teck Puat Advanced Surgery Training Centre
National University Hospital

Contents

DVD-ROM of Laparoscopic Procedures
Dmitrii Dolgunov, Wijerathne Sujith and Iyer Shridhar Ganpathi

Chapter 1

Role of the Accident & Emergency Department

Chiu Li Qi* and Malcolm R. Mahadevan*

Abdominal pain makes up 5% of all emergency department (ED) presentations. Despite our best efforts, a quarter of our patients are discharged and a third admitted with a label of undifferentiated abdominal pain. The challenges of evaluating an abdominal pain patient in the ED are multiple and include a heterogeneous population, benign conditions and life-threatening ones, intra-abdominal and even extra-abdominal ailments. This is compounded by the fact that most associated symptoms lack specificity and atypical presentations are not uncommon.

At the core of each evaluation is the question as to whether the patient has a life-threatening condition. The emergency physician EP is often placed in the untenable position of making a rapid assessment and instituting preliminary treatment with nothing more than clinical acumen and limited investigations. This makes rapid diagnosis and assessment of the critically ill patient quite challenging. Evaluation of the patient with abdominal pain usually proceeds along two lines — pain of traumatic or non-traumatic etiologies. The aims of this introductory chapter are: recognition of the sick patient, assessment of abdominal pain in trauma and non-traumatic conditions, and indications for surgical consultation.

Recognition of the Sick Patient

Recognition of the sick patient starts off with an awareness of the deceptively "well-looking" patient.

Young patients have larger physiologic reserves and may show little or no signs of haemodynamic instability when they first present. The elderly, on the other hand, partly because of communication challenges, atypical presentations and stoicism, may present with seemingly benign complaints while harbouring serious disease.

The fundamentals of recognising an ill patient should begin with an assessment of the vital signs. Hyperpyrexia (temperature >38.5°C), hypotension (relative hypotension) or orthostatic hypotension, tachycardia out of proportion to the expected, and tachypnoea are all causes of concern. Pain, commonly referred to as the fifth vital sign, should also be taken into serious consideration. Point-of-care testing is valuable in the unmasking of the ill patient. High base deficits in trauma patients at admission have been correlated with increased likelihood of early transfusion, increased ICU and hospital stays and an increased risk of shock-related complications.[1] Lactate, a product of anaerobic metabolism, is an indicator of hypoperfusion. It is useful to identify patients who present with apparent normal vital signs, such as in early phases of sepsis or trauma.[2] Serial measurement of lactate, assessing clearance, can be used to measure the effectiveness of resuscitation and prediction of mortality reduction.[3] Special attention should be given to abdominal pain in specific populations, namely paediatric, the elderly, immunocompromised and obstetrics. It is not uncommon for these unique groups to present with subtle and unusual presentations.

*L.Q. Chiu, MBBS, MCEM (UK), M Med (Emerg Med) Registrar and M.R. Mahadevan, MBBS, FRCP(Ed), FRCS(Ed), FAMS Chief & Associate Professor, Department of Emergency Medicine, National University Hospital, Singapore.

Approach to Non-traumatic Abdominal Pain

In the ED assessment of patients presenting with abdominal pain, the origin remains unknown in half of the patients despite evaluation. This is the diagnosis provided the workup has ruled out life-threatening diagnoses. Figure 1.1 is a schematic representation of one approach to abdominal pain.

In the traditional approach to abdominal pain, the physician proceeds with a history and physical examination. Contrary to the belief that there is a fixed history template for abdominal pain, each physician's "script" for abdominal pain is expected to constantly evolve as the patient encounters progress.

Four key concepts would include:

i) Nature of pain and its characteristics
ii) Other medical and surgical history (inclusive of medication history)
iii) Associated symptoms
iv) Pertinent negatives

It is important to discern somatic from visceral pain. Pain originating from intra-abdominal organs is crampy and dull. It originates from capsules of solid organs and stretching of hollow viscera due to distension, ischaemia or inflammation. Patients are unable to localise it well. Associated symptoms are that of autonomic response that cause diaphoresis, nausea, pallor, etc. Somatic pain arises from the parietal peritoneum that is inflamed. The patient is able to localise it well and frequently describes it as a sharp pain exacerbated by movement. Other key concerns regarding pain include the timing of onset, mode of onset, severity, location and migration, and progression.

The medical and surgical history should focus on important co-morbidities (which might suggest an extra-abdominal source of pain), history of previous surgeries, sexual activity, occupation, immunosuppression and psychosocial history. Having obtained a focused history, the attending physician is likely to reach a preliminary diagnosis. At this point, pertinent negatives should also be sought, further narrowing down the list of differentials.

A focused physical examination is often all that can be done in a resuscitation. It serves to confirm suspicions from the history, localise the area of disease and to avoid missing extra-abdominal causes of pain. The main focus is to rapidly rule out possible life-threatening causes of abdominal pain. Important findings sought

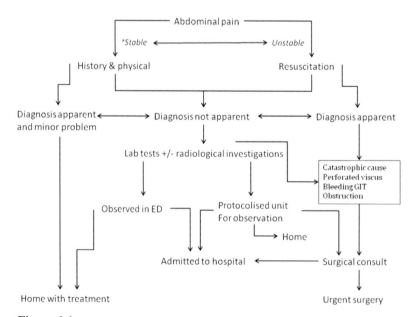

Figure 1.1.

Decision tree in the evaluation of abdominal pain in the ED.

*Stable: BP > 90/60 mmHg, no signs of shock/hyperlactaemia/severe metabolic acidosis.

include abdominal distension, guarding, rebound, pulsatile abdominal masses and blood on digital rectal examination. In the elderly and obese, findings of peritonism may be subtle and difficult to illicit. Some helpful manoeuvres include having the patient cough, jump or simply shaking the examination trolley. Examination of the cardiorespiratory system inclusive of peripheral pulses, as well as external genitalia of the patient are also important aspects of the physical examination and not to be missed.

Table 1.1 shows a possible schema of differential diagnoses.

Abdominal emergencies in the ED can be divided into a few major categories, namely: the catastrophic abdominal emergency, visceral perforation, bleeding gastrointestinal tract and intestinal obstruction. The next section provides an approach to identification, assessment and resuscitation of these patients.

Examples of catastrophic abdominal emergencies would be ruptured/leaking abdominal aortic aneurysm, ruptured hepatocellular carcinoma or other tumours. In such instances, the patient more often than not presents in extremis and severe pain. History

Table 1.1.

Etiologies of Abdominal Pain

Solid Organs	Hollow viscus
Includes: liver, spleen, pancreas, urogenital systems (including hernias), pregnancy and complications	Includes: stomach, small and large intestines, gall bladder
Causes: capsular stretch, inflammation, infection, and infarction	Causes: wall inflammation/erosion, infection, torsion or obstruction, distension
Vascular	**Extra-abdominal**
Causes: congestion, ischaemia e.g. hepatomegaly from venous congestion, abdominal aortic aneurysm, mesenteric ischaemia, solid organ infarction	Includes: cardiac, pulmonary, musculoskeletal system e.g. myocardial ischaemia, basal pneumonia, psoas abscess, herpes zoster, hip pathology
Others	**Trauma**
Acute porphyria	Traumatic causes
Diabetic ketoacidosis	Foreign bodies
Poisoning, e.g. lead poisoning	
Hypercalcaemia	

may be limited in these patients. Significant findings on examination include pallor, a distended, tender abdomen with/without guarding, unequal pulses, or a pulsatile abdominal mass. Patients with hepatocellular carcinoma often bear stigmata of chronic liver disease. Rapid assessment with bedside ultrasound allows visualisation of free intra-abdominal fluid, aortic dissection flap/false lumen, dilated abdominal aorta, liver parenchyma and significant hepatic lesions (Fig. 1.1). If the patient is stable enough, the diagnosis may be confirmed with a CT scan or CT aortogram, both of which are helpful in planning for surgery. Resuscitation is aimed at replacement of blood and blood products, ionotropic support and prompt surgical review.

In the assessment of a patient with possible perforation, a good history may reveal a change in nature and intensity of the patient's pain, accompanied by rapid development of new symptoms such as distension, fever, and generalised abdominal pain. In fact, some of these patients present to the ED with undifferentiated abdominal pain but develop a perforation during assessment or observation. This emphasises the importance of periodic review of patients even after initial assessment. Classical teaching is that of a tender, rigid and "board-like" abdomen on examination. However, this is not always present, especially if the patient is elderly or obese. Bowel sounds may also appear absent or sluggish. Contrary to traditional teaching in which analgesia is withheld with the belief that it would mask the pain from an acute abdomen, it has now been shown that adequate analgesia improves patient comfort, facilitates abdominal examination and does not result in misdiagnosis. Occasionally, erect chest X-rays or abdominal X-rays might reveal free intra-peritoneal air. These findings are fairly specific but not sensitive. In patients where clinical suspicion is high, but plain X-rays do not reveal any abnormalities, the EP may decide on further imaging, usually in the form of CT scans. The sensitivity of CT scan in picking up free intra-peritoneal air is much greater. At this juncture, where there is a diagnostic dilemma, a surgical consult is usually obtained.

Significant bleeding from the gastrointestinal tract (GIT) is usually obvious. However, in patients where a bleeding GIT is suspected, there are two issues — identification of the presence and source of bleeding, and estimation of the risk of significant re-bleeding. A digital rectal examination may be beneficial in differentiating fresh or stale melaena (indicative of upper GIT bleeding) from haematochezia (indicative of lower GIT bleeding). The insertion of a gastric tube, followed by aspiration, may be used to assess the significance of upper gastrointestinal tract bleeding, though this is neither sensitive nor specific. The risk of re-bleeding and the need for an early endoscopy can be assessed by the Rockall and Glasgow-Blatchford scores, respectively. The management of the haemodynamically unstable bleeding patient is a challenge. Apart from resuscitation with fluids and blood products, administration of medications such as intravenous proton-pump inhibitors and somatostatin, the definitive step is early activation of the surgical team for emergent endoscopy or operative intervention, or the interventional radiologist for angiogram and embolisation.

Intestinal obstruction and its complications of gangrene and perforation is the fourth major group of abdominal emergencies. The history may reveal patients with risks factors for intestinal obstruction, e.g. those with previous abdominal surgery, the elderly with megacolon, etc., who present with symptoms of abdominal distension, vomiting or obstipation. Physical examination may also reveal a distended abdomen with hyperactive bowel sounds. In cases of subacute obstruction, signs and symptoms may be more subtle. Examination should focus on the aetiology of the obstruction and determine if complications such as perforation have occurred. Examination of the hernial orifices for incarcerated hernias is a vital part of patient assessment. The most useful investigation is erect and supine abdominal films which can confirm the diagnosis and sometimes reveal the underlying cause of obstruction. Management of such patients involves fluid resuscitation, gut decompression, parenteral antibiotics, determination of cause of obstruction and identification of any complications. Most uncomplicated intestinal obstructions secondary to post-operative adhesions, or pseudo-obstruction due to electrolyte imbalances, may be managed conservatively. However, cases of mechanical obstruction, especially with bowel ischaemia or perforation will require early surgical review, further imaging and operative intervention.

In a resuscitation scenario, the traditional approach is abandoned for a "treat-first, then assess" approach. Resuscitation is carried out parallel to a focused physical examination with minimal supplementary history. The EP must be cognizant of rapidly changing patient conditions and work with ever changing probabilities. If a given treatment does not work, then the EP needs to consider that his diagnosis is wrong or that the patient is still decompensated. This is perhaps the greatest challenge for the EP. Figure 1.2 shows an approach towards the unstable patient with abdominal pain.

The observational unit, a short stay ward, is the third disposition possible for a select group of patients. An example is a patient with right iliac fossa pain. If the

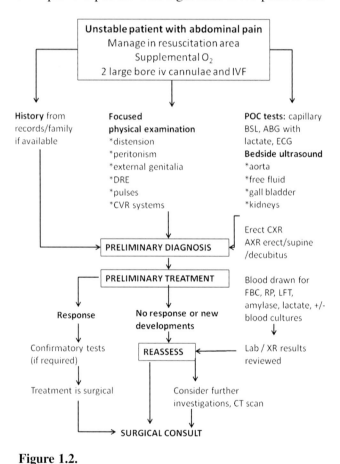

Figure 1.2.

An approach towards an unstable patient with abdominal pain.

ABG: arterial blood gas; BSL: blood sugar level; DRE: digital rectal examination; FBC: full blood count; IVF: intravenous fluids; LFT: liver function test; RP: renal panel.

patient has low to moderate probability of acute appendicitis based on the Alvarado scoring, they are observed with serial abdominal examinations. When symptoms progress, the patients are either scheduled for a CT scan of the abdomen, or referred to the surgeon for review. These pathways allow the physician to determine who to hospitalise while still maintaining patient safety.

Approach to Traumatic Abdominal Pain

An approach to abdominal pain in trauma is embodied in the principles of Advanced Trauma Life Support (ATLS). This is a team based approach comprising of often more than one EP, trauma surgeons, nurses, radiographers and hospital porters. This ensures maximal resources to facilitate assessment and management of the trauma patient. The principles of ATLS include primary and secondary surveys. Although described sequentially, evaluation, identification of injuries and resuscitation is almost always performed simultaneously. Approach to traumatic abdominal pain focuses on two issues: haemodynamic status of patient and nature of injury i.e. blunt vs. penetrating injury.

Important immediate investigations include a Focused Assessment with Sonography for Trauma (FAST) examination for any free fluid in the abdominal cavities, blood gas analysis for base excess, lactate levels, and a trauma series of X-rays (Fig. 1.3). Other important investigations include a full blood count, group and cross match, coagulation profile, blood biochemistries and urinalysis. Based on clinical suspicion, other modalities such as CT-scans and CT-angiograms may also be utilised.

Interventions for all trauma resuscitations focus on preventing the "triad of death" — hypothermia, acidosis and coagulopathy. Most EDs are equipped with warmed saline and warming blankets. Most have massive transfusion protocols in place to allow rapid activation and retrieval of blood and blood products. Expeditious care may also require anaesthetists to standby to receive the trauma patient for surgery.

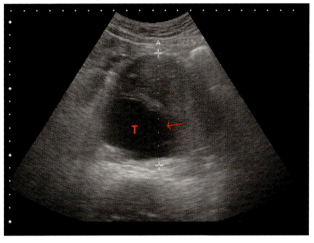

"T" showing true lumen for the abdominal aorta

Figure 1.3.

Bedside ultrasound of a 77-year-old presenting with hypotension and abdominal pain, showing a dissecting abdominal aortic aneurysm.

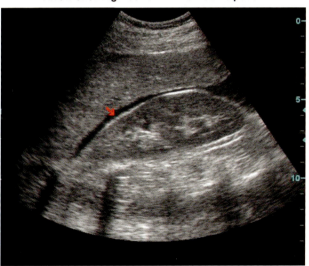

Arrow showing free fluid in Morrison's pouch

Figure 1.4.

FAST examination in a 24-year-old motorcyclist who skidded and hit the road barrier, showing free fluid in Morrison's pouch.

Ancillary Investigations in the ED

Tests ordered in the evaluation of the patient with abdominal pain should focus on confirming or excluding specific diagnoses on the working differential. Apart from the usual tests of full blood count and its differentials, liver and metabolic panels, amylase, etc., other useful tests include blood gas analysis with/without lactate, capillary blood glucose levels, electrocardiogram, X-rays and bedside ultrasound. An ECG may very well be the first investigation alluding to myocardial ischaemia as a cause of the patient's complaints. In summary, the EP selects only investigations of immediate and pertinent value, which will aid in diagnosis of his patient and rule out potential life-threatening differentials.

Indications for Referral

The EP must be aware of the extent of his and the department's capabilities. The surgical and emergency departments with their respective specialties and experiences, often complement each other. Therefore, there should be no hesitation in obtaining a surgical consult should there be a need. Such instances arise in three circumstances: i.e. the need for therapeutic expertise, diagnostic dilemmas, and any trauma resuscitation. In all patients with conditions where a surgical procedure is expected, an early liaison with the surgical team leads to earlier treatment and better outcomes. In patients where preliminary examination and investigations do not yield any obvious findings but who have suspected surgical aetiologies of pain, a surgical review may shed light on the underlying pathology. In all trauma resuscitations, there is strong evidence of improved outcomes with a team-based approach.

The EP who is prudent and well-informed of epidemiology and clinical presentations of patients will be successful in the evaluation of most patients with abdominal pain. This should be supported by up-to-date knowledge of the strengths and limitations of laboratory and imaging investigations, to ensure timely diagnosis and effective management of the patients.

References

1. Davis JW, Parks SN, Kaups KL, *et al.* (1996) Admission base deficit predicts transfusion requirements and risk of complications. *J Trauma* **41**: 769–74.

2. Asimos AW, Gibbs MA, Marx JA, *et al.* (2000) Value of point-of-care blood testing in emergent trauma management. *J Trauma* **48**(6): 1101–08.

3. Shapiro NI, Howel MD, Talmor D, *et al.* (2005) Serum lactate as a predictor of mortality in emergency department patients with infection. *Ann Emerg Med* **45**(5): 524–28.

Chapter 2

Perioperative Management of Patients with Complicated Abdominal Emergencies

Ngiam Kee Yuan*

Patients with complicated abdominal emergencies invariably present with sepsis and/or shock due to the perforated bowel contents and haemorrhage, respectively. Resuscitation and perioperative management aim to restore the physiology of the patient in preparation for surgery and hence to optimise the outcomes of intervention.

Assessment and resuscitation may be carried out according to the Basic Cardiac Life Support (BCLS) algorithm and Advanced Trauma Life Support (ATLS) as the default management algorithm for trauma patients.

The end point of all algorithms is to stabilise the patient sufficiently for definitive surgical management in patients who need it. The end points of resuscitation need to be defined and met in order to give the patient the best opportunity to undergo and survive, an emergency abdominal surgery. Sometimes it may not be possible to meet these end points of resuscitation, and this therefore dictates the operative approach (for example, damage control surgery vs. definitive surgery).

Shock and Organ Perfusion

In patients who present with shock, it is important to distinguish the type of shock (distributive or obstructive) and the severity of shock (Table 2.1). Typically, all patients with shock will receive 1–2 litres of crystalloids as an initial resuscitation and be assessed for response.

In hypovolaemic shock secondary to haemorrhage, the severity of shock dictates the use of fluids or blood products for resuscitation. Matched blood products are indicated for Class III shock, and unmatched products (Type O-) are indicated for Class IV shock.

Cardiogenic shock is another cause of low-output shock and often is a complication of severe hypovolaemia and anaemia from haemorrhage. The aims are to improve preload, increase contractility, decrease after load and decrease myocardial work. A combination of fluid resuscitation, inotropic agents, beta-blockers and nitrates isused to support the heart's functions.

Septic shock needs to be recognised and treated emergently with fluid resuscitation, empirical antibiotics and inotropic agents (such as noradrenaline). Definitive intervention can then be carried out to decompress pyogenic collections.

Outcomes of Resuscitation

The outcome of resuscitation may be divided into responders, transient responders and non-responders according to changes in blood pressure and heart rate to fluid resuscitation. This outcome of resuscitation will determine the urgency of intervention or the appropriate location to continue resuscitation.

* K.-Y. Ngiam, MBBS (Lond), MMed (Surg) FRCS (Edin), Associate Consultant, Department of Surgery, Khoo Teck Puat Hospital, Singapore.

Table 2.1

Classes of Shock

	Class I	Class II	Class III	Class IV
Blood loss, mL	Up to 750	750–1500	1500–2000	>2000
Blood loss, % blood volume	Up to 15%	15–30%	30–40%	>40%
Pulse rate, bpm	<100	>100	>120	>140
Blood pressure	Normal	Normal	Decreased	Decreased
Respiratory rate	Normal or Increased	Decreased	Decreased	Decreased
Urine output, mL/h	>30	20–30	5–15	<5
CNS/mental status	Slightly anxious	Mildly anxious	Anxious, confused	Confused, lethargic
Fluid replacement	Crystalloid	Crystalloid	Crystalloid and blood	Crystalloid and blood

Stable patients who require a period of resuscitation before surgery should be brought to the ICU/HD where invasive monitoring (CVP, intra-arterial lines and urinary catheters) may be inserted to optimise the delivery of fluids and drugs.

Clinically, signs of adequate end-organ perfusion would include normalisation of blood pressure, stabilisation or improvement of mental state, increased urine output and progressive warming and pinking up of peripheries (in hypovolaemic patients). In patients with central venous line inserted, the CVP readings provide a surrogate marker of right atrial filling (normal range 2–8 mmHg) although transoesophageal Doppler (where available) is the current modality of choice for estimating cardiac filling and function.

Non-responders and unstable patients with obvious abdominal pathology should be brought to the operating theatre immediately for laparotomy to stop bleeding, control contamination and to allow for further resuscitation. The operating theatre should be warmed in advance and required equipment prepared. The anaesthetist should be informed early to assist in the management of the airway and resuscitation. Damage control surgery should be performed in unstable trauma patients or patients with severely contaminated abdominal cavity from a perforated viscus.

Biochemically, a decreasing trend of lactate may be used as a surrogate endpoint to resuscitation. High initial and 24-hr lactate (> 2.0 mmol/L) is highly suggestive of significant metabolic derangement and is an independent predictor of hospital mortality.

Arterial blood gas analysis can help determine the severity of tissue hypoxia and level of metabolic insult and hence determine the level and urgency of treatment. A patient with pH of < 7.00 on presentation has a less than 50% chance of surviving the hospital stay.

Normalcy of haematological and biochemical markers facilitates the progress to surgery and reduces post-operative complications, but it must be remembered that these biochemical abnormalities may be a result of a surgically reversible condition and can only be reversed by surgical treatment. Therefore, it may not be realistic to expect normalisation of biochemical markers before surgery as many can be concurrently corrected intra-operatively.

How to Optimise a Patient Preoperatively

Goal-directed therapy has been studied extensively as a way to improve the outcomes of surgery. Maintaining blood pressure and decreasing tachycardia are crude indicators of the adequacy of resuscitation. Some of the earliest observational studies by Shoemaker and colleagues have described the use of oxygen delivery as a surrogate indicator to optimise patients for surgery.

In a normal patient, increased metabolic demand of surgery results in increase in cardiac output (CO) and increasing oxygen delivery. However, this does not always happen, and these patients would develop an oxygen debt, the magnitude and length of which is associated with an increased incidence of complications.

Of those who survived, the median values of the measured physiological parameters were:

- Cardiac index (CI) > 4.5 L min^{-1} m^{-2}
- Oxygen delivery (DO$_2$I) > 600 mL min^{-1} m^{-2}
- Oxygen consumption (VO$_2$I) > 170 ml min^{-1} m^{-2}

The use of intravenous fluids and inotropic agents to achieve these values with pulmonary artery catheter (PAC) as a guide resulted in a mortality reduction from 33% to 4%.

However, the use of PAC has fallen out of fashion in some countries and the availability of expertise to insert PACs has declined. There are newer, and perhaps safer, indicators of CI and DO$_2$I that may be obtained through transoesophageal Doppler or invasive pulse pressure waveform analysis via an arterial line (e.g. FloTrac/Vigileo devices).

Simpler indicators of adequacy of resuscitation may be obtained by estimating the CI using the formula:

$$CI = \frac{HR \times 1.74 \times Pulse\ pressure}{BSA},$$

where BSA (body surface area) is 1.9 in men and 1.6 in women.

Investigations

Investigations should be targeted and help direct management. Apart from essential baseline tests, investigations should not harm your patient, as this might compromise the surgical outcome. A CT scan with intravenous contrast in a patient with borderline renal impairment potentially requiring surgery might adversely impact the outcome of your surgery due to post-operative acute renal failure. Use alternatives such as decubitus plain abdominal radiographs to look for free air. Non-contrast CT scans may be employed in some conditions to look for mass effect, free fluid or air.

Use routine tests to prepare the patient for surgery and to look for any complications that might have occurred post-operatively. Examples of some baseline tests include full blood count, electrolyte panel, coagulation profile, infective profile, liver panel, serum enzymes (e.g. amylase, LDH, cardiac enzymes), serum lactate levels and arterial blood gas analysis. This list is not exhaustive and investigations should be tailored to the needs of the patient. The decision between group and save or cross-matched blood is dependent on the immediacy of blood product requirements. For relatively minor surgery (e.g. open appendicectomy in an otherwise healthy patient) no blood products need to be prepared. For most major surgical procedures, cross-matched blood would be necessary.

Fluid and Electrolyte Replacement

The SAFE and Australian ICU trials have established that there is no difference in mortality between the use of crystalloids and albumin in resuscitation of hypotensive or critically ill ICU patients. However, only 1/6 of crystalloid given intravenously remains in the vascular compartment (e.g. 6 L of crystalloid needs to be given to increase 1 L of intravascular volume), and such large volumes may not be given sufficiently quickly to meet ongoing intravascular losses via haemorrhage.

Furthermore, large volume resuscitation with 0.9% normal saline alone might worsen an already acidotic and renal-impaired patient due to the supraphysiologic amounts of chloride in normal saline (154 mmol/L compared to serum levels, normal range 95–105 mmol/L) resulting in hyperchloraemic metabolic acidosis. Resuscitate with balanced crystalloid solutions (e.g. Hartmann's solution) and correct coagulopathy with fresh frozen plasma and other products. Colloids may be given if blood products and fresh frozen plasma is not available and there is ongoing bleeding that is not sufficiently corrected with large volume crystalloid infusions.

Electrolyte replacement should be performed concurrently with fluid replacement. In particular, sodium, potassium and calcium are key components in many essential physiological functions, and their levels must be monitored carefully. These may be obtained quickly via point-of-care arterial blood gas analysis. In particular, for patients who are receiving large-volume blood transfusions, calcium levels should be checked regularly to avoid hypocalcaemia due to citrate chelation of calcium in packed red cell transfusions.

The principle of pre-operative fluid replacement is to ensure that the patient is fluid replete before the commencement of surgery in order to meet the haemodynamic fluctuations of anaesthesia and demands of blood loss during surgery. However, this is confounded by a multitude of pre-operative presentations, from septic, dehydrated patients to those with congestive cardiac failure. Hence, the amount of fluid to be given pre-operatively should be tailored to the patient as accurately as possible, taking into consideration the volume of fluid for resuscitation, maintenance, and to replace ongoing losses according to the goal-directed therapy described earlier.

Haematological Therapy

In patients who suffer from acute massive blood loss and who are hypotensive (e.g. severe trauma, ruptured abdominal aortic aneurysm and massive gastrointestinal bleeding), it is often necessary to request unmatched blood (Group O, Rhesus negative) to be warmed and transfused within 15–20 min of arrival at the emergency department. Early transfusion of unmatched packed cells or whole blood has been shown to improve the outcomes of trauma patients.

Beyond initial resuscitation with crystalloids, an actively bleeding, hypotensive patient should not continue to receive large-volume crystalloid-based resuscitation until blood or blood products are available. This would lead to severe haemodilution and coagulopathy and further exacerbate the haemorrhage. Therefore, it is imperative that unmatched blood be requested early in the resuscitation of these patients. The risk of death due to massive haemorrhage greatly outweighs the risk of antibody reaction from the use of unmatched blood in such circumstances, but cross-matched blood should be made available as soon as possible.

Patients who are having ongoing haemorrhage, permissive hypotension may be employed to prevent further blood loss yet prevent end-organ damage. This

may be achieved by modulating fluid resuscitation according to the blood pressure, which should be targeted at about 100 mmHg systolic and 50 mmHg diastolic. In patients with a contained leaking abdominal aortic aneurysm, high systolic blood pressures must be controlled with intravenous labetalol at 20 mg titrated over 2 min followed by 0.5–2 mg/min up to 300 mg aiming for blood pressure of 100 mmHg systolic and 50 mmHg diastolic. This should yield a mean arterial pressure of approximately 66 mmHg, which would be adequate to maintain cerebral, cardiac and renal perfusion.

In the setting of massive blood loss, a massive transfusion protocol, consisting of the ideal ratio of 1:1:1 of packed red blood cells, fresh frozen plasma and platelets, should be activated if available. Activation of the protocol allows for rapid release of multiple blood products and streamlines the work processes between the anaesthetist, blood bank staff, portering staff, perfusionist (for cardiac bypass) and the surgeon. The required equipment must be made available (e.g. large-volume infusion devices, blood product warmers and autologous cell savers).

Secure and adequate intravenous access must be obtained in a safe and appropriate setting. For example, it would be inappropriate to obtain central venous access in the emergency department when there is adequate peripheral access and an anaesthetist available in the operating theatre to perform this procedure. The level of access depends on the severity of hypotension; it can range from large-bore intravenous cannulae in bilateral antecubial fossae to large-bore central access for extracorporeal membrane oxygenation (ECMO) in patients with heart–lung failure.

Coagulopathy

Coagulopathy is a dreaded enemy of surgery. The lethal triad of coagulopathy, acidosis and hypothermia in trauma has a direct bearing on bleeding during subsequent surgery. The best efforts in surgical haemostasis would fail without coagulating factors and platelets, hence these should be obtained early in the setting of massive blood loss.

Correct acidosis by treating the source of acidosis (e.g. treat infection with antibiotics, with blood products if hypotensive, improve ventilation, etc.). The use of sodium bicarbonate is controversial, but it can be used in the setting of cardiac arrest or severe acidosis (pH < 7.1) as acidaemia decreases myocardial contractility.

Warm the operating theatre to avert hypothermia — this should be arranged before the patient arrives in the operating theatre. Meanwhile, keep the patient warm by warming fluids and blood products, and through the use of body warming devices (air warmers, radiant heaters) and warm saline wash during laparotomy.

Do not delay emergent surgery for moderate coagulation dysfunction as it may be corrected intra-operatively. Any decision not to operate must be a summation of the patient's physiologic factors and surgical need rather than being based on one condition alone.

Antibiotics

Prophylactic antibiotics should be given to most patients undergoing emergency abdominal surgery as many of these operations would result in at least clean contaminated wounds (Class II and above) or have an underlying septic pathology. Broad-spectrum antibiotics with Gram-negative activity and an anaerobic agent such as a third-generation cephalosprins (e.g. cefazoline, ceftrixone) with metronidazole should be routine used in most abdominal surgeries.

These antibiotics should be given just before the incision is made or when a septic process is suspected pending surgery. They should not be continued beyond 24 hrs in surgeries performed for minor infections (e.g. mildly inflamed appendicitis), as this would result in bacterial resistance with prolonged use. In contaminated operations, three doses of intravenous antibiotics are commonly given and may be converted to equivalent oral antibiotics for an additional week.

Apart from culture-proven organisms with sensitivities to specific antibiotics, certain circumstances mandate the use of specific empiric antibiotic therapy:

1. Recurrences of previous septic pathology with known antibiotic flora (e.g. recurrent cholangitis post-ERCP due to *Klebsiella pneumoniae*)
2. Operations which require the use of implants (e.g. gentamicin or rifampicin when using

vascular grafts in the repair of abdominal aortic aneurysms)
3. Patients with valvular heart disease requiring amoxicillin to prevent bacterial endocarditis
4. Necrotising pancreatitis (e.g. Carbapenems for their improved penetration into pancreatic tissue)
5. Patients who are infected with MRSA requiring emergent surgery (e.g. vancomycin)
6. *Clostridium-difficile*–associated diarrhoea or pseudomembranous colitis (e.g. oral metronidazole, intravenous metronidazole or vancomycin)
7. Empirical triple therapy (amoxicillin, clarithromycin and a proton pump inhibitor, omeprazole) in patients with bleeding antral or duodenal ulcers suspicious for *H. pylori* infection
8. Female patients with possible or diagnosed pelvic inflammatory disease would require empiric intravenous cephalosporins (*Neisseria*, *gonorrhoea*) and oral doxycycline (*Chlamydia trachomatis*)
9. Chronic wet wounds often grow *Pseudomonas aeruginosa* and may be treated empirically with ciprofloxacin
10. Dirty traumatic wounds with soft tissue or bone involvement (e.g. cefazolin)

The use, dose and duration of these empiric antibiotics should be adjusted according to the clinical context and upon consultation with the hospital's microbiologist, especially in complex cases where features of sepsis are not resolving despite empirical antibiotic therapy. Many hospitals now have antibiotic stewardship programs and have hospital guidelines for antibiotic use. In hospitals with electronic prescription systems, antibiotic prescription guidelines are incorporated into these programs with tracking and compliance features to monitor resistance patterns in the hospital.

Emergency Laparoscopic Surgery

Surgeons with mature laparoscopic skill sets might offer emergency laparoscopic surgery to optimise outcomes of patients who would otherwise be subject to the morbidity of conventional laparotomy. However, careful selection of patients together with the usual precautions of laparoscopy must exercised to ensure the success of such an endeavour.

Patient selection

1. Younger patients who would be able to withstand CO_2 pneumoperitoneum and steep Trend e len burg positions that are required in certain laparoscopic surgeries
2. Early presentation to hospital following the onset of symptoms (e.g. within 6 hours of onset of pain in perforated gastric ulcers)
3. Female patients with unconfirmed abdominal pathology requiring initial diagnostic laparoscopy and possible definitive surgery (e.g. RIF pain in a female with possible appendicectomy)

Contraindications

1. Severe abdominal distension due to dilated loops of small bowel or large bowel making pneumoperitoneum creation difficult
2. Hypertrophic obstructive cardiomyopathy (HOCM) or severe hypotension
3. Severe restrictive lung disease (e.g. COPD) or hypercarbia which would limit the extent of CO_2 pneumoperitoneum
4. Large abdominal scars or multiple previous abdominal surgeries indicating the possibility of dense adhesions
5. Blunt abdominal trauma with hypotension due to possible bleeding from viscus
6. Multiple injuries or abdominal pathology requiring major resectional surgery (e.g. total colectomy for ischemic bowel)
7. Unstable patient with intra-abdominal haemorrhage refractory to resuscitation

It is prudent to assess each patient carefully and to know your abilities before you undertake emergency laparoscopic surgery, taking into consideration the time of the day, the availability of equipment and the experience of your assistant. Always take consent for conversion to open surgery, as it is more important to be safe than it is to have a smaller wound.

The usual precautions of laparoscopy must be adhered to despite the emergent nature of surgery.

CO_2 insufflation pressures should be kept to the minimum where possible (10–12 mmHg). The patient must be adequately supported on the operating table to prevent nerve injuries due to excessive compression of nerve plexuses when tilting the patient.

Risk Factors for Surgery

ASA score

The most common scoring system used to stratify preoperative risk using co-morbid conditions is the American Society of Anaesthesiologist Score (ASA score). In uni-variate and multi-variate analyses of emergency surgical patients and mortality, ASA has consistently been shown to be a good predictor of death postoperatively, in spite of its subjective nature and the inter-observer variation in measuring ASA.

Cardiovascular risk

The most established scoring system devised to estimate the perioperative cardiac risk for emergent non-cardiac surgery is the Goldman Cardiac Risk Index used since 1977. It was based on nine independent risk factors and was subsequently revalidated and simplified in 2009 to the Revised Cardiac risk index (RCRI), which identified six independent predictors of major cardiac complications (CCF, CRF, CVA, CAD, DM and type of surgery).

Trauma

The most widely used anatomical trauma scoring system is the Injury Severity Score (ISS). Each injury is assigned an Abbreviated Injury Scale (AIS) score, allocated to one of six body regions (head, face, chest, abdomen, extremities and external). Only the highest AIS score in each body region is used. The three most severely injured body regions have their score squared and added together to produce the ISS score. The ISS takes values from 0 to 75 and correlates linearly with mortality, morbidity, hospital stay and other measures of severity.

Boey's Score for Perforated Gastric Ulcers

Boey and colleagues validated a three-factor score to predict the mortality of surgery on patients with perforated gastric ulcers:

- Number of hours since perforation (< 24 hr)
- Preoperative systolic BP (100 mmHg)
- Any one or more systemic illness (DM, liver, heart, lung failure)

Risk factor	Mortality (%)
One	10.0
Two	45.5
Three	100.0

Postoperative Care

Intensive Care/High Dependency

Many patients with emergency abdominal surgery will require a period of intensive care unit or high dependency ward stay. You should be familiar with factors that influence surgically related outcomes, such as nutrition, infection control, ventilator management, haemodialysis and cardiac optimisation. These are outside the scope of this chapter and may be learnt in specialised courses (e.g. critical care courses) or from reference books. Specific issues in post-operative care of complicated abdominal emergencies and traumatic injuries relate to sepsis, haemorrhage and end organ failure.

Sepsis Syndromes

Systemic Inflammatory Response Syndrome (SIRS) is the characteristic clinical response to a variety of insults manifested by two or more of the following:

- Body temperature < 36°C or >38°C
- Heart rate > 90 beats per minute

- Tachypnoea > 20 breaths per minute; or, an arterial partial pressure of carbon dioxide < 4.3 kPa (32 mmHg)
- White blood cell count <4000 cells/mm³ (4×10^9 cells/L) or > 12,000 cells/mm³ (12×10^9 cells/L)

Sepsis is SIRS with documented infection. Septic shock is sepsis with hypotension despite adequate fluid resuscitation with the presence of perfusion abnormalities.

SIRS is the imbalance of local inflammatory response vs. anti-inflammatory response resulting in the spillover of inflammatory mediators into the systemic circulation causing cardiovascular compromise, disruption of homeostasis, apoptosis, organ failure and suppression of immune function.

Multiple organ dysfunction syndrome (MODS) is the presence of altered organ function in acutely ill patients such that homeostasis cannot be maintained without intervention. It is associated with widespread endothelial and parenchymal cell injury with the presence of endotoxinaemia. It usually involves two or more organ systems and is the end point of a cascade of syndromes:

SIRS + infection → sepsis → severe sepsis → MODS

Risk factors include APACHE score, age and comorbidities. Supportive therapy is aimed at ameliorating initial insult (remove source, control sepsis, haemostasis) and preventing second hit (nosocomial infection, bacterial translocation toxins, hypovolaemia, repeat operations and intra-abdominal complications). There is currently no evidence for use of Activated Protein C (APC) in septic shock.

Acute respiratory distress syndrome (ARDS)

ARDS is a life-threatening lung condition that prevents enough oxygen from getting into the blood. It is characterised by:

- Acute onset
- Bilateral pulmonary infiltrates

- Pulmonary artery wedge pressure < 18 mmHg (obtained by pulmonary artery catheterisation); if unavailable, then lack of clinical evidence of left ventricular failure suffices
- PaO_2/FiO_2 < 200 implies ARDS [PaO_2/FiO_2 < 300 implies ALI, which is a less severe form of ARDS]

Causes include sepsis, burns, pancreatitis, massive blood transfusions, drugs, DIVC, cardiopulmonary bypass, near drowning and O_2 toxicity.

Treatment principles consist of the following:

Early diagnosis, judicious resuscitation, remove reversible causes, intubate and paralyse, increase FiO_2 acutely then wean, pressure-regulated volume control ventilator O_2 support (to keep PaO_2 > 60 mmHg) with minimum volume, permissive hypercapnoea, increase PEEP inverse I:E ratio (1:1 or 2:1), nutritional support, high-frequency ventilation, prone position, steroids, nitric oxide, surfactant, diuresis and ECMO.

Blood transfusion and blood component therapy

Massive blood transfusion is defined by complete replacement of circulating volume in < 24 hr or 10 pints of blood in < 24 hr. Some hospitals have a massive transfusion protocol which supplies packed cells, platelets and FFP in the ratio of 1:1:1 (by volume).

Complications of blood transfusions include the following:

Immediate: Allergic/febrile/haemolytic transfusion reactions, haematoma

Early: Hypocalcaemia, hyperkalemia, hypothermia, coagulapathy, TRALI, poor O2 carrying capacity, low pH, microemboli, fluid overload

Late: Infections, jaundice (haemolysis), haemosiderosis, immunosuppression

Postoperative Oliguria

Oliguria is defined as < 400 mL/day of urine, and anuria is < 100 mL/day. Look for distended bladder when examining the patient and flush the catheter in catheterised patients. The aetiology may be divided into pre-renal, renal and post-renal causes:

- **Pre-renal:** Renal hypoperfusion (usually due to under-resuscitation, check CVP), cardiogenic shock, ongoing intra-abdominal bleeding, septic shock and distended bowel causing abdominal compartment syndrome (ACS).
- **Renal:** Rhabdomyolysis in the setting of trauma, vasculitis, glomerulonephritis, tubular/interstitial nephritis, pyelonephritis, malignancy, nephrotoxic medications and hepatorenal syndrome.
- **Post-renal:** Solitary kidney with stone, stricture or trauma (iatrogenic).

Renal Replacement Therapy (RRT)

Indications for RRT

- Pulmonary oedema (diuretic resistant)
- Ureamic complications (pericarditis, neuropathy, encephalopathy)
- K^+ > 6.5 mmol/L or rapidly raising
- Uncompensated metabolic acidosis (pH < 7.1)
- Creatinine >400 μmol/L, urea >35 mmol/L (azotemia)
- Na < 115 mmol/L or > 160 mmol/L

Types of RRT

- **Haemofiltration:** Extracorporeal filtration of blood across a semi-permeable membrane down a hydrostatic gradient (requiring a pump), resulting in non-selective passage of substances. Fluids and electrolytes need to be replaced before infusing back to the patient. This is beneficial for cardiac patients as filtration pressure is not dependent on cardiac output.
- **Haemodialysis:** Extracorporeal filtration across a semipermeable membrane down an osmotic gradient (ultrafiltration).
- **Continuous Ambulatory Peritoneal Dialysis (CAPD):** Intracorporeal passive dialysis across peritoneal membrane with exchange of dialysate via Tenckhoff catheter.

Abdominal compartment syndrome (ACS)

ACS is a clinical entity caused by an acute increase in intra-abdominal pressure to >20 mmHg, and it is the end result of untreated intra-abdominal hypertension (IAH) (12–19 mmHg). It adversely affects the function of the renal, pulmonary and cardiovascular systems and is commonly encountered in multiply injured patients who were given massive fluid resuscitation.

The abdominal pressure is measured via the urinary catheter using a manometer at the level of the symphysis pubis at end expiration. Non-operative management of ACS includes decompressing the upper GI tract with NGT suction, fleet enemas, judicious fluid resuscitation with diuresis as necessary, removing constrictive dressings, adequate analgesia, and ventilation with paralysis. Surgical management is indicated if the IAP > 25 mmHg and the patient has failed non-operative management. Temporary abdominal closure is fashioned after the abdomen is opened to release the pressure and continued efforts are made to reduce the oedema to allow definitive closure of the abdomen in the next few days.

Nutrition

In patients who are otherwise well but with poor physiological reserve, nutritional status can affect the outcome of surgery. Nutritional status may be estimated by anthropometry (BMI <18.5 or > 10% weight loss in six months), triceps skinfold thickness and bioelectric impedance. Serum albumin, transferrin and pre-albumin are used as surrogate markers of nutrition, but they are decreased by sepsis, trauma and malignancy despite normal nutrition and should be interpreted with caution in these settings.

Malnutrition has an impact on healing, complication rate, hence ongoing sepsis and prolonging the catabolic state post-surgery. Nutrition should be given enterally where possible as it is more physiological, immunological, with less risk of hyperglycaemia, biliary stasis, and is cheaper. However, many parenteral with emergency abdominal surgery have impaired bowel function, necessitating the use of total parenteral nutrition (TPN). A brief outline on what to give in TPN is as follows:

- Caloric requirement: (25–30 kcal/kg/day), give 30% in fat (up to 1 g/kg/day maximum)
- Protein requirement: 1 g/kg/day
- Volume requirement: 30–50 mL/kg/day with other replacement as required
- Electrolyte requirement: Na^+–2 mmol/kg/day, K^+–1 mmol/kg/day
- Other requirements: Zn, Cr, Mn, Cu, vitamins, etc. in standard RDA amounts

Pros and cons of TPN

Pros: reliable delivery goals, independent of enteric function.

Cons: complications related to insertion of lines (air embolism, pneumothorax, brachial plexus injury, retained hardware), use of lines (infection, embolism), metabolic (hyperglycaemia, cholestatic liver dysfunction, gallstones, increased septic morbidity in trauma) and high cost.

Chapter 3

Non-Variceal Upper Gastrointestinal Haemorrhage and Endoscopic Management

Eric Wee Wei Loong* and Christopher Khor Jen Lock**

Introduction

The rate of annual hospitalisation for acute upper gastrointestinal bleeding is estimated to be as high as 160 admissions per 100,000 population.[1] In patients presenting with upper gastrointestinal bleeding, 80–90% are due to non-variceal bleeds. The majority of non-variceal bleeds are due to peptic ulcer disease.

Other causes of non-variceal bleeding are non-acid related ulceration (e.g. tumours, viral infections, and inflammatory disease), Mallory–Weiss tears, erosions, esophagitis, Dieulafoy's lesions, angiodysplasias, gastric antral vascular ectasia and portal hypertensive gastropathy. Even rarer causes are hemobilia, hemosuccus pancreaticus and aorto-enteric fistulas.

Upper gastrointestinal bleeding is defined as bleeding proximal to the ligament of Treitz. This may manifest as hematemesis or melena. Occasionally, hemoptysis may be confused with hematemesis when the history is unclear. Bleeding can also come from the oral pharynx.

Melena is typically described in upper gastrointestinal bleeding. However melena is also a feature of small bowel bleeding and can also present in bleeding from the right-sided colon. When the rate of upper gastrointestinal bleeding is rapid, fresh blood may be seen per rectum instead of melena.

The mortality of upper gastrointestinal bleeding is between 5% and 10%.[2] The majority of patients with an episode of upper gastrointestinal bleeding will not re-bleed once treated. Endoscopy is the best modality to investigate upper gastrointestinal bleeds as it is effective and safe. Unfortunately, up to 25% of patients will have persistent bleeding or episodes of re-bleeding during their admission.[3]

Management of Non-Variceal Upper Gastrointestinal Bleeding

Initial Management

In patients with upper gastrointestinal bleeding suspected to be of non-variceal origin, the initial management should be resuscitation of the patient by stabilising the airway, breathing and circulation.

Patients who are hypoxemic should be given supplemental oxygen. Those who have high oxygen flow requirements might require intubation before endoscopy can be performed. Alternatively, specially

*Eric Wee WL, MBBS, MRCP, M. Med (Int Med), Consultant, Gastroenterology, Department of General Medicine, Khoo Teck Puat Hospital, Singapore.
**Christopher Khor JL, MBBS, FRCP (Edin), FAMS, FASGE, Department of Gastroenterology & Hepatology, Singapore General Hospital, Singapore.

designed endoscopy masks with one way valves for endoscopes to be inserted are available. These can provide ventilation during endoscopy and are suitable for short periods of use.

Hypotensive patients should be resuscitated with volume expanders. Fluids such as normal saline or blood products may be given. Correction of hypotension is important not only to maintain organ perfusion, but also to allow conscious sedation with drugs such as midazolam during endoscopy.

Coagulopathy should be corrected with blood products. Patients on anticoagulation (e.g. warfarin) or antithrombotic therapy (e.g. aspirin, dipyridamole or clopidogrel) should have their medications stopped temporarily, as the risk of continued bleeding usually outweighs the risk of thrombosis.

In patients who are taking warfarin for a mechanical cardiac valve, high doses of vitamin K (10 mg) should not be given. Rather, fresh frozen plasma with or without low-dose vitamin K (1–2 mg) is preferred.[4] The optimal international normalised ratio (INR) target for a bleeding patient has not yet been determined in clinical trials, but INR levels below 1.5 are generally accepted to be adequate.

Patients who are over anticoagulated and have supra-therapeutic INR values (INR > 3–3.5) should have endoscopy delayed till the coagulopathy is corrected. Patients with therapeutic INR (INR = 2–3) and below do not necessarily need to wait for coagulopathy to be corrected before endoscopy is performed.[5]

For patients on anti-platelet therapy, these medications should be stopped and platelets can be transfused if needed to correct the functional platelet defect. Patients with recently inserted cardiac stents (within one year) should have their case discussed with the cardiologist as well.

Risk stratifying upper gastrointestinal bleeding

Risk stratification scores allow the doctor to assess the urgency of treatment and to predict the risk of mortality and re-bleeding in an objective manner. There are several scores, amongst which the Rockall and the Glasgow–Blatchford scores are frequently used.[6,7]

Table 3.1.

Rockall Score

Criteria	Points
Age	
< 60 years	0
60–79 years	1
≥ 80 years	2
Shock	
No shock	0
Heart rate >100 beats/min	1
Systolic blood pressure <100 mmHg	2
Coexisting illness	
Nil	0
Ischemic heart disease, congestive heart failure, other major illness	2
Renal failure, hepatic failure, metastatic cancer	3
Endoscopic diagnosis	
No lesion observed, Mallory–Weiss tear	0
Peptic ulcer, erosive disease, esophagitis	1
Cancer of upper gastrointestinal tract	2
Endoscopic stigmata of recent haemorrhage	
Clean base ulcer, flat pigmented spot	0
Blood in upper gastrointestinal tract, active bleeding, visible vessel, clot	2

Rockall score

The Rockall score was developed to determine the risk of re-bleeding and death (Table 3.1). This score is based on the patient's age, presence of shock, co-existing illness, diagnosis and stigmata of haemorrhage. Therefore, endoscopy must first be performed, so that the score can be completed.

Patients with a low score of 2 or below are at low risk of re-bleeding and death. The Rockall score predicts mortality with greater accuracy than re-bleeding. However, one validation study found the prediction of re-bleeding to be unsatisfactory with the Rockall score.[8]

Glasgow–Blatchford score

The Glasgow–Blatchford score (Table 3.2) is calculated by tallying up the points for each of the following criteria: systolic blood pressure, blood urea nitrogen, haemoglobin and the presence of tachycardia, melena, syncope, liver or cardiac diseases.

Table 3.2.

Glasgow–Blatchford Score

Criteria on admission	Score
Blood urea (mmol/L)	
6.5 to < 8.0	2
8.0 to < 10.0	3
10.0 to < 25.0	4
≥ 25.0	6
Hemoglobin for men (g/dL)	
12.0 to < 13.0	1
10.0 to < 12.0	3
< 10·0	6
Hemoglobin for women (g/dL)	
10.0 to < 12.0	1
< 10.0	6
Systolic blood pressure (mmHg)	
100–109	1
90–99	2
< 90	3
Other markers	
Pulse ≥ 100 (per min)	1
Presentation with melena	1
Presentation with syncope	2
Hepatic disease	2
Cardiac failure	2

High scores carry a worse prognosis and require intervention, as compared to lower scores. One advantage of this score is that it can be calculated at the presentation of the bleed. In addition, unlike the Rockall score, both endoscopy and the diagnosis are not required for calculation of the score.

The Glasgow–Blatchford score has been used successfully to stratify patients into different risk groups. Those with low scores can be safely discharged. The Glasgow–Blatchford score has also been used to determine the need for intervention and the risk of mortality.

Medical Therapy

Intravenous proton pump inhibitors (PPI) should be initiated in all patients with suspected upper gastrointestinal bleeding. Intravenous PPI are available as various preparations (e.g. omeprazole, pantoprazole,

esomeprazole), and there is no current evidence to favour the use of one drug over the other.

Proton pump inhibitors (such as omeprazole) are given as an infusion. The loading dose of 80 mg of PPI is administered first, followed by an infusion of 8 mg/hour of PPI. PPI therapy should be started even before the endoscopy is performed, but it should not delay the endoscopy.[5] Starting PPI infusion before endoscopy has been shown to downstage the high-risk stigmata seen at endoscopy and result in faster resolution of bleeding. Therefore, even though no mortality benefit is seen in early PPI initiation, it is beneficial to the endoscopist since therapy is less likely to be required.[9]

During endoscopy, bleeding lesions are graded based on the Forrest classification (Table 3.3).[10] Lesions which are Forrest IIb and above should continue with PPI infusion, while lesions which are Forrest IIc and below can be treated with oral PPI therapy.

The doses of PPI are:

IV omeprazole 80 mg as a loading dose, followed by IV omeprazole 8 mg/hr infusion.
IV pantoprazole 80 mg as a loading dose, followed by IV pantoprazole 8 mg/hr infusion.
IV esomeprazole 80 mg as a loading dose, followed by IV esomeprazole 8 mg/hr infusion.

PPI infusion is continued for 72 hr before it is converted to an oral formulation. High-risk lesions take 72 hr to become low-risk lesions. This regimen of PPI

Table 3.3.

Forrest Classification

Class		Bleeding Stigmata
I		(Active bleeding)
	Ia	Spurting vessel
	Ib	Oozing vessel (Fig. 3.1)
II		(Stigmata of recent haemorrhage without bleeding)
	IIa	Visible vessel (Fig. 3.2)
	IIb	Adherent clot (Fig. 3.3)
	IIIc	Haematin spot on ulcer base (flat pigmented spot) (Fig. 3.4)
III		Clean ulcer base with no bleeding (Fig. 3.5)

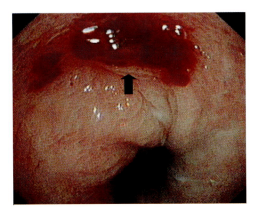

Figure 3.1.

Gastric antrum ulcer with oozing vessel (Forrest Ib).

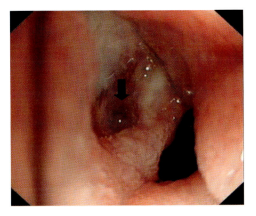

Figure 3.2.

Duodenal bulb ulcer with a visible vessel — the reflection of the white light (from the endoscope) on the protruding vessel is a clue that the spot is elevated and not a flat lesion (Forrest IIa).

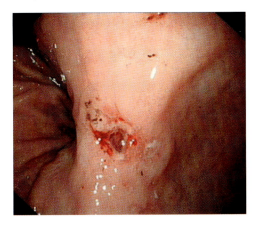

Figure 3.3.

Gastric incisural ulcer with a small adherent blood clot (Forrest IIb).

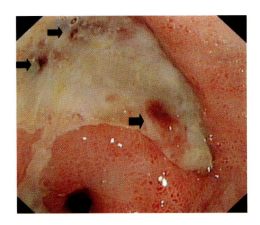

Figure 3.4.

Gastric antrum ulcer with multiple flat haematin spots (Forrest IIc).

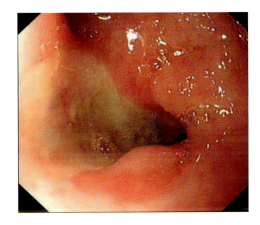

Figure 3.5.

Clean-based ulcer in the gastric antrum — Biopsy revealed malignant signet ring cells (Forrest III).

administration is supported by a randomised controlled trial which showed that patients receiving PPI infusion had lower re-bleeding rates, transfusion requirements and hospitalisation stay after endoscopic therapy.[11]

The risk of re-bleeding is highest in the first 72 hr. Hence, should a patient have further episodes of bleeding, it is recommend that the PPI infusion should be continued for at least 72 hr from the time of the most recent gastrointestinal bleed before it is converted to an oral formulation.

In the rare patient with an allergy to PPI, histamine-2 receptor antagonists such as intravenous ranitidine can be given, although the acid suppression of histamine-2 receptor antagonists is inferior to that of PPI infusion.

This was illustrated in a multi-centre randomised controlled trial, where intravenous pantoprazole was shown to be superior to intravenous ranitidine in the treatment of upper gastrointestinal arterial spurters.[12]

Prokinetic therapy is useful in the preparation of patients for endoscopy. It is useful in patients who are suspected to have a large number of blood clots in the stomach or in patients who have recently consumed a meal and require urgent endoscopy. Prokinetic therapy should be used only when indicated and not routinely.

Drugs such as intravenous metoclopramide or erythromycin can be given.

Intravenous metoclopramide is prescribed as a bolus dose of 10 mg.

Erythromycin can be given as a dose of 3 mg/kg of body weight, usually 150–250 mg of intravenous erythromycin in 100 mL of saline over 15 min. Erythromycin should be avoided in patients with prolonged QTc due to the risk of triggering tachyarrhythmias such as Torsade de pointes.

Endoscopic Therapy

Timing of endoscopy

After the initial resuscitation and medical therapy, endoscopic therapy should be performed. It should be done early, rather than late. A systematic analysis suggested that early endoscopy (within 24 hr) for non-variceal upper gastrointestinal bleeding led to a reduction in the length of hospitalisation, lower costs, lower transfusion requirements and better patient outcomes.[13]

The appropriate endoscopic management depends on the stigmata of haemorrhage seen. This can be graded according to the Forrest classification (Table 3.3).[10]

Endoscopic therapy is necessary in lesions which present with:

  Active bleeding (spurting or oozing)
  Non-bleeding visible vessels
  Adherent clots (Fig. 3.6)

These are lesions graded as Forrest IIb and above. A randomised controlled trial showed that treating non-bleeding lesions such as a visible vessel or

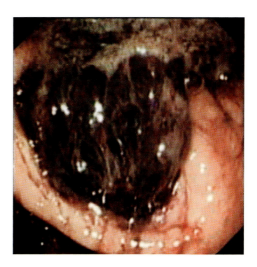

Figure 3.6.

Large adherent clot (Forrest IIb).

adherent clot with endoscopic therapy and PPI was superior to just PPI therapy alone in the prevention of re-bleeding.[14]

However, the evidence for removal of adherent clots is weak, although it has been advocated in an international consensus meeting.[5] When an adherent clot is seen, it is advisable to inject epinephrine at four quadrants around the clot before removing it.

The clot is then removed after epinephrine injection. Clot removal can be performed by:

  Flushing vigorously
  Displacing it with an instrument
  Sucking at it
  Snaring the clot away[14,15]

The latter is a relatively safe and atraumatic method. Guillotine cold snaring is performed by gently opening and closing the snare over the clot (Fig. 3.7). This fragments the clot and may reveal an underlying vessel. One should be cautious not to snare a protuberant vessel. Once the clot is successfully removed, endoscopic therapy is applied to the underlying lesion.

In addition, lesions with persistent oozing without a clot or vessel should also be treated with endoscopic therapy, although clinical trials to support this practice are lacking.

Otherwise, clean-based ulcers and those with a flat red spot or necrotic base do not require endoscopic therapy, and are at a very low risk of re-bleeding.

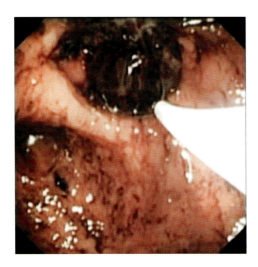

Figure 3.7.

Cold snare removal of the adherent clot.

These lesions (graded Forrest IIc and below) can be treated solely with medical therapy.

Once the bleeding source is identified, haemostasis is applied through one or more of the following methods as described below.

Epinephrine injection

Epinephrine injection is a useful method to induce haemostasis for both arterial and venous bleeding. However, the effects and duration of action of epinephrine are temporary.

A meta-analysis of randomised controlled trials has indicated that when epinephrine injection therapy is combined with a second modality of haemostatic therapy (see below), the re-bleeding, emergency surgery and mortality rates are reduced. This benefit is irrespective of the type of second modality used with epinephrine. Hence, it is recommended to combine epinephrine injection therapy with another haemostatic method.[16, 17]

Epinephrine injection is performed by injecting a solution of epinephrine (1:10,000 concentration) in aliquots of 1–2 mL at four quadrants around the bleeding source. Larger volumes of epinephrine may be required if the bleeding persists.

Epinephrine is drawn out into a 10 mL syringe and attached to the injection cannula. The injection cannula is inserted through the therapeutic channel of the endoscope and the tip is placed abutting the mucosa near to, but not at the bleeding source.

The assistant is instructed to insert the needle out of the cannula and slowly inject the epinephrine. The assistant should verbalise the amount of epinephrine injected so that the endoscopist, whose attention is on the monitor, is aware of the amount delivered. The needle is then withdrawn and another quadrant selected. This is performed in four quadrants before assessing for a response.

A response is indicated by cessation of bleeding and blanching of the surrounding mucosa into a pale whitish-red colour. This is indicative of successful vasospasm induced by epinephrine (Fig. 3.8).

The endoscopist should avoid injecting epinephrine into the vessel or bleeding point as this may result in epinephrine being delivered directly into the systemic circulation, cumulating in sudden tachycardia, hypertension and a restless patient.

Thermal therapy

The aim of thermal therapy is to coagulate the vessel. This can be performed with bipolar/multipolar electrocoagulation, heater probe, argon plasma coagulation or laser.

Thermal therapy with heater probe and electrocoagulation works through the mechanism of coaptive coagulation of the vessel. Therefore it is important to apply firm pressure against the vessel when using these thermal therapies.

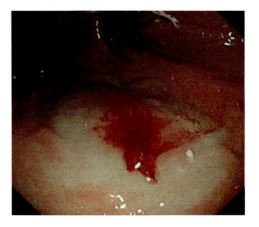

Figure 3.8.

Post-epinephrine injection. The mucosa blanches almost immediately (pale white) due to vasoconstriction by epinephrine.

The heater probe is used with low power settings of 15–30 Joules. Sometimes several pulses of the heater probe are required before the vessel is ablated. Power settings in the duodenum (15 Joules) should be lower than settings in the stomach, where the walls are thicker.

The heater probe also comes with a water jet, which prevents the tip from sticking to the charred tissue. After coagulation, the water jet is activated before the probe is withdrawn. A shallow depression is left at the spot where therapy is applied, and the vessel will be absent (Figs. 3.9–3.11).

Further therapy is needed if bleeding persists, but it will lead to deeper depressions within the ulcer. Hence, thermal therapy is unsuitable in deep ulcers,

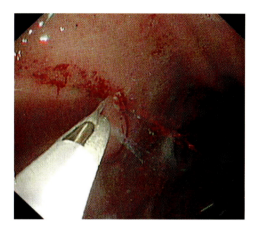

Figure 3.11.

The water jet of the heater probe can be used to wash the blood away without removing the catheter.

especially in the duodenum or small bowel, as there is a risk of causing perforation.

Bipolar/multipolar electrocoagulation probes are safer than the older monopolar probes. This is because the depth of thermal therapy is shallower and more predictable. In these probes, electrocoagulation generates heat when electricity conducts through tissues with electrical resistance. Multipolar probes are usually large 10 French probes and used at 30–40 watts for a duration of up to 10 seconds.

Thermal therapy is particularly useful in treating lesions with oozing edges or surfaces. It is also useful in areas of the gastrointestinal tract where limited distance between the endoscope and the vessel hampers the successful deployment of a clip. However, coagulation probes may not be useful in targeting vessels when the plane of the lesion is almost parallel with the probe, since this might not allow sufficient pressure to tamponade the vessel during coagulation.

Argon plasma coagulation

Unlike other thermal therapies, the argon plasma coagulation does not require tissue contact. Argon plasma coagulation causes tissue coagulation when electricity is conducted across argon gas emitted by the catheter.[18] As such, the tissue damage is superficial, up to a depth of 2–3 mm.

To perform argon plasma coagulation, the catheter needs to be placed within several millimetres of the

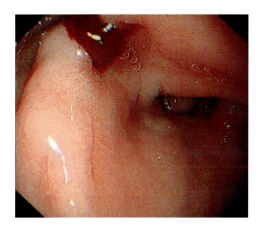

Figure 3.9.

Forrest 1b oozing gastric antrum ulcer.

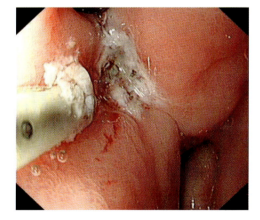

Figure 3.10.

After coaptive coagulation with a heater probe, the typical white charred mucosa is seen with no further bleeding.

lesion, but not in contact with it. One or more brief pulses of argon plasma coagulation (usually stepping on the foot pedal for less than 1 second) are applied and the outcome assessed. Because contact is not needed, argon plasma coagulation can be applied tangentially to the lesion.

Argon plasma coagulation is not useful when bleeding is originating from a spurting vessel. In these cases, coaptive thermal coagulation or clipping is required. Argon plasma coagulation is useful for lesions which ooze, such as the raw surface of a gastric tumor, edges of an ulcer or a vascular lesion such as an angiodysplasia or gastric antral vascular ectasia (Fig. 3.12). Argon plasma coagulation is also useful for haemostasis in areas where the gastrointestinal wall layer is thin, such as in the small bowel and oesophagus (Figs. 3.13–3.15).

As argon plasma coagulation involves unipolar cautery, one should be cautious in patients with implantable cardio-defibrillators and pacemakers.[19]

Endoscopic clipping

The hemoclip is used for endoscopic clipping. These clips come in various sizes. Some are rotatable and some have prongs which can open and close repeatedly before release. The assistant who is manipulating the clip should be familiar with its loading and deployment. Clips are available as preloaded sets as

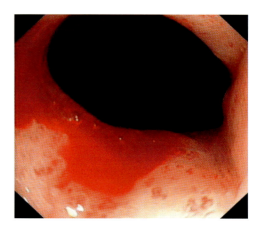

Figure 3.13.

Multiple small angiodysplasia at the gastro-oesophageal junction with active oozing. Note the numerous dilated vessels in a corkscrew pattern.

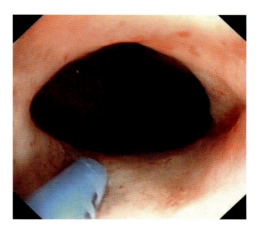

Figure 3.14.

Argon plasma coagulation to the oozing angiodysplasia.

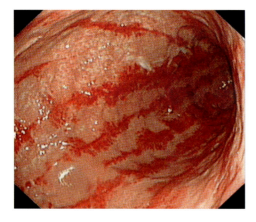

Figure 3.12.

Gastric antral vascular ectasia (also known as a watermelon stomach) in a patient with cryptogenic liver cirrhosis. Argon plasma coagulation can be applied to these lesions, but multiple sessions will be required.

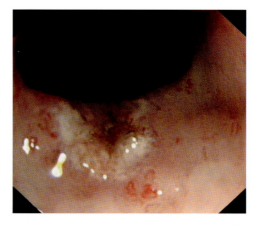

Figure 3.15.

Post argon plasma coagulation with cessation of bleeding.

well. These might be more convenient to use in the setting of an actively spurting lesion. Often, more than one clip is used as it may be fired in a poor position or the lesion may require multiple clips before the bleeding is controlled.

It is crucial to obtain good positioning before deployment of the clip, and the lesion should always be visible. Application of the clip blindly with blood obscuring the lesion is invariably a futile process. To obtain good positioning, a few centimetres of distance between the endoscope and the lesion are required for the clip to be advanced and opened fully.

Frequently, both the endoscope and the clip require rotation before the vessel can be targeted. The clip should be firmly opposed against the mucosa with the vessel centred between both prongs before it is deployed. If bleeding persists, further clips can be placed or coaptive thermal therapy applied (Figs. 3.16–3.18).

Endoscopic clipping has been shown to be superior to epinephrine injection alone in treating non-variceal upper gastrointestinal bleeding. However, endoscopic clipping is neither superior nor inferior to thermal therapy in terms of re-bleeding, surgical rates or mortality.[20]

In addition, endoscopic clipping may be difficult in locations such as the posterior wall of the gastric body, lesser curve and the posterior wall of the duodenal bulb. Hence, the choice of applying endoscopic clipping over thermal therapy should be based on the following factors:

1. Ease of application of therapy (which may be determined by the site of the bleeding).
2. Endoscopist familiarity with the modality of therapy.
3. Potential contraindication to further thermal injury (e.g. deep ulceration in the duodenum with concerns of inducing perforation).
4. Type of stigmata of haemorrhage (oozing edges may be more appropriately treated with thermal therapy).
5. Coagulopathic patient (endoscopic clipping may be less traumatic to the mucosa than thermal therapy).

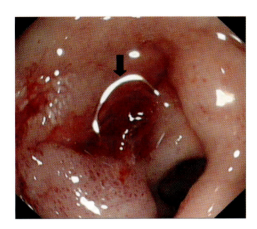

Figure 3.16.

Duodenal bulb ulcer with visible vessel after epinephrine injection. Note the pale mucosa. (Arrow: visible vessel)

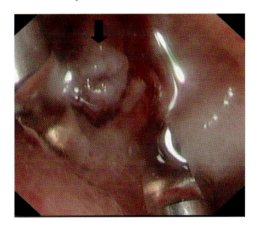

Figure 3.17.

Clipping of the duodenal ulcer. (Arrow: visible vessel)

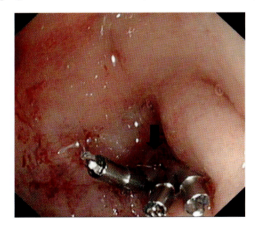

Figure 3.18.

Completion of hemostasis with three clips over the vessel site. This patient had no further episodes of bleeding. (Arrow: visible vessel)

Failure of endoscopic therapy

In patients who re-bleed after the initial endoscopy, there is a role to repeat endoscopy.[5] Endoscopic retreatment has been shown to be as good as surgical intervention in patients who re-bleed in terms of hospitalisation duration, blood transfusion requirements and mortality. In the absence of re-bleeding, there is usually no need for a re-look endoscopy.

Surgical therapy is indicated when non-variceal upper gastrointestinal bleeding cannot be controlled with endoscopic therapy or if the patient is actively bleeding with persistent hemodynamic instability.[21] Patients with hypotension or large ulcers more than 2 cm are likely to fail repeat endoscopy and may benefit from surgery.[22] Surgery is also indicated if a surgical complication such as a perforation is present as well.

In patients who are unsuitable for surgery, an alternative therapy is percutaneous angiogram and selective embolisation. Embolisation is performed with the use of coils, alcohol, cyanoacrylate glue, gelatin sponges or polyvinyl.[23] However, complications of embolisation include bowel ischemia, infarction of the stomach, liver and spleen and subsequent duodenal stenosis.[24,25]

References

1. Lewis JD, Bilker WB, Brensinger C, Farrar JT, Strom BL. (2002) Hospitalization and mortality rates from peptic ulcer disease and GI bleeding in the 1990s: relationship to sales of nonsteroidal anti-inflammatory drugs and acid suppression medications. *Am J Gastroenterol* **97**: 2540–2549.

2. Lim CH, Vani D, Shah SG, Everett SM, Rembacken BJ. (2006) The outcome of suspected upper gastrointestinal bleeding with 24-hour access to upper gastrointestinal endoscopy: a prospective cohort study. *Endoscopy* **38**: 581–585.

3. Kovacs TOG, Jensen DM. (1997) Therapeutic endoscopy in upper gastrointestinal bleeding. In: Tayler MB, Gollan JL, Steer ML, Wolfe MM (eds). *Gastrointestinal Emergencies.* 2nd ed. Baltimore: Williams & Wilkins, pp. 181–198.

4. Bonow RO, Carabello BA, Chatterjee K, *et al.* (2008) Focused update incorporated into the ACC/AHA 2006 guidelines for the management of patients with valvular heart disease: a report of the American College of Cardiology/American Heart Association Task Force on Practice Guidelines: endorsed by the Society of Cardiovascular Anesthesiologists, Society for Cardiovascular Angiography and Interventions, and Society of Thoracic Surgeons. *Circulation* **118**(15): e523–661.

5. Barkun AN, Bardou M, Kuipers EJ, *et al.* (2010) International Consensus Upper Gastrointestinal Bleeding Conference Group. International consensus recommendations on the management of patients with nonvariceal upper gastrointestinal bleeding. *Ann Intern Med* **152**(2): 101–113.

6. Blatchford O, Murray WR, Blatchford M. (2000) A risk score to predict need for treatment for upper-gastrointestinal haemorrhage. *Lancet* **356**(9238): 1318–1321.

7. Rockall TA, Logan RF, Devlin HB, Northfield TC. (1996) Risk assessment after acute upper gastrointestinal haemorrhage. *Gut* **38**: 316–321.

8. Vreeburg EM, Terwee CB, Snel P, *et al.* (1999) Validation of the Rockall risk scoring system in upper gastrointestinal bleeding. *Gut* **44**(3): 331–335.

9. Dorward S, Sreedharan A, Leontiadis GI, *et al.* (2006) Proton pump inhibitor treatment initiated prior to endoscopic diagnosis in upper gastrointestinal bleeding. *Cochrane Database Syst Rev* **2006**: CD005415.

10. Forrest JA, Finlayson ND, Shearman DJ. (1974) Endoscopy in gastrointestinal bleeding. *Lancet* **2**: 394–397.

11. Lau JY, Chung SC, Leung JW, *et al.* (1998) The evolution of stigmata of hemorrhage in bleeding peptic ulcers: a sequential endoscopic study. *Endoscopy* **30**: 513–518.

12. Van Rensburg C, Barkun AN, Racz I, *et al.* (2009) Intravenous pantoprazole vs. ranitidine for the prevention of peptic ulcer rebleeding: a multicentre, multinational, randomized trial. *Aliment Pharmacol Ther* **29**(5): 497–507.

13. Spiegel BM, Vakil NB, Ofman JJ. (2001) Endoscopy for acute nonvariceal upper gastrointestinal tract hemorrhage: is sooner better? A systematic review. *Arch Intern Med* **161**(11): 1393–1404.

14. Jensen DM, Kovacs TO, Jutabha R, *et al.* (2002) Randomized trial of medical or endoscopic therapy to prevent recurrent ulcer hemorrhage in patients with adherent clots. *Gastroenterology* **123**(2): 407–413.

15. Laine L, Stein C, Sharma V. (1996) A prospective outcome study of patients with clot in an ulcer and the effect of irrigation. *Gastrointest Endosc* **43**: 107–110.

16. Laine L, McQuaid KR. (2009) Endoscopic therapy for bleeding ulcers: an evidence based approach based on meta-analyses of randomized controlled trials. *Clin Gastroenterol Hepatol.* **7**: 33–47.

17. Vergara M, Calvet X, Gisbert JP. (2007) Epinephrine injection versus epinephrine injection and a second endoscopic method in high risk bleeding ulcers. *Cochrane Database Syst Rev* **2007**: CD005584.

18. Farin G, Grund KE. (1994) Technology of argon plasma coagulation with particular regard to endoscopic applications. *Endosc Surg Allied Technol* **2**(1): 71–77.

19. Petersen BT, Hussain N, Marine JE, *et al.* (2007) Endoscopy in patients with implanted electronic devices. *Gastrointest Endosc* **65**(4): 561–568.

20. Sung JJ, Tsoi KK, Lai LH, *et al.* (2007) Endoscopic clipping versus injection and thermo-coagulation in the treatment of non-variceal upper gastrointestinal bleeding: a meta-analysis. *Gut* **56**(10): 1364–1373.

21. Imhof M, Ohmann C, Röher HD, Glutig H. (2003) Endoscopic versus operative treatment in high-risk ulcer bleeding patients — results of a randomised study. *Langenbecks Arch Surg* **387**: 327–336.

22. Lau JY, Sung JJ, Lam YH, *et al.* (1999) Endoscopic retreatment compared with surgery in patients with recurrent bleeding after initial endoscopic control of bleeding ulcers. *N Engl J Med* **340**(10): 751–756.

23. Kim S, Duddalwar V. (2005) Failed endoscopic therapy and the interventional radiologist: non-variceal upper gastrointestinal bleeding. *Tech Gastrointest Endosc* **7**: 148–155.

24. Ljungdahl M, Eriksson LG, Nyman R, Gustavsson S. (2002) Arterial embolization in management of massive bleeding from gastric and duodenal ulcers. *Eur J Surg* **168**: 384–390.

25. Poultsides GA, Kim CJ, Orlando R 3rd, *et al.* (2008) Angiographic embolization for gastroduodenal hemorrhage: safety, efficacy, and predictors of outcome. *Arch Surg* **143**: 457–461.

Chapter 4

Upper Gastrointestinal Variceal Haemorrhage and Endoscopic Management

Eric Wee Wei Loong* and Christopher Khor Jen Lock**

Introduction

Oesophageal and gastric varices occur with portal hypertension when the Hepatic Venous Pressure Gradient (HVPG) is more than 12 mmHg (normal HVPG = 3–5 mmHg).[1]

Varices can occur in any part of the gastrointestinal tract from the pharynx to the rectum. Varices can also occur within the peritoneal cavity. In most patients, bleeding varices develop in the distal oesophagus (oesophageal varices) or proximal stomach (fundal varices).

In patients with isolated gastric fundal varices, splenic vein thrombosis should be considered as a possible etiology, especially if the liver is not cirrhotic on imaging such as ultrasound, CT scan or magnetic resonance imaging.

Bleeding varices are associated with high mortality rates, and up to 70% of the survivors of variceal bleeding will re-bleed again within one year of their index bleed.[2]

The management of upper gastrointestinal varices starts from the primary prophylaxis of varices detected on screening, to the management of acute variceal haemorrhage, to the secondary prophylaxis of varices (after a bleed) and finally to the management of subsequent variceal re-bleeding.

When decompensated liver cirrhosis is the underlying cause of variceal bleeding, a liver transplant will correct the underlying pathophysiology and disease. However in some patients, liver transplantation is not a suitable option due to various contraindications (such as age, advanced liver cancer, underlying comorbidities, e.g. significant ischemic heart disease, etc.).

In addition, there is frequently a lag, from the time of listing for liver transplant to the time of surgery. During this interim period, variceal haemorrhage can be managed by endoscopy (preferably) or a transjugular intrahepatic portosystemic shunt (TIPS) procedure. Portosystemic shunt surgery is discouraged if the patient is a transplant candidate as it will increase the technical difficulty of the liver transplant surgery.

Grading and Nomenclature of Varices

Oesophageal varices usually occur in the lower half of the oesophagus. Based on current recommendations, they can be divided into small or large. Large varices are more than 5 mm in diameter.[3]

*Eric W. L. Wee, MBBS, MRCP, M. Med (Int Med), Consultant, Gastroenterology, Department of General Medicine, Khoo Teck Puat Hospital, Singapore.
**Christopher J. L. Khor, MBBS, FRCP (Edin), FAMS, FASGE, Department of Gastroenterology & Hepatology, Singapore General Hospital, Singapore.

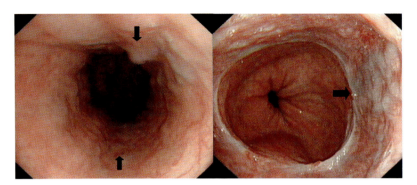

Figure 4.1.   **Figure 4.2.**

Small grade I varices in the distal oesophagus (*arrows*).

Some centres grade varices into three grades of small, medium and large based on their morphology and size.

○ Grade I — Small varices (< 5 mm in diameter) which are minimally elevated and run a fairly straight course (Figs. 4.1 and 4.2).

○ Grade II — Medium varices (> 5 mm in diameter) which are tortuous and occlude *less* than one-third of the oesophageal lumen (Fig. 4.3).

○ Grade III — Large varices (> 5 mm in diameter) which are tortuous and occlude *more* than one third of the oesophageal lumen (Figs. 4.4 and 4.5).

In the two-grade classification (of small and large varices), medium-sized varices are considered to be large varices. The advantage of grading varices into only small and large is that it is less ambiguous and subjective than a three-grade classification (of grades I, II and III). Both two- and three-grade classifications

are able to dictate management effectively. Small varices, or grade I varices, are treated medically, while large varices, or grade II and III varices, are amenable to endoscopic therapy.[3]

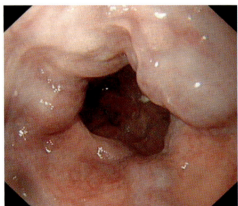

Figure 4.4.

Large grade III oesophageal varices.

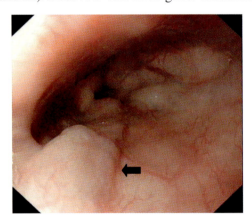

Figure 4.3.

Medium-sized grade II oesophageal varix (*arrow*).

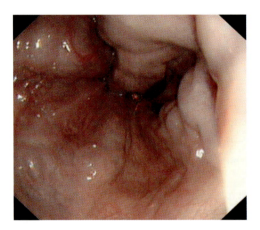

Figure 4.5.

Large grade III oesophageal varices.

Gastric varices can be divided into gastro-oesophageal varices (GOV), which drain into oesophageal varices, and isolated gastric varices (IGV), which are not in continuity with oesophageal varices.

Gastro-oesophageal varices can be subdivided into gastro-oesophageal varices type 1 (GOV1) and gastro-oesophageal varices type 2 (GOV2).[4]

GOV1 are gastric varices which originate along the lesser curve of the stomach and drain into the oesophageal varices. These are more common and occur in 70% of all gastric varices (Fig. 4.6).

GOV2 are gastric varices which originate along the fundus and drain into the oesophageal varices. These are less common and occur in 20% of all gastric varices (Fig. 4.7).[5]

For all gastro-oesophageal varices which are not actively bleeding (regardless of subtype), therapy is targeted at the oesophageal portion. However, if the gastric varix is bleeding, then therapy is targeted directly at the gastric portion (bleeding source).[5]

Isolated gastric varices can be subdivided into two types.[4]

1) Isolated gastric varices type 1 (IGV1) are located at the fundus and do not drain into oesophageal varices. These occur in 10% of all gastric varices.[5]
2) Isolated gastric varices type 2 (IGV2) are located anywhere in the stomach, except the fundus. They may be along the corpus or antrum of the stomach

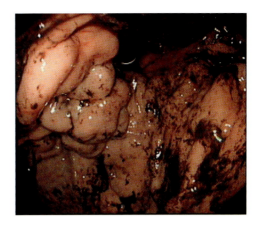

Figure 4.7.

Endoscope in retroflexed position showing large gastrooeso phageal varices type 2 (GOV2) along the fundus with coffee-ground blood. No varices were seen on the lesser curve.

and are not associated with oesophageal varices. These occur very infrequently.

Varices with red signs (red wale, cherry red spots, hematocystic spots), regardless of size, and large varices (which have thin walls) are at an increased risk of bleeding.

Stigmata of recent variceal haemorrhage include the white nipple sign (which represents a fibrin clot), hematocystic spot, adherent clot and ulceration (Fig. 4.8). In a patient with an episode of hematemesis,

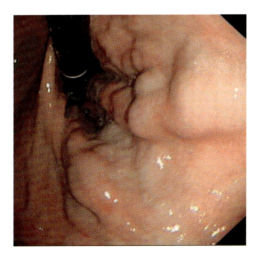

Figure 4.6.

Endoscope in retroflexed position showing large gastro-oesophageal varices type 1 (GOV1) traversing from the lesser curve and into the oesophagus.

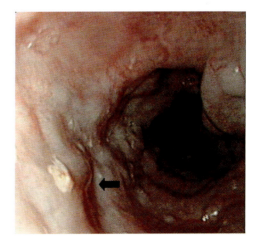

Figure 4.8.

White nipple sign (arrow). This small elevated white lesion represents a fibrin plug overlying the site of bleeding. Endoscopic variceal ligation should be targeted on that particular column of varix, either distal to the lesion or at the level of the lesion, since the flow of blood is from distal to proximal in oesophageal varices.

variceal bleeding should be presumed if only varices are found on endoscopy (even if stigmata of recent haemorrhage is absent) and no other potential source is present (e.g. Mallory–Weiss tear, ulcer, cancer, Dieulafoy's lesion, etc.) (Figs. 4.9–4.12).

Management of Variceal Bleeding

During an episode of acute variceal haemorrhage, the treatment involves resuscitation, pharmacotherapy, endoscopic management, TIPS and surgery. Liver transplantation has no role in the acute management of a variceal bleed.

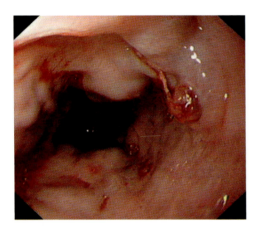

Figure 4.9.

Another patient with hematemesis and a fibrin plug on the esophageal varix indicating the site of bleed.

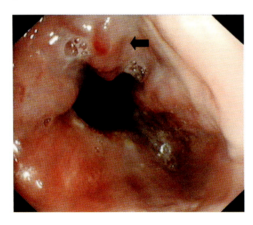

Figure 4.10.

The hematocystic spot (arrow) on a column of oesophageal varix is seen as a protuberant red lesion. This is opposed to a cherry red spot, which is represented by a flat red spot on a varix.

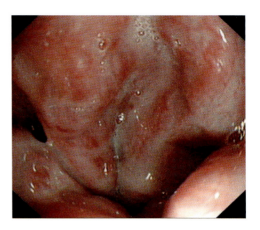

Figure 4.11.

Red wale sign on large grade III oesophageal varices. The red wale sign is a depicted by erythematous streaks on the surface of a varix. Varices with red wale signs are at high risk of bleeding.

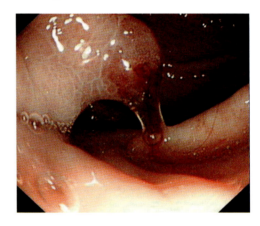

Figure 4.12.

Active oozing from a gastric fundal varix.

Medical Management and Resuscitation

Patients with acute variceal haemorrhage may present with hypovolemic shock. In these cases, resuscitation with crystalloids and blood is the priority, aiming for a systolic blood pressure above 90 mmHg. One should not over resuscitate, as excessively high intravascular volumes may exacerbate portal hypertension and aggravate the bleeding.[6]

Coagulopathy (thrombocytopenia, clotting factor deficiency) should be corrected with the relevant blood products:

1. Platelet transfusion for thrombocytopenia.
2. Fresh frozen plasma for prolonged prothrombin (PT) and partial thromboplastin times (PTT).
3. Cryoprecipitate for hypofibrogenemia.

Patients with underlying liver cirrhosis have an increased risk of bacteremia during an acute variceal haemorrhage. They should receive an antibiotic with activity against gram negative organisms which are colonisers of the gastrointestinal tract (e.g. intravenous ceftriaxone or ciprofloxacin).

Antibiotics should be continued for one week's duration. Once the patient is allowed to eat, intravenous antibiotics can be switched to an oral preparation (e.g. ciprofloxacin).

Non-selective beta-blockers such as propranolol are frequently prescribed for primary and secondary prophylaxis of variceal bleeding. These drugs should be stopped during variceal bleeding due to the risk of aggravating hypotension. Beta-blockers can be restarted when there is certainty that re-bleeding will not occur. This is usually upon discharge or 3–5 days after securing haemostasis.

Intravenous drugs constrict the splanchnic circulation and reduce portal venous inflow and pressure.

These drugs should be administered early. They are continued for at least 3–5 days with the exception of vasopressin (see below), which should not be given for more than 24 hr.[3]

Vasopressin is the most potent vasoconstrictor and has to be used with a nitrate infusion. However, it is rarely used due to the risk of inducing myocardial ischemia, bowel gangrene and peripheral limb ischemia, especially when alternative drugs are available with fewer side effects.[7] Vasopressin is given as an intravenous infusion titrated from 0.2 units/min to a maximum of 0.8 units/min. Intravenous nitroglycerin is given at a starting dose of 40 mcg/min, titrated up to as high as 400 mcg/min. Nitrites cause veno-dilatation, thereby reducing systemic blood pressure, while portal pressures are only mildly reduced. Nitroglycerin is titrated against the systolic blood pressure aiming to maintain it above 90 mmHg.[3] Because of the risk of ischemia, vasopressin should not be used for more than 24 hr at high infusion doses.

Terlipressin is a long-acting synthetic analogue of vasopressin. It is associated with significantly fewer peripheral side effects and is therefore safer to use. However ischemia such as myocardial infarction and peripheral gangrene has been known to occur.[8,9] It is given as a dose of 2 mg every 6 hr, rather than as an infusion due to its long half-life. Terlipressin is not readily available in some countries and its high cost may prohibit its use.

Somatostatin is a very commonly used drug and has a short half-life of 1–3 min. It inhibits the release of glucagon, causing splanchnic vasoconstriction, reducing azygous flow and therefore reducing the portal pressure.[6] Somatostatin is given as a slow-loading bolus of 250 mcg, followed by an infusion of 250 mcg/hr for 3–5 days.

Octreotide is an analogue of somatostatin and has a longer half-life of 80–120 min. Octreotide is given as a slow-loading bolus of 50 mcg, followed by an infusion of 50 mcg/hr. Infusions are typically given for 3–5 days because this is the period of greatest risk of re-bleeding. Both octreotide and somatostatin have minimal side effects and can be used continuously for several days without any concern of precipitating an ischemic event.

Endoscopic Management

Endoscopy should not be delayed in a patient with an acute variceal haemorrhage. The ideal time is once the patient is hemodynamically stable.

Attempts to correct any coagulopathy (e.g. fresh frozen plasma, platelet transfusions) are best done before endoscopy. Occasionally, intravenous erythromycin infusion before endoscopy may be useful as a prokinetic agent to empty the stomach of food and blood. This ensures better visualisation and reduces the risk of aspiration, but has never been shown to alter survival rates.

If the patient is hemodynamically unstable, drowsy or having active hematemesis, then endoscopy is best performed in the intensive care unit where close monitoring and a high level of medical support is available.

Patients who are at high risk of aspiration (drowsy, confused, active hematemesis) can be intubated prophylactically and sedated before the procedure to protect their airway. One advantage of airway protection is that it facilitates repositioning of the patient when the source of bleeding is submerged under or obscured by blood. Positioning the patient's body 45 degrees head up, rotating to supine or right lateral may sometimes improve visibility by pooling blood and clots away, revealing the source of the bleeding. These manoeuvers, with the exception of positioning the patient's head up, should be performed only after intubation.

There are a variety of endoscopic techniques for obtaining hemostasis during a variceal bleed. Endoscopic variceal band ligation is the treatment of choice in oesophageal varices, while the injection of cyanoacrylate glue is preferred in gastric fundal varices.[3]

Endoscopic sclerotherapy, which was performed commonly in the past, has been superseded by the previous two methods due to the complications of oesophageal stricture formation, ulceration and mediastinitis. Cyanoacrylate glue appears to be superior to sclerotherapy in the treatment of gastric fundal varices in terms of hemostasis, variceal obliteration and reducing re-bleeding rates.[10] For bleeding oesophageal varices, endoscopic variceal band ligation is superior to injection sclerotherapy in reducing re-bleeding and mortality rates, and has a lower risk of causing oesophageal strictures.[11]

Other endoscopic hemostatic modalities such as endo-loop ligation and clipping have been described in small clinical trials.[12] However, clinical data is limited and it cannot be recommended.

Variceal band ligation

Variceal band ligation is commonly used to treat bleeding oesophageal varices.[13] The multi-band ligator consists of a plastic barrel, which is usually transparent or translucent and slotted into the tip of the scope like a sleeve. Along the outer edges of the plastic barrel are several rubber bands. These rubber bands are attached to a cord that is threaded in a retrograde fashion through the instrument channel of the adult gastroscope. At the operator end, the cord is secured to a dial, which tugs the cord when turned and fires the bands.

Before assembling the multi-band ligator, we recommend surveying the upper gastrointestinal tract with the gastroscope. If it is confirmed that the bleeding is from oesophageal varices, only then should the multi-band ligator be applied. This is because endoscopic visibility with the band ligator is reduced by the plastic barrel.

Before commencing endoscopic variceal ligation, it is important to ensure the following:

1. The plastic barrel is firmly attached to the endoscope tip.
2. The barrel is turned till the cords are not obscuring the view of the endoscopist (Figs. 4.13 and 4.14).
3. The barrel needs to be well lubricated on the exterior surface before insertion.

Once the multi-band ligator has been inserted successfully, the oesophageal varix with the stigmata of recent haemorrhage should be targeted first.

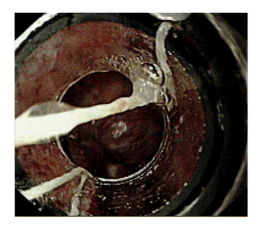

Figure 4.13.

Poor orientation of the variceal ligator barrel resulting in cords obscuring the view.

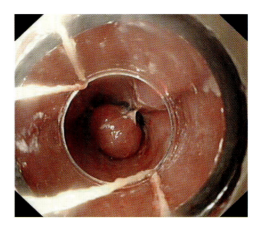

Figure 4.14.

Anti-clockwise rotation of the barrel results in good orientation of the variceal ligator barrel with cords not obscuring view.

Endoscopic band ligation is performed from the lower oesophagus starting from the bleeding varix. Band ligation need not always be applied at the exact spot of the bleed, since strangulation of the varix distally near the gastro-oesophageal junction would stop the bleeding proximally. Many endoscopists would also place a band at the site of bleeding as well.

To perform band ligation, the endoscope tip is placed directly on the varix and continuous suction is applied. When the varix has been sucked into the barrel and occupies the entire lumen (a complete red-out of the screen may occur), then the band ligator is fired. This may require several seconds of suctioning and a little jiggling of the endoscope to coax the varix into the lumen (Figs. 4.15–4.17).

Endoscopic banding is subsequently performed in a spiral fashion on the other cords of varices, moving

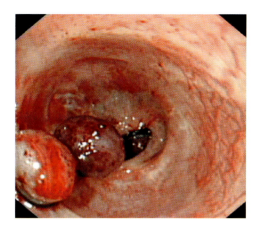

Figure 4.17.

Post band ligation. No further active bleeding is seen.

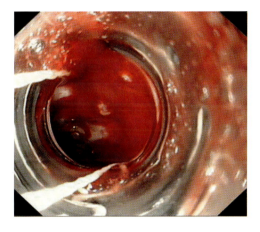

Figure 4.15.

Active bleeding from an oesophageal varix.

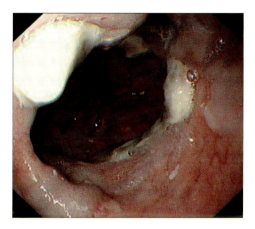

Figure 4.18.

Post-endoscopic variceal ligation ulcers in the distal oesophagus (commonly seen in the first few weeks after ligation). Delayed bleeding can occur from these ulcers.

slightly proximally with each banding. Successful banding will result in flattening of the proximal column. It is important to note that only large varices are amenable to band ligation. Bands will not hold well on small varices and may slip off soon after (Figs. 4.18 and 4.19).

Cyanoacrylate glue

Cyanoacrylate glue injection is useful in treating an acute variceal haemorrhage and can lead to variceal obliteration. The drug used is N-butyl-2-cyanoacrylate (Histoacryl; B.Braun, Dexon, Spangenberg, Germany).

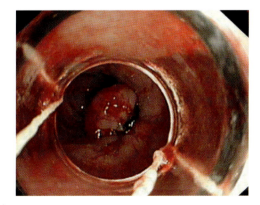

Figure 4.16.

Endoscopic variceal band ligation of oesophageal varices.

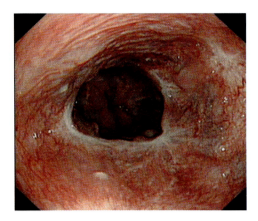

Figure 4.19.

Post-oesophageal endoscopic variceal ligation scaring at 4 o'clock. Varices have collapsed.

Cyanoacrylate glue is particularly useful in the treatment of gastric fundal varices.[6] It can also be used in oesophageal and intra-gastric varices when endoscopic band ligation is not feasible.

When oesophageal varices are actively bleeding, cyanoacrylate glue maybe preferred by some endoscopists as the visibility with the endoscopic band ligator may be poor in such situations. Once haemostasis is obtained with cyanoacrylate glue, endoscopic band ligation can be performed on the non-bleeding oesophageal varices.

Cyanoacrylate glue has been compared to endoscopic band ligation for gastric varices, and both therapies are effective in controlling an acute haemorrhage. However cyanoacrylate glue injection therapy is associated with lower re-bleeding rates.[14] In addition, it is usually easier to target gastric fundal varices with an injector rather than with banding because of the limitations in retroflexion of the endoscope.

Cyanoacrylate glue is a liquid which can be delivered via a standard injection catheter. It polymerises almost instantly on contact with blood, becoming a solid. This plugs the gastric varix immediately, stems the bleeding and thromboses the vein. After injection, the varix will shrivel up weeks later and the glue will be extruded naturally into the stomach. This will leave an ulcer, which will heal spontaneously. Re-bleeding from this ulcer rarely occurs.

There are numerous minor variations in the technique of cyanoacrylate injection. However, the basic principles are universal.

To prepare the glue injection, 0.5 mL of cyanoacrylate is mixed with 0.8 mL of Lipiodol (Guerbet, Roissy, France). This ratio is kept constant in the mixture. Lipiodol prevents premature polymerisation of the cyanoacrylate glue. Lipiodol is also radio-opaque and allows the cyanoacrylate glue to be visualised radiologically. This mixture is aspirated into a 2-mL syringe and kept with the assisting nurse.

Next, the dead space in the injection catheter should be determined. This is measured by filling the injection catheter with saline and noting the volume retained in the catheter. This volume may be 1–2 mL of saline or more. A syringe filled with 10 mL of saline is then kept with the assisting nurse. Syringes used should be of the Luer-lock fitting type or equivalent to prevent accidental spillage of cyanoacrylate during injection.

During endoscopy, gastric varices are targeted at the site of active oozing or at areas with stigmata of recent haemorrhage (e.g. adherent clot, hematocystic spot, white nipple sign, ulceration).

With the endoscope in retroflexion, the tip of the injection catheter is placed at the site of the fundal varix. Cyanoacrylate/lipiodol filled syringes and saline syringes should be ready.

With the injector needle inserted into the varix, 1 mL of the cyanoacrylate/lipiodol mixture is injected.[12] Immediately after that, saline is injected. The volume of saline used is slightly more than the dead space of the catheter (usually in the range of 1–2 mL). This ensures that the entire cyanoacrylate/lipiodol mixture is delivered into the varix and does not remain in the catheter. The needle is retracted, catheter withdrawn, and this is followed immediately with saline flushing of the catheter to ensure its continued patency. If the catheter is felt to be partially occluded, it should be changed for a new one (Figs. 4.20–4.22).

Further injections can be performed until the bleeding has stopped. The varix can be prodded with the catheter (needle retracted) to look for any areas which dimple on compression. These areas can also be targeted at the same session or at subsequent endoscopies.

Of note, the assisting nurse should be wearing gloves and eye shields for protection. The endoscopist and any other assistant should also do likewise. This is

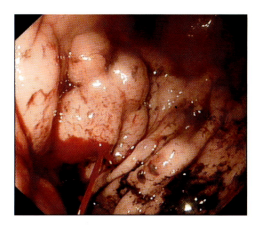

Figure 4.20.

Large fundal varices (GOV2) with active bleeding seen.

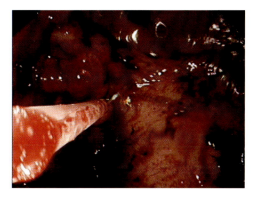

Figure 4.21.

Saline flushing of the injection catheter after delivery of cyanoacrylate glue. This is important to prevent occlusion of the needle after injection and to confirm patency before the next injection.

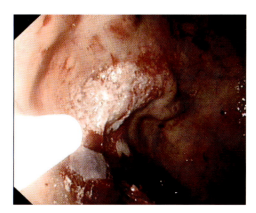

Figure 4.22.

Post-cyanoacrylate glue injection with cessation of bleeding of the fundal varix.

because cyanoacrylate may be accidentally squirted out of the syringe during delivery. Also, the endoscopist should refrain from excessive suction during glue injection as glue may be aspirated into the endoscope and occlude the channel permanently.

Complications of cyanoacrylate/lipiodol injection include bleeding, pulmonary embolism of the glue, cerebral embolism of glue, splenic infarction, portal vein and splenic vein thrombosis.[15] Glue injection should be avoided in patients with large gastro-renal shunts, hepato-pulmonary syndrome and intra-cardiac shunts due to embolic risks. Also, the risk of glue embolism can be reduced by injecting aliquots of not more than 1 mL each time.[12]

Other complications related to cyanoacrylate glue injection include needle adherence to the varix, catheter occlusion, and adherence of glue to the endoscope (particularly the lens and suction channel).

Endoscopic sclerotherapy

Since injection sclerotherapy is used infrequently due to other alternatives, we shall describe it briefly. Endoscopic sclerotherapy, which was frequently used in the past, is effective in controlling variceal bleeding.

Injection sclerotherapy is used to treat oesophageal varices. It has also been used in the management of gastric varices. However, isolated gastric varices are better treated with cyanoacrylate glue injection.

Sclerotherapy is performed by either intra-variceal (into the varix) or para-variceal (around the varix) injection of a sclerosant. Intra-variceal injections lead to endothelial damage and thrombosis with collapse of the varix, while para-variceal injections cause mechanical tamponade of the varix.

Agents such as sodium tetradecyl sulfate, sodium morrhuate, ethanolamine oleate, polidocanol and ethanol have all been used.

However, injection sclerotherapy is not widely practiced anymore due to its higher incidence of complications such as fever, retrosternal pain, dysphagia, bleeding, oesophageal ulceration, perforation, mediastinitis, fistula and infections as compared to other methods of variceal endoscopic therapy.[16]

Subsequent endoscopy

After the initial episode of acute variceal bleeding has resolved, endoscopy for variceal eradication and further therapy is recommended two weeks later.

Endoscopy should continue at this interval until the varices have been eradicated or are too small to treat endoscopically. After which, it is suggested that a screening endoscopy is performed three months later and if only small varices are present, the next endoscopy can be performed annually for life.[3]

Insertion of the Sengstaken–Blakemore tube

The Sengstaken–Blakemore tube (SB tube) is a useful tool in the initial control of variceal bleeding (both gastric cardia and oesophageal varices) when endoscopic therapy fails.[17]

It is successful in up to 80% of the time.[18] The SB tube applies mechanical tamponade on the varices, thereby preventing further bleeding. This provides ample time to correct any haematological derangements and to organise a definitive plan of treatment (such as portal systemic shunt therapy or repeat endoscopy).

The SB tube consists of a gastric balloon which compresses on the fundal/cardia varices and an oesophageal balloon which compresses on the oesophageal varices.

At the proximal end are 3 ports:

1. One port which drains the distal lumen of the SB tube and is for gastric decompression.
2. One port for inflating the gastric balloon.
3. One port for inflating the oesophageal balloon.

A modification of the SB tube is the Minnesota tube, where there is another port that allows the evacuation of secretions above the oesophageal balloon (Fig. 4.23).

Expertise and training is recommended before inserting a SB tube. This is because improper placement can lead to persistence of bleeding or fatal complications.

Before the insertion of an SB tube, one should have the following accessories ready: two pairs of artery forceps, a 1 kg weight such as a 1 L bag of saline, a pulley and cord to suspend the weight, lubricating gel,

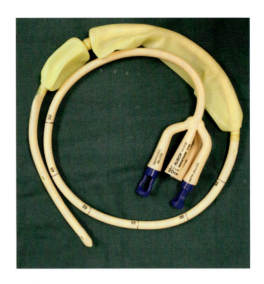

Figure 4.23.

The four-port Minnesota tube, a modified SB tube with an additional port for the aspiration of oesophageal secretions above the oesophageal balloon. The other three ports are the oesophageal balloon inflation port, gastric balloon inflation port and the distal lumen port.

pressure gauge or a blood pressure manometer set, and a 50 ml syringe.

All patients should be intubated and possibly sedated, as aspiration may occur in an actively bleeding patient and the SB tube is usually poorly tolerated in an agitated, sometimes encephalopathic patient.

The gastric and oesophageal balloons should be tested before insertion by inflating them. Placing the balloon underwater briefly is useful to check for any bubbling, which would suggest a leak.

During inflation of the balloons, the manometer or pressure gauge is connected between the desired port and the syringe. A trial inflation of the gastric balloon before insertion is useful. The pressure of the gastric balloon should be noted as it distends progressively with air. For instance, the corresponding inflation pressures as measured by the manometer at 50 mL, 100 mL, 200 mL, 300 mL and 400 mL of air are noted.

The SB tube is then copiously lubricated with jelly and inserted through the nostril after anaesthetising the nasal passage with a local anaesthetic spray. One should be careful to avoid coiling the tube in the oropharynx as it may give an inaccurate estimation of the depth of insertion. The aim is to insert the SB tube as far in as possible, usually past the 50 cm mark, such that the gastric balloon is well past the gastro-oesophageal junction.

Once deep in the stomach, the position is confirmed by aspirating blood or gastric secretions and the air insufflation test. Testing the gastric pH may not be useful as the bloody aspirate may stain the testing strip.

The gastric balloon is inflated first, noting the pressure measurement on the manometer. Based on the volume of air infused, the pressure should correspond in a similar fashion to the recorded pressures noted earlier. If the gastric balloon is positioned within the oesophagus, the pressure will be drastically higher than previously noted, indicating incorrect positioning. With proper positioning, the gastric balloon is inflated to a total volume of 400 mL before the gastric port is clamped with a pair of artery forceps.

The SB tube is tugged so that the gastric balloon is compressed against any fundal varices at the gastro-oesphagal junction, then the oesophageal balloon is inflated to a pressure of 30–35 mmHg. Inflation to a pressure greater than 35 mmHg increases the risk of oesophageal wall ischemia and pressure necrosis. Once the optimal pressure is achieved, the port is clamped with the second pair of artery forceps.

The external end of the SB tube is attached via the cord to a weight (e.g. saline bag) and suspended from a pulley at the foot of the bed. This ensures that the gastric balloon applies constant pressure against the fundal varices. The gastric aspiration port can be connected to low intermittent suction as required.

The position of the SB tube should be confirmed with a chest radiograph. Every four hours, the oesophageal balloon should be deflated for five minutes before re-inflating it to the optimal pressure of 30–35 mmHg. The gastric balloon is never deflated (Fig. 4.24).

If the SB tube appears to be migrating out of the nose, it usually indicates that the gastric balloon could be leaking air. In the event that the patient has respiratory distress, one possibility is that the gastric or oesophageal balloon may have migrated proximally and compressed on the airway. During deflation, the

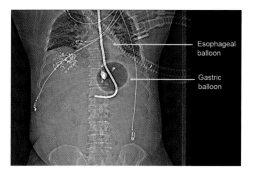

Figure 4.24.

CT scan showing Sengstaken–Blakemore tube inserted in a patient with uncontrolled oesophageal variceal bleeding. Outlines of the oesophageal and gastric balloons are visible as hypodense shadows. Lipiodol injected into a hepatocellular carcinoma is present as a hyperdense speckled lesion in the right hypochondrium.

oesophageal balloon is always deflated first, followed by the gastric balloon.

The most dreaded complication of SB tube insertion is the inflation of the gastric balloon within the oesophagus, resulting in oesophageal rupture.[19] Other complications of SB tube insertion include migration of the tube with upper airway obstruction, trauma to the pharynx and oesophagus, mucosal ischemia from prolonged inflation, and accidental insertion of the tube into the airway.[20] Generally, SB tubes should not be left inflated for more than 24 hr due to the risk of oesophageal ischemia caused by the oesophageal balloon.

Portosystemic shunts: TIPS and surgery

Endoscopic management is successful in the majority of variceal bleeds. However, there are occasionally patients who continue to bleed. Patients who fail two attempts of endoscopic therapies and continue to bleed should be considered for other non-endoscopic therapies. In the interim period, the variceal bleeding can be arrested temporarily with a SB tube, while plans on a definitive procedure are contemplated.

In such cases, either TIPS or surgical portosystemic shunts are indicated. In gastric variceal bleeds, a TIPS procedure may be combined with embolisation of the varix.

Portosystemic shunts include selective and non-selective shunts: portocaval, interposition mesocaval, and splenorenal shunts. Portosystemic shunts are very effective in reducing portal pressures. However they increase the risk of postoperative hepatic decompensation and hepatic encephalopathy. A study showed that both TIPS and distal splenorenal shunts are equivalent in the prevention of re-bleeding, and there was no difference in survival rates or hepatic encephalopathy.[21]

Another option other than shunt surgery is to perform surgical oesophageal transaction or devascularisation. However this is associated with a high risk of late re-bleeding, as portal hypertension is not resolved. This procedure is usually reserved for patients who are not candidates for a shunt procedure.

One should bear in mind that TIPS is the preferred treatment rather than surgery if the patient is a candidate for liver transplant surgery. Surgical shunts may cause subsequent scarring and can make the liver transplant surgery more complicated.[22]

A TIPS procedure is performed by the interventional radiologist under fluoroscopic guidance and involves decompressing the portal venous system by creating an artificial shunt between a branch of the portal vein and the intrahepatic vein. The aim is to decrease the portal pressure to less than 12 mmHg, and this should be achieved in 90% of all cases.[23] Decreasing the portal pressure leads to a cessation of acute variceal bleeding in up to 93% of the patients. However, performing TIPS for an acute variceal bleed is an independent predictor of mortality, and despite controlling the bleed, short-term mortality rates are high.[24]

Not all patients are suitable for a TIPS procedure. Absolute contraindications to TIPS include a patient with congestive heart failure, multiple liver cysts, uncontrolled sepsis, biliary obstruction with dilated intrahepatic ducts, severe pulmonary hypertension (mean pulmonary pressures more than 45 mmHg) and poorly controlled hepatic encephalopathy.[25]

Complications of a TIPS procedure include infection, hepatic capsular puncture, hepatic encephalopathy, bleeding, hemobilia and stent occlusion.[26] Of note, the rates of stent occlusion have decreased with the introduction of newer polytetrafluoroethylene covered stents as opposed to the older bare metal stents.[27]

References

1. Garcia-Tsao G, Groszmann RJ, Fisher RL, *et al.* (1985) Portal pressure, presence of gastroesophageal varices and variceal bleeding. *Hepatology* **5(3)**: 419–424.
2. Chalasani N, Kahi C, Francois F, *et al.* (2003) Improved patient survival after acute variceal bleeding: A multicenter, cohort study. *Am J Gastroenterol* **98**: 653–659.
3. Garcia-Tsao G, Sanyal AJ, Grace ND, *et al.* (2007) Prevention and management of gastroesophageal varices and variceal hemorrhage in cirrhosis. *Hepatology* **46(3)**: 922–938.
4. Sarin SK, Lahoti D, Saxena SP, *et al.* (1992) Prevalence, classification and natural history of gastric varices: A longterm follow-up study in 568 portal hypertension patients. *Hepatology* **16**: 1343–1349.
5. Zaman A. (2006) Portal hypertension-related bleeding: management of difficult cases. *Clin Liver Dis* **10(2)**: 353–70, ix.
6. Hadengue A. (1999) Somatostatin or octreotide in acute variceal bleeding. Digestion **60 Suppl 2**: 31–41.
7. Bolognesi M, Balducci G, Garcia-Tsao G, *et al.* (2001) *Complications in the medical treatment of portal hypertension. Portal Hypertension III. Proceedings of the Third Baveno International Consensus Workshop on Definitions, Methodology and Therapeutic Strategies.* Oxford, UK: Blackwell Science, pp. 180–203.
8. Lee MY, Chu CS, Lee KT, *et al.* (2004) Terlipressin-related acute myocardial infarction: A case report and literature review. *Kaohsiung J Med Sci* **20(12)**: 604–608.
9. Lee JS, Lee HS, Jung SW, *et al.* (2006) A case of peripheral ischemic complication after terlipressin therapy. *Korean J Gastroenterol* **47(6)**: 454–457.
10. Sarin SK, Jain AK, Jain M, *et al.* (2002) A randomized controlled trial of cyanoacrylate vs. alcohol injection in patients with isolated fundic varices. *Am J Gastroenterol* **97**: 1010–1015.
11. Laine L, Cook D. (1995) Endoscopic ligation compared with sclerotherapy for treatment of esophageal variceal bleeding. *Ann Intern Med* **123**: 280–287.
12. Seewald S, Ang TL, Imazu H, *et al.* (2008) A standardized injection technique and regimen ensures success and safety of N-butyl-2-cyanoacrylate injection for the treatment of gastric fundal varices (with videos). *Gastrointest Endosc* **68(3)**: 447–54.
13. Van Stiegmann G, Cambre T, Sun JH. (1986) A new endoscopic elastic band ligating device. *Gastrointest Endosc* **32(3)**: 230–233.

14. Tan PC, Hou MC, Lin HC, *et al*. (2006) A randomized trial of endoscopic treatment of acute gastric variceal hemorrhage: N-butyl-2-cyanoacrylate injection versus band ligation. *Hepatology* **43**: 690–697.

15. Chang PN, Sheu BS, Chen CY, *et al*. (1998) Splenic infarction after histoacryl injection for bleeding gastric varices. *Gastrointest Endosc* **48**: 426–427.

16. Higashi H, Kitano S, Hashizume M, *et al*. (1989) A prospective randomized trial of schedules for sclerosing esophageal varices. 1-versus 2-week intervals. *Hepatogastroenterology* **36(5)**: 337–340.

17. Sengstaken RW, Blakemore AH. (1950) Balloon tamponage for the control of hemorrhage from esophageal varices. *Ann Surg* **131(5)**: 781–789.

18. Avgerinos A, Klonis C, Rekoumis G, *et al*. (1991) A prospective randomized trial comparing somatostatin, balloon tamponade and the combination of both methods in the management of acute variceal haemorrhage. *J Hepatol* **13(1)**: 78–83.

19. Chojkier M, Conn HO. (1980) Esophageal tamponade in the treatment of bleeding varices. A decadel progress report. *Dig Dis Sci* **25(4)**: 267–272.

20. Kelly DJ, Walsh F, Ahmed S, *et al*. (1997) Airway obstruction due to a Sengstaken–Blakemore tube. *Anesth Analg* **85**: 219–221.

21. Henderson JM, Boyer TD, Kutner M, *et al*. (2006) Distal splenorenal shunt versus transjugular intrahepatic portal systemic shunt for variceal bleeding: A randomized trial. *Gastroenterology* **130**: 1643–1651.

22. Rikkers LF, Jin G. (1994) Surgical management of acute variceal hemorrhage. *World J Surg* **18(2)**: 193–199.

23. Haskal ZJ, Martin L, Cardella JF, *et al*. (2003) Quality improvement guidelines for transjugular intrahepatic porto-systemic shunts. *J Vasc Interv Radiol* **14**: S265–S270.

24. Vangeli M, Patch D, Burroughs AK. (2003) Salvage tips for uncontrolled variceal bleeding. *J Hepatol* **37**: 703–704.

25. Boyer TD, Haskal ZJ (2010) American Association for the Study of Liver Diseases. The Role of Transjugular Intrahepatic Portosystemic Shunt (TIPS) in the Management of Portal Hypertension: update 2009. *Hepatology* **51(1)**: 306.

26. Rossle M, Siegerstetter V, Huber M, *et al*. (1998) The first decade of the transjugular intrahepatic portosystemic shunt (TIPS): state of the art. *Liver* **18**: 73–89.

27. Bureau C, Garcia-Pagan JC, Otal P, *et al*. (2004) Improved clinical outcome using polytetrafluoroethylene-coated stents for TIPS: Results of a randomized study. *Gastroenterology* **126**: 469–475.

Chapter 5

Interventional Radiology in the Management of Gastrointestinal Haemorrhage

Lenny Tan*

Introduction

Gastrointestinal bleeding is divided into:

Upper GI bleed — occurring proximal to the ligament of Treitz, i.e. the oesophagus, stomach and duodenum.
Lower GI bleed — from the rest of the small bowel and colon.

Bleeding may be:

Direct into the lumen from a primary pathology in that segment of bowel.
Indirect as in transpapillary bleeding through biliary or pancreatic ducts. It may be inflammatory, malignant or postoperative in origin.

There are no reliable Singapore figures for frequency and causes of GI bleeding. In the US and UK, it is estimated that the incidence of upper GI bleeding is 100/100 000 adults/year with a mortality of 5%–14%. For those under age 60 with no co-morbidities, it is much lower at 0.6%.

Lower GI bleed occurs in 24.4/100 000 adults/year in similar publications.

It is significant that the majority of gastrointestinal bleeding will stop on its own without direct treatment but may recur. Often, fluid and/or blood replacement is all that is required.

It is particularly important to first determine if the patient is still bleeding at the time of presentation before any investigation or intervention is considered.

Various parameters have been used.
Published data indicate that:

1) when BP is < 90 mmHg, positive angiography rate is 87% vs 12% if BP higher
2) if patient requires transfusion of 5 units of blood, positive rate is 84% vs 16% if less
3) if hemoglobin falls more than 5 gm/ml, positive rate is 85% vs 26%
4) heart rate, BP are useful clinical indicators

Patient will likely be in shock when > 40% of blood volume is lost.[1]

Management Options

The current practice is first to perform upper GI endoscopy to exclude upper GI bleed and to institute appropriate treatment if found.

If endoscopy is negative, CT angiography and possibly catheter angiography with a view to embolisation or surgery are options.

---
*Lenny Tan, MD, FSIR, Emeritus Consultant, Department of Diagnostic Imaging, National University Hospital and Professor, National University of Singapore, Singapore.

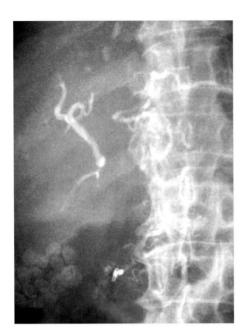

Figure 1.

Inadvertent endoscopic injection of glue into hepatic artery.

In a series of 163 patients with upper GI bleed over 11 years, *Shenker et al.*[2] found that if embolisation was successful and no further bleeding occurs, mortality is 11%. This compares with 68% if unsuccessful. These figures closely parallel other published series from different institutions.

Bleeding on endoscopy or angiography may be diffuse over a wide area as in haemorrhagic gastritis, duodenitis and is a clinical dilemma. It would be difficult to embolise completely, and equally difficult to treat by endoscopy or surgery.

Endoscopy provides both diagnostic and therapeutic potential in the upper GI tract. However, care should be exercised particularly in the use of liquid embolic material which could be inadvertently injected (Fig. 1).

Catheter Angiography

Angiography must be selective and preferably subselective. All potential supply vessels must be studied and include the Coeliac Axis, Superior and Inferior Mesenteric Arteries and their branches with the use of microcatheters in more peripheral vessels (Figs. 2 and 3).

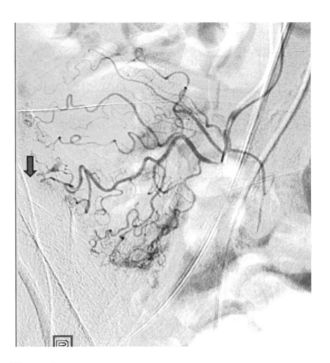

Figure 2.

Subselective injection into caecal artery showing site of bleeding.

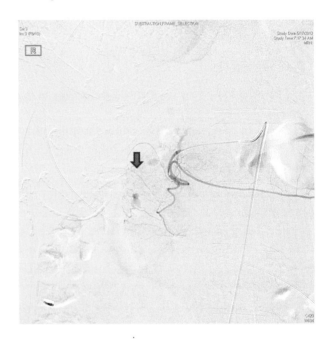

Figure 3.

Bleeding site shown in injection close to bleeding artery.

It is significant to mention that there are extensive collaterals around the stomach and duodenum and flow patterns should be fully understood before intervention in this area. It may be necessary to occlude several arteries to reduce perfusion and encourage thrombosis to develop before bleeding ceases.

Angiography has been variously estimated as likely to be positive when the bleeding rate is at least 0.5 mL/min. The advent of good digital subtraction angiography greatly enhances its sensitivity, which may be increased, tremendously (by a factor of 5 to 9) depending on various factors, including patients ability to cooperate and the equipment available.

The use of microcatheters and very selective catheterisation of suspected bleeding vessels further improve successful detection and management.

CT Angiography

MDCT has high contrast sensitivity and plays a very important role especially in post-trauma patients.

Publications on its role in GI bleeding confirm its value. It demonstrates active bleeding, the exact site and possible pathology by way of extravasation of contrast injected.

In published series, the cohorts are usually small but results consistent. The patient, however, must be bleeding at the time of scan. So do not delay the study to stabilise the patient as bleeding may have stopped by then.

All studies indicate that the inclusion of arterial and delayed phases with MDCT reformation in at least coronal/sagittal planes are helpful (Figs. 4 and 5).

Delayed scans are particularly useful to detect very small bleeds.

Direct signs of bleeding are seen as extravasation of contrast into the lumen of bowel or attached organs (Figs. 6 and 7). Indirect signs such as false or true aneurysms, irregularity of vessels, vessel cut-off and shunting may be seen in patients without extravasation (Fig. 8).

CO_2 angiography is utilised to take advantage of its low viscosity compared with contrast media. There are many reports published comparing its value with contrast angiography. In properly equipped centres, the detection rate is favourable with reported comparisons of 44 % vs 14%.[3]

Its value lies in its lack of toxicity and being less viscous than contrast media, hence its ability to exit a small bleeding point is greatly enhanced. However, there are some difficulties in this technique and it carries a larger dose of radiation.

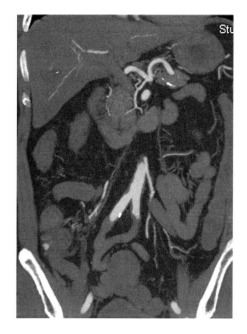 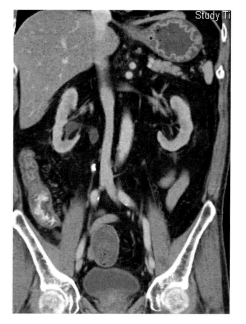

Figure 4.

CT angiogram showing delayed — accumulation of contrast in caecum.

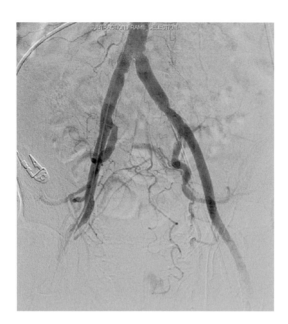
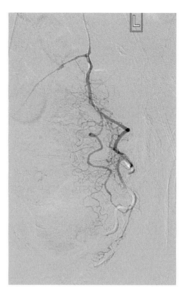

Figure 5.

Angio shows bleeding artery and post embolism.

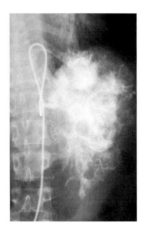
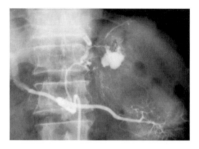
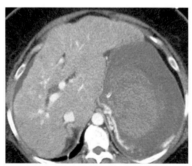

Figure 6.

Demonstrates bleeding into lumen of stomach.

There may be no nephrotoxicity associated with medical CO_2 but technical problems may arise if segmentation or break-up of the column of gas occurs.

Other variations include CT angiography with carbon dioxide given through a selectively placed catheter amongst others.

Many variations and combinations of the above techniques have been tried but none have gained general acceptance.

Radioisotope imaging, either by way of RBC scintigraphy, sulphur colloid, is seldom used in acute bleeding because of the longer time taken for the

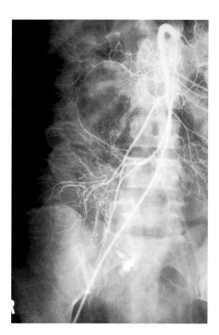

Figure 7.

Bleeding into ileum in typhoid enteritis.

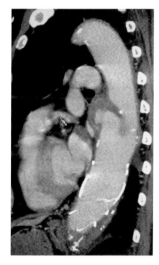
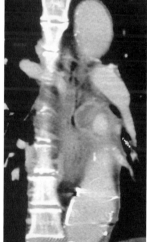

Figure 8.

Aorto-esophageal fistula on CT.

procedure. Its value lies in very slow and intermittent bleeds as in Meckels diverticulum.

Vasopressin perfusion has been used previously as a vasoconstrictor to encourage thrombosis at the bleeding point.

It is hardly used today because of its cardiovascular effects as well as the longer time taken to effectively control bleeding if at all. The additional disadvantage is the long duration the catheter is maintained in the vessel with the potential hazards of dislodgement, thrombus formation and ischemia. The patient will need careful monitoring and outcomes are uncertain.

Success with vasopressin occurs in 52% as compared with 88% in embolisation.[4]

Embolic Agents

Which embolic agent should be used?

Embolisation must be carried out with absolute accuracy. There is no option for flow directed delivery as the potential for unintended embolisation and its consequences are no longer acceptable.

All particulate material must be accurately deployed as they may be impossible to retrieve.

Unfortunately, there has never been any randomised trial on embolic material available.

Various types, including gel foam particles, PVA particles, microcoils, have been used. It is not advisable to use liquid embolic material as it is difficult to control its delivery.

If microcoils are used, it must be accurately deployed and if one cannot advance beyond the marginal artery, it should be avoided (Figs. 9–12).

Difficulties

Technical difficulties are often an issue. Sometimes, it is not possible to get close enough to the bleeding vessel or in the process of advancing the guidewire/catheter system, and the vessel is traumatised (Fig. 13). This should always be borne in mind when conducting such procedures.

Contraindications to Angiography/CT/Embolisation

1) Sensitivity to contrast media is an absolute contraindication and CO_2 angiography would then be the preferred alternative.

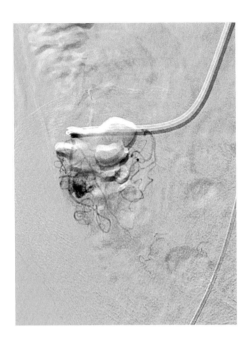
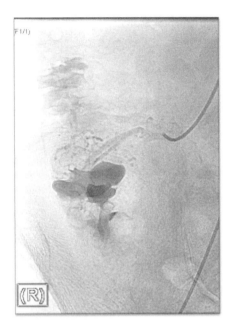

Figure 9.

Catheter is very peripheral to deliver embolic material.

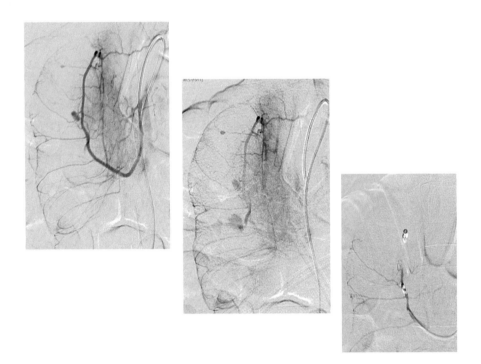

Figure 10.

Duodenum bleed with coils at both ends of artery.

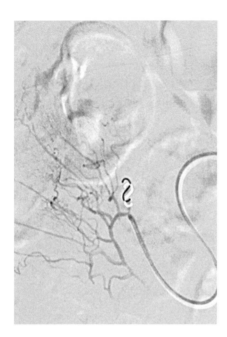

Figure 11.

Coil delivered peripherally.

2) Renal failure is another relative contraindication depending on the severity of bleeding and need for intervention. Appropriate rehydration is important.

3) Previous extensive surgery or radiotherapy may have altered the circulation and the risk of infarction is greatly increased. This should be borne in mind.

Complications of Angiography

Complications are usually related to the puncture site, i.e. haematoma. Other possibilities include true/false aneurysms and a/v fistula.

Trauma to the arterial/venous structures in the process of manipulating the catheter/guidewire system is particularly likely as small vessels are involved.

Contrast media sensitivity and contrast nephropathy have been mentioned previously.

Unintended embolisation can occur if particles are too small, if injection had been too forceful or the catheter badly placed.

Liquid sclerosants are difficult to control and may lead to necrosis. It is preferable not to use them.

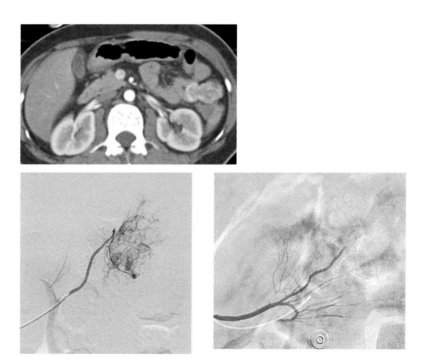

Figure 12.

Tumour presented with bleeding embolised.

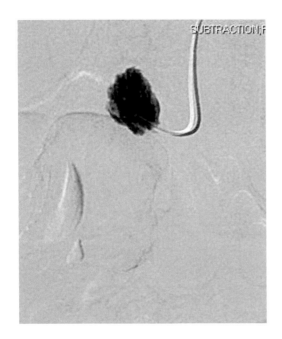

Figure 13.

Trauma to vessel during catheter angiography.

Outcomes

Technical success rates are very high — varying from 80%–100% in various series.

Initial control of bleeding occurs in 71%–86% in various series.

It is significant that if embolisaton is performed distal to the marginal artery in the colon, recurrence is almost 0% vs 52% if delivered more proximally.[5,6]

Technical failure is often due to vessel spasm or tortuosity preventing adequate access close to the bleeding point.

Clinical success is more difficult to measure as it cannot predict collateral vessels that may open up and coagulopathies after severe blood loss.

Indirect Bleeding

These include haemobilia often from previous surgery and treatment in the first instance is usually conservative. If that fails, embolisation of the abnormal vessels demonstrated at angiography is the treatment option available.

Pancreatic aneurysms/pseudoaneurysms, particularly associated with pancreatitis, warrants separate consideration. Mortality exceeds 90% with conservative management.

Aneurysms commonly involve the splenic artery and the pancreatico-duodenal arcades, and should be managed surgically. Radiology may facilitate by reducing the likelihood of bleeding with appropriate embolisation (Fig. 14).

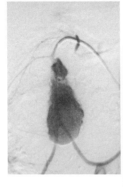
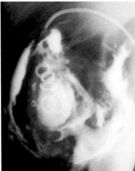
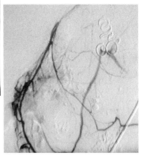

Figure 14.

Pancreatitis with aneurysm-embolised before surgery.

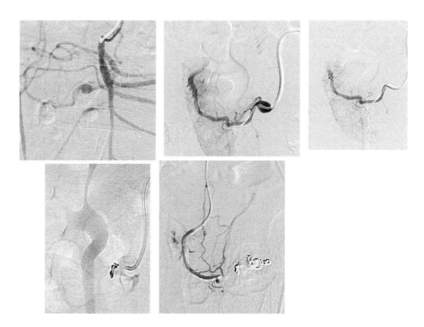

Figure 15.

Aneurysm embolised — arteries coiled at both sides.

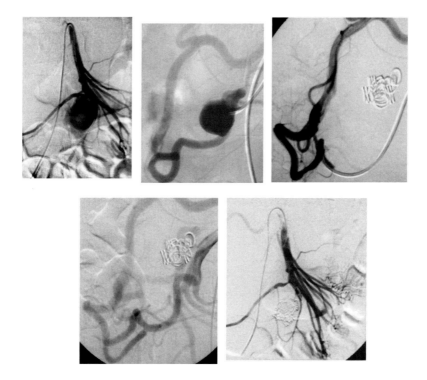

Figure 16.

Larger aneurysm — coils in aneurysm only.

True aneurysms are best treated with either proximal and distal embolisation or covered stents may be used, depending on the aetiology (Figs. 15 and 16).

The ultimate choice of management options depends on the pathology, urgency, available expertise, facilities, equipment and overall ancillary support at that point in time.

References

1. Abbas *et al.* (2005) *Aust NZ J Surg* **75**: 953–957.
2. Shenker *et al.* (2001) *JVIR* **12**: 1269–1271.
3. Back *et al.* (1998) *Surg Clin North America* **78**: 575–591.
4. Gomes *et al.* (1986) *AJR* **146**: 1031–1037.
5. Nicholson *et al.* (1998) *Gut* **43**: 79–84.
6. Peck *et al.* (1998) *JVIR* 747–751.

Chapter 6

Bleeding Peptic Ulcer — Surgical Management

Ti Thiow Kong*

I. Indications

As described in Chapters 3–5, modern endoscopy and interventional radiology services provide effective and less invasive alternative procedures to surgery in the management of upper gastrointestinal haemorrhage. Surgery is now a stand-by for the dwindling numbers of patients in whom endoscopy and interventional radiology have failed to *arrest life-threatening haemorrhage*. Nevertheless, the challenge for the surgeon has become all the greater as these patients, exsanguinated by complicated bleeding lesions, are also frequently old and in poor condition from systemic disease and possibly organ failure.

Besides peptic ulcer disease, a diverse group of gastro-duodenal conditions can bleed massively, necessitating emergency surgery.

1. Dieulafoy's lesion, in which an aberrant vessel in the mucosa bleeds through a pinpoint ulcer in the proximal stomach occasionally re-bleeds even after repeated endoscopic clipping. Haemostasis is easily accomplished by suture-ligation through gastrostomy.
2. Local surgical treatment also arrests the occasional severe bleeding from duodenal diverticulum or Mallory–Weiss tear.
3. Gastroduodenal tumours — carcinoma, lymphoma, stromal tumour and carcinoid — all have

necessitated urgent resection for life-threatening haemorrhage.
4. Bleeding stress gastritis/ulcer in ventilator-dependent patients is best prevented by appropriate prophylaxis. The role of surgery when massive bleeding occurs in this condition is uncertain.
5. Variceal haemorrhage, most commonly from portal hypertension in liver cirrhosis, is best managed by endoscopic ligation/sclerotherapy and, if this fails, by transjugular intrahepatic portasystemic shunt (TIPS). Surgical oesophago-gastric devascularisation and emergency porto-caval shunting have perhaps outlived their role.

To a large extent too, advances in medical treatment, endoscopy and interventional radiology have diminished the role of surgery in peptic ulcer disease. Elective surgery for peptic ulcer is virtually extinct, its role being confined to the treatment of complications of the disease.

Operative Strategy for Bleeding Peptic Ulcer

The primary aim of surgery is to identify the lesion and arrest bleeding expeditiously, and prevent recurrent bleeding. Thus in all patients, suture-ligation of the bleeder should be performed soonest. With the availability of PPI and anti-*Helicobacter pylori*

*T. K. Ti, MD. FRCS, FRACS, FRCSE *ad hominen*, Emeritus Consultant, Department of Surgery, National University Hospital, and Professorial Fellow, National University of Singapore, Singapore.

treatment, many surgeons nowadays do not proceed to definitive ulcer surgery after arresting haemorrhage.

The secondary aim of ulcer cure by surgery has a stronger argument in gastric ulcer than in duodenal ucer. While PPI and anti-Helicobacter medication heal the majority of duodenal ulcer, gastric ulcer healing has a failure rate of 30–40%.

As ulcer curative surgery increases the magnitude of the procedure, it should be offered only to fit patients by experienced gastric surgeons.

*The present author's selective operative strategy on bleeding peptic ulcer is along the following guidelines:

1. Suture-ligation only is performed on a patient with a short history of ulcer disease, operative findings of small or non-fibrotic duodenal or gastric ulcer, or who is in a poor general condition.
2. Definitive ulcer surgery is performed on a patient with a long ulcer history, failed medical treatment, has a large fibrotic duodenal ulcer or NSAID related giant ulcer (GDA) and is in a good general condition. Curative surgery is usually by vagotomy with a drainage procedure. It is however imperative that the surgeon has the skills to convert from over-sewing to a salvage gastrectony should operative complications arise.
3. A large bleeding fibrotic gastric ulcer is treated by excision of the ulcer when a patient is in a poor condition. Hemigastrectomy is performed in a patient who is fit.
4. Definitive surgery for peptic ulcer disease would also be advantageous in poor communities where cost and distance make continual follow-up care not always feasible.

II. Preoperative Preparation

1. Ensure adequate infusion of fluids and blood components to restore and maintain blood volume and circulation as outlined in Chapter 2.
2. Insert a large-bore nasogastric tube and apply suction to help empty the stomach.

3. To avert mortality in patients with advanced age and/or with severe systemic disease, provide maximal supportive peri-operative care in ICU.
4. In patients with massive bleeding, it is imperative that endoscopy be performed in the operation theatre, thus facilitating, when necessary, immediate conversion to surgery.

III. Operative Procedures for Bleeding Peptic Ulcer

The anatomy of the stomach and upper abdomen is shown in Fig. 6.1.

A. Laparotomy and Identification of Site of Haemorrhage

1. **Exposure:** Upper mid-line incision from the xiphisternum to the umbilicus. This exposure is usually adequate without extending the incision below the umbilicus for all gastro-duodenal procedures. Limitation of exposure occurs when the incision does not reach the xiphisternal notch. Goligher retractors are helpful in improving exposure, especially in obese patients undergoing definitive ulcer surgery.
2. **Assessment:** Retract the liver and gallbladder. Massive bleeding is frequently evident in a stomach grossly distended by blood and clots. Identify the Vein of Mayo, which separates the pylorus from the duodenum. Note and feel the stomach, especially in the antrum and lesser curvature for induration and scarring suggestive of gastric ulcer. Assess extent of duodenal scarring and peri-duodenal fibrosis and fixity of the duodenal bulb to the pancreas and hilum of liver, the presence of which are features of advanced duodenal disease. Correlate with findings at gastroscopy.
3. **Anticipate** more technical difficulties when the duodenal bulb is distorted and fixed.

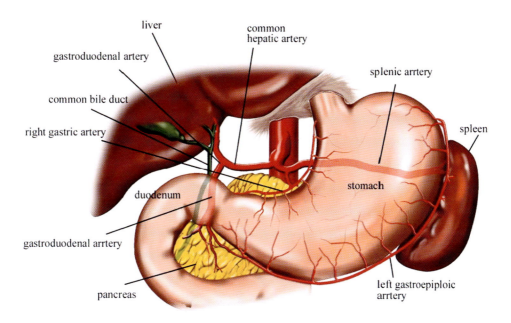

Figure 6.1.

Gross anatomy and blood supply of the stomach and duodenum.

B. Over-Sewing a Bleeding Ulcer

1. For duodenal ulcer, **Kocherisation** facilitates exposure of the duodenum, especially in obese patients with severe duodenal disease. The peritoneal reflection on the second part of the duodenum is divided by scissors or diathermy allowing the proximal part of duodenum with the pancreas to be lifted forward. The hepatic flexure of colon, when in the way, requires mobilisation and downward retraction before Kocherisation.

2. In **duodenal ulcer haemorrhage**, a 5–6 cm incision is made axially over the pylorus and first part of duodenum, centred at the Vein of Mayo, which is diathermised. Blood and clots are evacuated from the stomach.

3. With adequate retraction, the bleeder and ulcer are sought. Bleeding may be from a spurter or ulcer margin or may even have stopped. One or more figure-of-eight stitches of absorbable sutures (e.g. vicryl 3-0) are used to stop bleeding from a spurting vessel or prevent recurrent bleeding from clotted vessels at the base of the duodenal ulcer.

4. Unless the ulcer is very large and fibrotic, it is usually possible to appose the ulcer margins with several interrupted 3-0 vicryl sutures. This reduces the possibility of recurrent haemorrhage and expedites healing.

5. The gastro-duodenal incision is sutured longitudinally — inner continuous vicryl or PDS 3-0, and outer sero-muscular interrupted silk, 3-0. When vagotomy is anticipated, the gastro-duodenal incision is closed transversely as a **pyloroplasty**, with a single layer of interrupted absorbable 3-0 vicryl or PDS. The gaps between sutures are checked with the dissecting forceps and, where found, obliterated by a reinforcing suture (Fig. 6.2).

6. For a small **gastric ulcer**, a 5–6 cm incision is made over the anterior mid-stomach and the bleeding ulcer similarly sutured and over-sewn. Following suture-ligation of gastric bleeder, the gastrostomy is closed using a full thickness inner layer of continuous 3-0 vicryl or PDS followed by outer sero-muscular layer of 3-0 continuous silk sutures.

C. Techniques for Problematical Duodenal Ulcer Bleeding

Complicated duodenal ulcer disease is manifested as duodenal distortion and stenosis. Severe periduodenal fibrosis frequently indicates deep penetrating ulcers

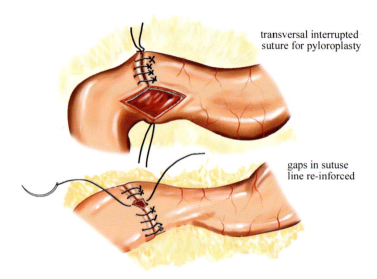

transversal interrupted
suture for pyloroplasty

gaps in sutuse
line re-inforced

Figure 6.2.

Pyloroplasty.

and duodenal ulcer extending into the second part of duodenum. Periduodenal oedema and emphysema is sometimes evident in deep penetrating ulcers that had undergone attempts at endoscopic sclerotherapy.

Problem 1

Extensive ulceration extending into second part of duodenum

Severe duodenal ulcer disease may present as extensive areas of deep ulceration and mucosal denudation extending into the second part of duodenum.

1. To deal with this, duodenostomy is extended after full Kocherisation.
2. The raw areas are covered over by approximating remnant adjacent epithelial margins with interrupted or a continuous running stitch of 3-0 vicryl (Fig. 6.3).
3. This could narrow the lumen considerably, in which case a gastro-enterostomy is performed after closing the duodenostomy longitudinally in two layers.

Problem 2

Bleeding main gastroduodenal artery

1. When torrential bleeding is found from the posterior wall at duodenostomy, it is impossible to

stitch the **bleeding gastroduodenal artery** without first slowing down the bleeding.
2. Direct gauze pressure over the bleeding vessel is applied by the assistant, while the surgeon applies, through the foramen of Winslow, the left index finger exerting pressure downwards and forward compressing on the origin of the gastro-duodenal artery.
3. If this fails to slow down bleeding to allow figure-of-eight suturing of the bleeding artery, the **gastroduodenal artery is ligated** at the superior and inferior border of the duodenum.

Problem 3

Inability to close duodenum

Deep irregular penetrating duodenal ulcer extending circumferentially with adjacent oozing and oedematous mucosa defy suturing. Gastro-duodenal dislocation may occur.

Conversion to salvage gastrectomy becomes necessary.

D. Key Points in Vagotomy-Drainage for Bleeding Duodenal Ulcer

Should the decision be made to perform an ulcer curative procedure for a patient with bleeding

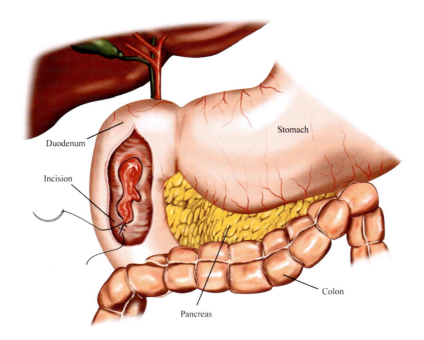

Figure 6.3.

Suturing of giant bleeding duodenal ulcer.

duodenal ulcer, choose vagotomy with drainage after over-sewing of bleeding ulcer. V-D has fewer complications and a lower operative mortality compared with gastrectomy. Unlike in the elective setting, vagotomy is done after completing the drainage procedure.

Pyloroplasty/gastroenterostomy

The drainage procedure is usually a pyloroplasty, and this has been described earlier and illustrated (Fig. 6.2).

When severe duodenal ulcer disease has resulted in gross duodenal distortion, or when an excessively long gastroduodenal opening has been made, the gastroduodenal opening is closed longitudinally using two layers of suture. A **posterior gastroenterostomy** is performed for gastric drainage (Fig. 6.4).

1. Identify the duodeno-jejunal junction just below the root of the mesocolon, to the left of the mid-line.
2. Make a 6–8 cm opening in an avascular part of the mesocolon to the left of the middle colic vessels.
3. The posterior stomach wall is grasped with Babcock forceps and brought down through the opening in the mesocolon.

4. It is convenient to use soft anastomotic clamps for gastro-enterostomy. One pair of clamps grasps the posterior wall of stomach and aligned with a similar length of jejunum, 6–8 cm held in an isoperistaltic position by the second clamp. The afferent jejunal loop should be comfortably positioned and not excessively long.
5. A standard two-layer anastomosis is performed — inner full thickness, using 3-0 absorbable running suture (e.g. vicryl or PDS), and outer seromuscular using 3-0 silk. Four stitches anchor the stomach to the mesocolon.

Truncal vagotomy

1. Exposure of the lower oesophagus is more difficult in obese patients, and in patients with large fatty left lobe of liver or cirrhosis. As a first step, ensure that the abdominal mid-line incision reaches to its maximal superior extent, i.e. the linea alba is divided up to the notch between the left or right side of the xiphistenum and the costal cartilage. Consider using a Goligher retractor to create more space in the upper abdomen.
2. If exposure of the lower oesophagus appears insufficient after anterior retraction of the left

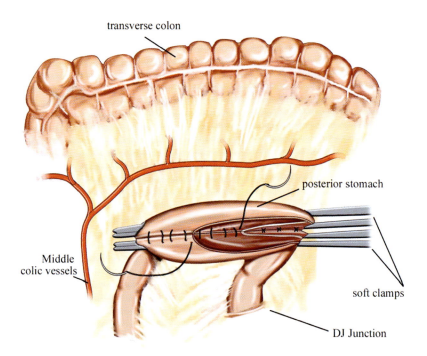

Figure 6.4.

Posterior gastro-jejunostomy.

liver lobe, divide the left triangular ligament with a long tip diathermy starting from the left free margin taking care not to traumatise the left hepatic vein near the mid-line. The left lobe can then be more easily retracted anteriorly. Folding of the left lobe of liver on to the right lobe further improves exposure, but would not be possible with a cirrhotic or fatty liver.

3. After transversely dividing the peritoneum over the lower esophagus, the right index finger works its way behind the oesophagus — the naso-gastric tube in place helping in its identification. The posterior vagal trunk, encountered as a cord a few millimeters behind the oesophagus, is pushed to the right and lifted up by a nerve hook (Fig. 6.5).

4. Robert arteries are applied on the nerve trunk 1 cm apart and following division; the intermediate segment of nerve is removed and sent for histological confirmation. The divided nerve is tied at both ends to prevent bleeding from an accompanying vessel.

5. The anterior vagus nerve is usually in two branches, and nerve segments are excised in the same way.

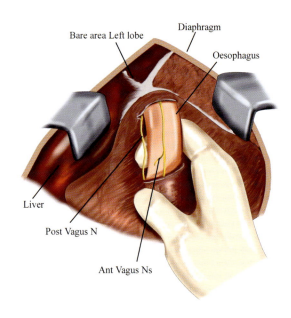

Figure 6.5.

Truncal vagotomy.

6. By careful inspection of the anterior surface of the oesophagus, smaller branches of the anterior trunk, including the criminal nerve of Grassi running from the left lower oesophagus to the gastric fundus, are picked up by the nerve hook and diathermised.

E. Key Points in Billroth II Gastrectomy/Vagotomy Antrectomy for Bleeding Duodenal Ulcer

In the heyday of surgery for duodenal ulcer bleeding, gastrectomy had a 20% operative mortality compared to 5% for vagotomy with drainage. Gastrectomy is a more stressful procedure for both patient and surgeon; the area of greatest concern — the Achilles' heel — is duodenal stump leakage.

Ensure safe duodenal stump closure

To ensure safe closure of duodenum, there must be a healthy duodenal cuff with its posterior wall ½ to 1 cm proximal to the gastro-duodenal artery.

This requires a great deal of patience and determination to achieve in the severely ulcerated duodenum, indicated by peri-duodenal fibrosis fixing down the duodenal bulb and pylorus.

1. Start freeing the duodenum by Kocherisation.
2. Isolate and divide the right gastric vessels between 2-0 silk sutures where they approach the lesser stomach curvature. The right gastro-epiploic vessels are similarly divided near their origin from the gastro-duodenal vessels, after 2-0 silk ligation (Fig. 6.6).
3. Free adhesions and fibrosis between the posterior wall of stomach, duodenal bulb and pancreas. By lifting up the distal stomach, the posterior wall of the duodenum is cleared of adhesions and fibrosis to the pancreatic head until the gastro-duodenal artery is exposed.
4. Frequently, the most challenging dissection is to free the superior border of the proximal duodenum without damaging the common hepatic artery and bile duct (Figs. 6.7 and 6.8).
5. Apply a crushing clamp to the pyloro-duodenal region and a non-crushing clamp distally to the duodenum just proximal to the gastro-duodenal artery. Cut clamped duodenum, leaving an adequate cuff for anastomosis.
6. The duodenal stump is closed as a first all-coats layer with 3-0 vicryl or PDS running suture. Check for gaps in the suture line that are reinforced with figure-of-eight stitches. The second layer is sero-muscular, inverting the two corners with a half purse-string 3-0 silk suture, together with two or three interrupted silk between the half purse-strings (Fig. 6.9).

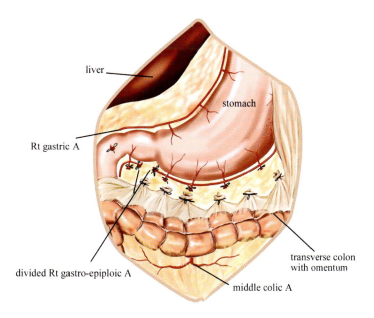

Figure 6.6.

Gastrectomy — gastro-duodenal dissection.

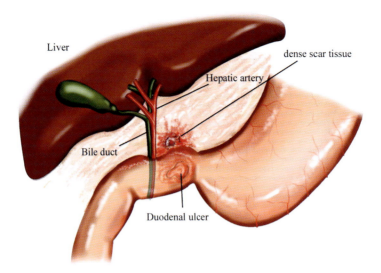

Figure 6.7.

Dense scar tissue in severe duodenal ulcer disease.

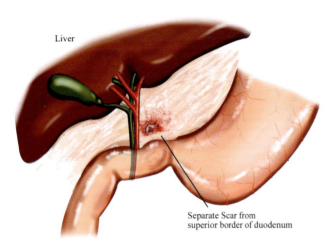

Figure 6.8.

Separating scar tissue from superior border of duodenum.

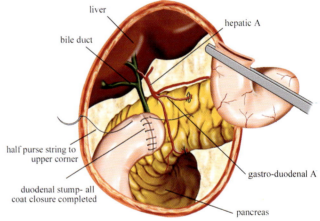

Figure 6.9.

Duodenal stump closure.

7. If the short cuff of the posterior duodenal wall has not allowed complete inversion of the mucosal suture line, the closure is reinforced by a third row of interrupted silk sutures from the anterior duodenal wall to the pancreatic capsule.

Dealing with problems related to the posterior duodenal ulcer penetrating into the pancreas

1. Meticulous dissection to free the duodenal wall distal to the ulcer is done to obtain a small cuff of

posterior duodenal wall to facilitate subsequent duodenal closure. Lahey's suggestion of placing a Bakes dilator into the common bile duct could help in preventing inadvertent division of the bile duct (Fig. 6.10).[1]

Closure of the duodenal stump is as described previously, without use of intestinal clamp, and preserving more of the anterior duodenal wall.

2. However, should a small cuff of posterior duodenum not be available, Norman Tanner's technique[2] of three-layer interrupted sutures between

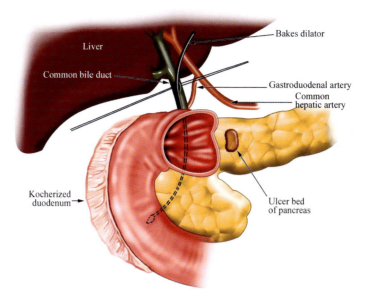

Figure 6.10.

Bakes dilator in common bile duct.

the duodenal stump and the fibrotic ulcer margin is an option. Figure 6.11 shows the posterior wall of the duodenal stump being sutured to the distal margin of the ulcer base on the pancreas. A second layer of interrupted vicryl stutures closes the duodenal stump by suturing the anterior wall of duodenum stump to the proximal margin of the ulcer base (Fig. 6.12). The third layer of suture is

sero-muscular from the anterior duodenal wall to fibrous capsule of pancreas.

3. Performing duodenostomy, i.e. closing the duodenal stump around a tube, is the last resort. Intraperitoneal leakage, frequently gross in amount, makes post-operative management difficult to manage successfully in these patients who are frequently poor operative candidates to start with.

Mobilisation of distal stomach

The extent of gastric resection for duodenal ulcer disease depends on whether vagotomy is also performed. With vagotomy, resection of the gastric antrum, which constitutes about one-third of the stomach, suffices. Without vagotomy, two-thirds of distal stomach is resected.

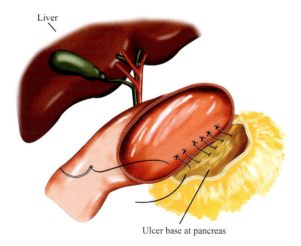

Figure 6.11.

Posterior wall of duodenum sutured to distal margin of ulcer base.

1. In **antrectomy**, following division of the avascular lesser omentum, the descending branch of the left gastric vessels near their junction with the main left gastric vessels is separated from the lesser curve of stomach and divided after ligation with 2-0 silk. Along the greater curvature, the gastro-colic omentum is divided progressively between sutures until at a point about one-third

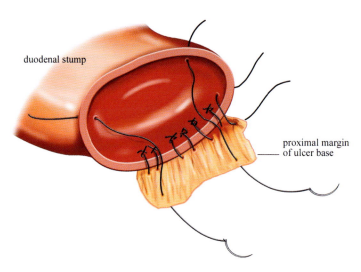

Figure 6.12.

Anterior wall of duodenum sutured to proximal margin of ulcer base.

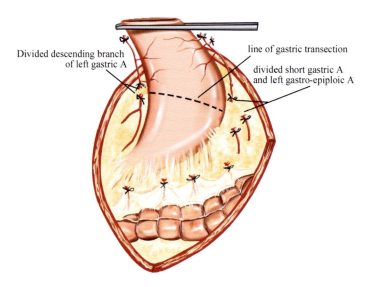

Figure 6.13.

Antrectomy and gastrectomy — mobilisation of distal stomach.

of its length from the pylorus when the gastro-epiploic vessels are isolated and divided between 2-0 silk ties.

2. In **gastrectomy**, for duodenal ulcer disease, it is necessary to mobilise two-thirds of the distal stomach for resection. Freeing the lesser curve requires ligation of the main gastric as well as the ascending branch of the left gastric vessels. On the greater curve, in addition to division

and ligation of the gastrocolic omentum, the left gastro-epiploic vessels, and the lower one or two short splenic vessels need ligation and division (Fig. 6.13).

*Caution: It is necessary to be particularly gentle in this part of the operation as excessive traction easily injures the spleen. Although mild tears of the spleen causing haemorrhage can be controlled by diathermy,

profuse bleeding necessitates splenectomy. A technique that is helpful in arresting surface bleeding from the spleen (and the liver) is to increase the coagulating diathermy to the maximal reading of 6 and apply it directly on the narrow inner tube of a sucker. With rapid movements, the tip of the sucker is applied intermittently and gently on the bleeding surface, superficially cauterising the vascular splenic tissue.

Billroth II gastroenteral anastomosis

Reconstruction may be hand-sewn or by use of stapling instruments.

Hand-sewn anastomosis is facilitated by the use of intestinal clamps and in particular, Lane's twin clamps.

1. In Billroth II anastomosis, a loop of jejunum is brought over the transverse colon and lined up in an isoperistaltic position to the stomach at the prepared line of resection between the upper third and lower two-thirds. The jejunal loop should just be long enough from the DJ junction to lie comfortably, without being too short either. The twin clamps are applied (Fig. 6.14).
2. Following completion of posterior running 3-0 silk sero-muscular sutures between stomach and jejunum, a strong crushing Payr's clamp is applied at the line of stomach resection. A knife using the crushing clamp as table top cuts off the distal two-thirds of stomach.
3. The right half of the stomach margins are sutured together with a running 3-0 vicryl or PDS suture, leaving 5 cm of stomach opening for anastomosis with jejunum, which is incised over a similar length.
4. Gastro-enteral anastomosis is performed (Fig. 6.15). It is well to remember that the inner continuous suture with absorbable material such as 3-0 vicryl or PDS is haemostatic and hence must be meticulously executed, making sure that the needle passes through full thickness of both stomach and intestine, and the sutures are close at 2–3 mm apart and held reasonably tight by the assistant. The outer anterior layer of 3-0 silk is sero-muscular, and sutures are applied further apart at 5–6 mm.

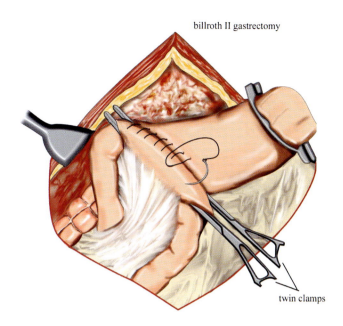

billroth II gastrectomy

twin clamps

Figure 6.14.

Billroth II gastrectomy.

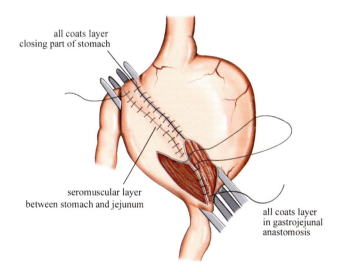

all coats layer
closing part of stomach

seromuscular layer
between stomach and jejunum

all coats layer
in gastrojejunal
anastomosis

Figure 6.15.

Billroth II gastrectomy with Hofmeister valve.

5. By closing off part of the stomach opening, a Hofmeister valve is created and the gastro-enteral stoma is limited to 5 cm wide. This has the theoretical advantage of preventing too rapid gastric emptying.

Stapling is preferred by some surgeons.

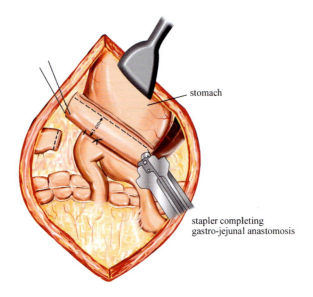

stomach

stapler completing
gastro-jejunal anastomosis

Figure 6.16.

Stapling in Billroth II gastrectomy.

Some precautions:

1. A margin of 2–3 cm between the gastro-enterostomy and the distal staple line of the gastric stump is necessary to prevent avascularity (Fig. 6.16).
2. Stapled anastomotic line bleeding could be more frequent than from a well hand-sewn anastomosis. The mucosal aspect of the anastomosis should be inspected and, if necessary, reinforced with figure-of-eight sutures before completion.
3. In severe duodenal ulcer disease, where the duodenum is distorted, hand-sewn closure is more reliable than stapling, which is best avoided.

   *Some surgeons have switched over from the traditional Billroth II gastro-enterostomy anastomosis to a **Roux-en-Y procedure** that reduces bile gastritis. However the clinical benefits have not been widely confirmed.

Surgical Techniques for Bleeding Gastric Ulcer

F. Local Excision of Gastric Ulcer

A large gastric ulcer with bleeding fibrotic edges in a relatively unfit patient can be treated by local excision of the ulcer.

1. To excise a gastric ulcer in its typical position at the lesser curve of the antrum distal to the incisura, the descending branch of the left gastric artery and accompanying vein and right gastric vessels need to be ligated, and wedge excision with a healthy margin performed.
2. The application of non-crushing intestinal clamps helps reduction of bleeding.
3. The stomach margins are sutured transversely in two layers.

Key Points in Billroth I Gastrectomy for Bleeding Gastric Ulcer

Fitter patients with large gastric ulcers with fibrotic bleeding margins or eroding into the pancreas are treated by Billroth I gastrectomy, with resection of half the stomach and much of its lesser curve. Resection is particularly valid when there is a suspicion of malignancy.

Reconstruction and gastro-duodenal anastomosis can be hand-sewn, using intestinal clamps, or by stapling.

1. Kocherisation of the duodenum, mobilisation of the distal stomach and division from the duodenum is similar to that described for Billroth II gastrectomy.
2. If a large gastric ulcer penetrates into the pancreas, its margins are pinched off, leaving behind its ulcer base, which is diathermised.
3. The traditional technique uses two straight intestinal clamps (soft on the proximal side) applied transversely for 5 cm from the middle of the greater curvature. Following division of the stomach between the clamps, a second set of curved clamps (soft on the proximal side) are applied obliquely across to the upper part of the lesser curvature which had earlier been cleared of omentum. A knife cut between this second pair of clamps excises the distal half and lesser curvature of the stomach (Fig. 6.17).
4. The new lesser curve of stomach is created by a two-layer closure of the stomach margin held by the proximal curved clamp.
5. An end-to-end anastomosis is made between the gastric margins held by the straight clamp and

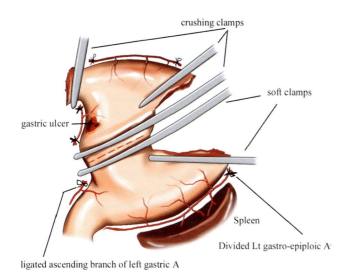

Figure 6.17.

Billroth I gastrectomy.

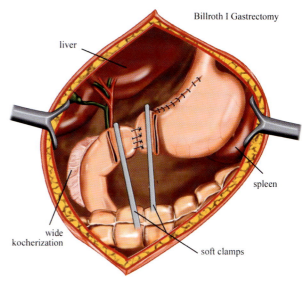

Figure 6.18.

Gastro-duodenal anastomosis in Billroth I gastrectomy.

the duodenum. A posterior 3-0 silk sero-muscular layer, an inner all-coats layer with continuous 3-0 vicryl or PDS and an anterior outer sero-muscular layer of interrupted 3-0 silk interrupted (Fig. 6.18).

6. An additional silk stitch augments the "angle of sorrow" where the suture lines meet. More important in preventing leakage is to avoid tension at the gastro-duodenal anastomosis by Kocherisation and freeing any adhesions between the gastric stump and the pancreas.

Incisional wound closure

The midline abdominal wound is closed by continuous 1-0 PDS suture. One or two drains, e.g. Redivac, are placed in the vicinity of opened viscera, especially after duodenal stump closure.

Postoperative care

1. The elderly, those with organ impairment and those who had received massive blood transfusion need to be monitored in the ICU. Post-operative mortality remains high in these high-risk patients.

2. The main concerns are:
    a) Haemodynamic stability
    b) Continued or recurrent haemorrhage
    c) Cardiovascular complication
    d) Sepsis from pulmonary complications or anastomotic leakage.

3. PPI and prophylactic antibiotics are routinely administered.

4. The nasogastric tube should be periodically checked for patency. If oral feeding is delayed, parenteral nutrition will have to be considered.

References

1. Lahey Technique, *Maingot's Abdominal Operations*, 9th ed., Volume I, Seymour I, Schwartz & Harold Ellis eds. (1990), Prentice-Hall International Inc.

2. Tanner NC. (1969) *Operations for Bleeding Peptic Ulcer, in-Operative Surgery. Abdomen and Rectum & Anus — Part I.* Charles Rob, Rodney Smith, Sir Clifford Naunton Morgan, Butterworths, London.

Chapter 7

Surgical Management of Upper Gastrointestinal Perforations

Surendra Kumar Mantoo* and Jimmy Bok Yan So**

Indications

1. Conservative Management or Surgery?

   A randomised trial comparing non-operative versus operative treatment in patients with perforated peptic ulcers showed that non-operative treatment was successful in about 70% of patients.[1] However in the elderly (age >70 years) and high-risk populations, this approach is associated with a prohibitive morbidity and mortality and not recommended. Patients in whom conservative treatment is being entertained should probably have a water-soluble oral contrast study to document that the ulcer perforation is contained. Non-operative treatment involves nasogastric suction, broad-spectrum antibiotics, and high-dose intravenous antisecretory agents (e.g. proton-pump inhibitor). Clinical improvement during a primary non-operative approach should be apparent within 12 hours, failing which surgical intervention is indicated.

2. Simple Closure or Definitive Ulcer Surgery?

   In the past, a controversy surrounding ulcer surgery was whether to perform a definitive ulcer operation, which generally involves an acid-reducing procedure (such as truncal, selective, highly selective or parietal-cell vagotomy). Prior to the development of acid-reducing medications and an understanding of the role of *H. Pylori* in the pathogenesis of PUD, acid-reducing surgical procedures were generally considered to be the standard approach because of an unacceptably high risk of ulcer recurrence without them. However such procedures have the potential to result in long-term adverse gastrointestinal sequelae such as diarrhoea and dumping syndrome. The appreciation of the role of *H. Pylori* has changed the importance of this distinction.

   Simple closure without acid-reducing procedure became a popular treatment once it became evident that eradication of *H. Pylori* alone substantially reduced ulcer recurrence. Furthermore, the availability of potent acid-suppressing drugs made long-term medical therapy a reasonable option even in patients without *H. Pylori*. However, the cause of the ulcer may not be evident at the time of surgery, particularly since there is no reliable, rapid test for *H. Pylori* that can be achieved during laparotomy. Some patients may not tolerate or be compliant with therapy. It has also become increasingly apparent that many ulcers are not caused by *H. Pylori*, and the natural history of

*S. K. Mantoo, MBBS (Rani Durgavati), MS, MRCS (Edin), MMed (Gen Surg), MS (Surg), General Surgery, Associate Consultant, Department of Surgery, National University Hospital, Singapore.

**Jimmy B. Y. So, MBChB, FRCS (Edin), FRCS (Glasg), FAMS, Senior Consultant and Surgeon, Upper Gastrointestinal & General Surgery, Department of Surgery, National University Hospital, Singapore.

such ulcers is incompletely understood. Thus, the controversy surrounding definitive acid-reducing procedures continues to be debated. These procedures may be most appropriate in patients whose ulcers are due to NSAIDs and who will require their continued use. On the other hand, such patients can also be potentially treated with COX-2 inhibitors or with concomitant proton pump blockers that reduce the incidence of recurrent PUD.

Preoperative Preparation

1. Set up an intravenous drip and insert a nasogastric tube for gastric aspiration.
2. Start broad-spectrum antibiotics.
3. Patients may require resuscitation and treatment of septic shock.
4. A Foley catheter should be inserted as some patients present with retention of urine and may need monitoring of urine output.

Operative Treatment

A. Benign Duodenal Ulcer Perforation

1. **Open closure:** A mid-line upper abdominal incision is made. Most perforated duodenal ulcers occur in the anterior wall of the first portion. They are usually less than 1cm, and the time-tested technique of primary closure with omental patch, first described by Roscoe Graham in 1935,[2] has not changed much (Fig. 1(a) and 1(b)). If the omentum is not available or not sufficient to close the perforation, the falciform ligament may be divided from the anterior abdominal wall and a flap mobilised based on its attachment to the liver. The same principle applies for perforated prepyloric ulcers, which should be treated as duodenal ulcers.

   The extent of peritoneal contamination varies with the size of the perforation, the duration of its occurrence and the last meal taken. Thorough peritoneal lavage is done with warm water before and after closure of perforation.

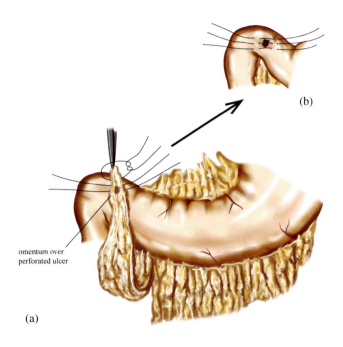

omentum over perforated ulcer

(a)

(b)

Figure 1(a) and (b)

Omental patch repair for perforated ulcer.

Ensure that the sub-phrenic spaces and the pelvis are clean before abdominal closure. Place one or more abdominal drains depending on the extent of peritoneal contamination.

Eradication of *H. pylori* significantly reduces the relapse of duodenal ulcer after simple closure of perforation.[3]

2. **Laparoscopic closure:** With the advent of minimally invasive surgery and increasing expertise in this field, laparoscopic repair of small anterior wall perforations is feasible, safe and results in faster recovery, less post-operative pain and earlier discharge.[4] Mid-line wound complications such as infection and dehiscence, which can occur with the open surgery, are also prevented. An additional advantage of the laparoscopic technique is the improved visualisation of the entire peritoneal cavity, which facilitates better lavage and drainage of loculated fluid collections, thereby reducing the incidence of post-operative abscesses in the abdominal cavity. The main disadvantage is the longer operating time and greater technical expertise required to perform this surgery.

   Patient selection, however, is the key to a good outcome. Most studies advocate that laparoscopic closure should be attempted in patients who are haemodynamically stable without ionotropic support and have early perforation of less than 6 hours duration. Laparoscopic repair is usually a 3-port technique. Various methods have been described in literature such as standard primary closure of the perforation with an omental plug, stapled omental plugs, use of gelatine sponge as a plug with fibrin glue, and a "single-suture closure" technique.[5,6,7] All these techniques should be accompanied by generous and thorough peritoneal toilet to avoid post-operative abscesses.

3. **Closure of complex or giant duodenal ulcer perforations:** The size of "giant" perforated duodenal ulcers has arbitrarily been defined by various authors as more than 2 cm. These perforations are considered particularly hazardous because of the extensive duodenal tissue loss and surrounding tissue inflammation, which preclude simple closure using omental patch.

There is a paucity of data in the literature regarding giant duodenal ulcers with some case reports and very few series. There has not been a single randomised control study for the management of this severe variant of duodenal ulcer disease. One of the reasons for this is that giant duodenal ulcers are an uncommon entity. In a series of 1,434 patients with peptic ulcers, giant duodenal ulcers were found in 2.4%.[8] The different techniques described include resectional and non-resectional procedures.

i) **Omental Plug Technique[9]:** The tip of the nasogastric tube is guided through the perforation. The free edge of the omentum is taken and sutured to the tip of the Ryle tube using 20 plain catgut. The nasogastric tube is gently withdrawn, pulling the plug of omentum into the stomach. Approximately a 5–6 cm length of omental plug suffices to occlude the perforation. The omentum is then fixed to the perforation site with five to six interrupted sutures of 2O chromic catgut taken between the omentum and the healthy duodenum, approximately 3–4mm away from the margins of the perforation. An abdominal drain is placed.

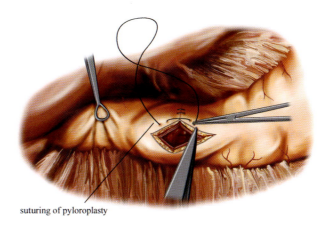

suturing of pyloroplasty

Figure 2.

Technique for pyloroplasty.

Post-operatively, a Gastrografin study is done before starting feeding on seventh day, and the nasogastric tube is removed if no leak is demonstrated.

ii) **Conversion of the Perforation into a Pyloroplasty[10]:** Closing the perforation transversly with omental reinforcement (Fig. 2).

iii) **Closure of the Perforation using a Serosal Patch or a Pedicled Graft of the Jejunum[11,12,13]:** A loop of jejunum is brought up to the perforation and sutured to the defect, using interrupted absorbable sutures.

iv) **Resection of the perforation bearing duodenum and the gastric antrum** in the form of a partial gastrectomy, with reconstruction as either a Billroth I or II anastomosis. Where there has been difficulty with duodenal closure, a lateral T-tube or an end duodenostomy tube is inserted to decompress the duodenal stump (Figs. 3 and 4).[14]

B. Benign Gastric Ulcer Perforations

The surgical treatment of a gastric ulcer depends on the ulcer size, the distance from the GE junction, and the degree of surrounding inflammation. However the most important decision to make is whether a gastric cancer can be excluded or not. Whenever possible, the ulcer should be excised in the form of ulcerectomy or wedge resection if a gastric cancer can be excluded or the situation warrants a more conservative approach.

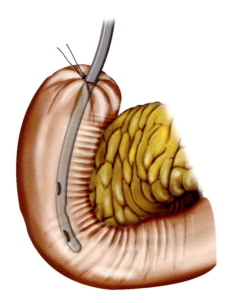

Figure 3.

Insertion of end duodenectomy tube.

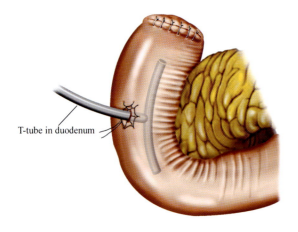

T-tube in duodenum

Figure 4.

Lateral duodenectomy with a T-tube.

The most aggressive approach for benign gastric ulcer is to perform a gastrectomy if the location of the ulcer like high gastric ulcers does not permit a lesser resection.[15]

C. Surgery for Malignant Gastric Ulcer Perforation

Perforation is a rare complication of gastric carcinoma, accounting for less than 1% of all gastric cancer cases. Most of these patients present with acute abdomen and preoperative diagnosis of malignancy is unusual, accounting for about 30% of cases. During surgery the gastric ulcer is often difficult to be characterised as benign or malignant by the surgeon. Therefore a biopsy and frozen section should be performed in all gastric perforations when a pathologist is available. Malignant gastric perforation is more often a manifestation of advanced cancer with serosal invasion (55–82%) and lymph node metastasis (57–67%). Nevertheless, as confirmed by different observations,[16,17] gastric cancer can perforate at an early stage as well. It is still debated. Several studies have noted free gastric cancer cells in the peritoneum to be associated with poor prognosis. However, viable free cancer cells have not been demonstrated in the peritoneal cavity of patients with perforated gastric cancer and the metastatic efficiency of gastric cancer cells possibly shed during perforation is uncertain in the presence of the peritonitis.

When a curative operation can be performed, survival rates after gastric cancer perforation appear similar to survival rates observed in elective patients.[18]

The most important factors in the management of a patient with histological diagnosis of perforated gastric carcinoma are: the presence of preoperative shock, the severity of peritoneal contamination, the resectability of the neoplasm and comorbidities of the patient. If a patient has a curable tumour and acceptable general condition, for example no signs of shock, localised peritonitis and no comorbidities, the treatment of choice is radical total or subtotal gastrectomy with associated D2 lymphadenotomy.[19] When general condition is good but the tumour is at an advanced stage with no possibility of R0 resection, a palliative gastrectomy, if technically possible, is recommended for better symptom control and lower risk of complications like bleeding and obstruction. Simple repair or omental patch are reserved only for those patients with advanced-stage disease and whose general condition is poor.[20] If a pathologist is not available and histologic examination is not possible during surgery, a gastric resection is recommended if surgical expertise is available and the patient is stable during surgery. Otherwise, the ulcer edge should be biopsied and lesser procedure should be performed. (When the postoperative histologic examination confirms malignancy a secondary radical gastrectomy is mandatory if feasible.)

References

1. Crofts TJ, Park KGM, Steele RJC, *et al.* (1989) A randomized trial of non-operative treatment for perforated peptic ulcer. *NEJM* **320**: 970–973.

2. Graham PR. (1937) The treatment of perforated duodenal ulcers. *Surg Gynaem Obstetric* **64**: 235–238.

3. Bose AC, Kate V, Ananthakrishnan N, Parija SC. (2007) Helicobacter pylori eradication prevents recurrence after simple closure of perforated duodenal ulcer. *J Gastroenterol Hepatol* **22(3)**: 345–348.

4. Bertleff MJ, Halm JA, Bemelman WA, *et al.* (2009) Randomized clinical trial of laparoscopic versus open repair of the perforated peptic ulcer: The LAMA trial. *World J Surg* **33**: 1368–1373.

5. Thompson AR, Hall TJ, Anglin BA, Scott-Conner CE. (1995) Laparoscopic placation of perforated ulcer. *South Med J* **88**: 185–189.

6. Matsuda M, Nishiyama M, Hanai T, Saeki S. (1995) Laparoscopic omental patch repair of perforated peptic ulcer. *Ann Surg* **221**: 236–240.

7. Siu WT, Leong HT, Law BK, *et al.* (2002) Laparoscopic repair for perforated peptic ulcer: A randomized controlled trial. *Ann Surg* **235**: 313–319.

8. Csendes A, Becker P, Valenzuela J, *et al.* (1991) Clinical characteristics of patients with multiple or giant peptic ulcers. *Rev Med Chil* **119**: 38–44.

9. Sharma D, Saxena A, Rahman H, *et al.* (2000) Free omental plug: A nostalgic look at an old and dependable technique for giant peptic perforations. *Dig Surg* **17**: 216–8.

10. Karanjia ND, Shanahan DJ, Knight MJ. (1993) Omental patching of a large perforated duodenal ulcer: A new method. *Br J Surg* **80**: 65.

11. Chaudhary A, Bose SM, Gupta NM, *et al.* (1991) Giant perforations of duodenal ulcer. *Ind J Gastroenterol* **10**: 14–5.

12. Mclrath DC, Larson RH. (1971) Surgical management of large perforations of the duodenum. *Surg Clin North Am* **51**: 857–61.

13. Cranford CA, Olson RO, Bradley EL III. (1988) Gastric disconnection in the management of perforated giant duodenal ulcer. *Am J Surg* **155**: 439–42.

14. Aoki T. (2000) Current status of and problems in the treatment of gastric and duodenal ulcer disease: Introduction. *World J Surg* **24**: 240–327.

15. Adachi Y, Mori M, Maehara Y, *et al.* (1997) Surgical results of perforated gastric carcinoma: An analysis of 155 Japanese patients. *Am J Gastroenterol* **92(3)**: 516–8.

16. Kitakado Y, Tanigawa N, Muraoka R. (1997) A case report of perforated early gastric cancer. *Nippon Geka Hokan* **66**: 86–90.

17. Bonenkamp JJ, Songun I, Hermans J, van de Velde CJ. (1996) Prognostic value of positive cytology findings from abdominal washing in patients with gastric cancer. *Br J Surg* **83**: 672–674.

18. Gertsch P, Yip SKH, Chow LWC, Lauder IJ: Free perforation of gastric carcinoma. Results of surgical treatment. *Arch Surg* 1995, **130**: 177–181.

19. Tsugawa K, Koyanagi N, Hashizume M, *et al.* (2001) The therapeutic strategies in performing emergency surgery for gastroduodenal ulcer perforation in 130 patients over 70 years of age. *Hepatogastroenterology* **48**: 156–162.

20. So JBY, Yam A, Cheah WK, *et al.* (2000) Risk factors related to operative mortality and morbidity in patients undergoing emergency gastrectomy. *Br J Surg* **87**: 1702–1707.

Chapter 8

Management of Complications Following Bariatric Surgery

Asim Shabbir* and Chih-Kun Huang†

Introduction

The rise in obesity and the efficacy of bariatric surgery in producing effective, sustainable and reproducible weight loss have brought bariatric surgery to the forefront of medicine. The increasing number of bariatric procedures mandates that surgeons are familiar with the management of complications of such procedures.

A proactive, vigorous surveillance after surgery for signs and symptoms of complications is the key to early detection and management.

General Complications

Thromboembolism

Obesity is a well-known risk factor for deep vein thrombosis and pulmonary embolism, though the incidence in Asia is apparently low. Preventive measures during and after surgery include adequate hydration, low molecular weight heparin, pneumatic calf compression, anti-embolic stockings, early ambulation and in very high risk cases, even using vena caval filters.

Atelectasis

Good pain control, incentive spirometry, nursing patients in 30° reverse Trendelenburg position and early ambulation enhance respiratory function and is key to preventing atelectasis.

Nausea and Vomiting

These are largely related to anaesthesia and administration of opioid analgesics.

Following sleeve gastrectomy, vomiting may occur from oedema at the gastroesophageal junction, stricture as a result of too close stapling near the incisura and/or gastric tube torsion. In most patients, resting the gastrointestinal tract, anti-emetics and IV hydration will be rewarding. When symptoms are intractable, upper gastrointestinal contrast study will help define the problem. After gastric bypass, a narrow gastrojejunostomy opening due to oedema will spontaneously, resolve. In intractable cases, endoscopic dilatation or surgical revision would be required.

*Dr Asim Shabbir, MBBS (Pak.), MMed (Surg.), FCPS (pak. FRCS (Edln.), FAMS (Surg), Consultant, Department of Surgery, National University Hospital.

†Dr Chih-Kun Huang, Chairman, International Excellence Federation for Bariatric & Metabolic Surgery; President, Taiwan Obesity Support Association; Director, Bariatric & Metabolic International Surgery Center, E-Da Hospital, Taiwan; Director, Minimally Invasive Surgery Training Center, E-Da Hospital, Taiwan.

Wound Complications

The laparoscopic approach has significantly diminished the rates of major wound complications which have been frequent after open bariatric surgery.

To further reduce the risk of incisional hernia, it is our practice to suture all port sites that are greater than 5 mm, especially those that employ tissue cutting rather than splitting blades.

Acute Abdominal Complications

1. Bleeding

The incidence of gastrointestinal haemorrhage ranges between 0.5 and 5 percent. The use of buttress material has been shown to decrease the incidence of postoperative bleeding in bariatric surgery. However, it cannot be stressed enough that meticulous haemostasis needs to be achieved prior to closing the abdomen. Perioperative management of bleeding disorders and hypertension is important in preventing bleeding tragedies.

In 50–70%, bleeding is self-limiting following blood transfusion or fluid resuscitation. When re-exploration is necessary after sleeve or gastric bypass, a thorough survey of the entire operative field including the staple line, omentum and sutured areas is necessary. Bleeding points can be secured by using clips, suturing, or an energy device. The peritoneal cavity is cleared of blood and a drain left near the bleeding site. Early intra-luminal GI haemorrhage has not been reported after sleeve resection but is well documented after gastric bypass. It commonly occurs either at the gastrojejunostomy or jejunojejunostomy site and the presence of luminal clots may make localisation difficult. Surgery is required when endoscopic localisation or therapeutic attempt fails. Oversewing the entire anastomosis is preferred over opening the anastomosis to look for the bleeder.

An option to detect acute GI haemorrhage is to do a CT angiography followed by angioembolisation of the bleeding site. Chronic GI bleeding could occur after bariatric surgery. Endoscopy, capsule endoscopy and radioactive labelled isotope scan may be diagnostic. For patients suspected to have gastric cancer after gastric bypass, access to the remnant stomach would require a gastrostomy under general anaesthesia.

2. Leaks

The aetiology of a leak is multifactorial, most commonly involving local factors like tension on the anastomosis and poor blood supply. Systemic patient factors include diabetes and the use of steroids, etc. During surgery, special attention should be paid to ensure a good blood supply and judicious use of energy devices. For gastric bypass, proper orientation of intestinal loops, tension-free anastomosis and checking the anastomosis for integrity at the end of surgery using an underwater air leak test would reduce unpleasant outcomes. For patients undergoing sleeve gastrectomy, ensure the use of an appropriate staple height, prevent an hour glass gastric tube and remember not to staple the oesophagus.

Prompt identification and early detection of leakage are pivotal in preventing long-term morbidity. Patients with leaks may present with decrease level in haemoglobin resulting from intra-luminal or intraperitoneal bleeding, abdominal pain or subtle signs of sepsis like tachycardia, pyrexia, hypotension and tachypnoeia.

If a drain is *in situ*, then a simple methylene blue test may confirm a leak. If clinical findings are suggestive of a leak, then a computerised tomography scan with contrast can supplement clinical suspicion. But if the scan is negative, it should not be used to make a decision to abandon re-exploration as clinical findings take precedence.

The principles of treatment of a leak include early re-operation, decompression, peritoneal lavage, drainage, fluid replacement, broad spectrum antibiotics and enteral feeding through a gastrostomy or jejunostomy tube, depending on site of leak. Dealing with a GJ leak after gastric bypass is not easy but as this is a low pressure system with no bile, it heals better in comparison with leaks from sleeve gastrectomies.

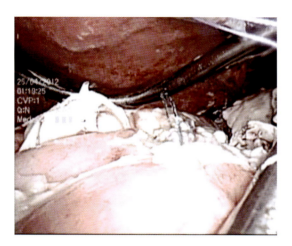

Figure 1.

Loose suture at site of gastrojejunostomy leak on laparoscopic exploration.

Treatment options for GJ leak

a) Sometimes the leak is very small and the site cannot be identified even with an intraoperative endoscopy, in this case, drainage and feeding mechanism would suffice and healing would occur.

b) If the site of leak can be identified (Fig. 1), most surgeons would attempt to repair it primarily but the majority of these primary repairs would fail and result in formation of a fistula that would eventually close with conservative management.

c) The use of omental or falciform patch similar to Ghram's omental patch for perforated ulcer yields better results.

For perforated chronic marginal ulcer, redoing the enteric anastomosis may be warranted.

In more complex cases the use of retrievable stents or tissue glues or redoing the whole anastomosis has been reported.

Managing sleeve leak

1. The principles of management remain the same. In addition, rule out the presence of stenosis that is creating a high pressure zone. This can be done by an upper GI contrast study.

2. Minor leaks with localised sepsis: conservative management with drainage, feeding mechanism and control of infection with antibiotics would suffice.

3. For major leaks, in addition to the above, a retrievable covered stent that spans from gastroesophageal junction to across the pylorus may be necessary. This stent bridges the leak area, thus limiting leak associated sepsis and promotes healing. It also harmonises pressure across the gastric tube that increases the chances of early healing. If a long stent is not available, a stent over a stent may be necessary.

4. Conversion of a leak into a controlled fistula by placing a T-tube through the leak site and exteriorising it is another option.

5. In certain cases the leak becomes chronic with fistula formation-consider the following options of treatments:

   a) for distal staple line leaks, conversion to gastric bypass and resection of distal stomach
   b) jejunal Roux loop diversion, i.e. creating an anastomosis between the leak and a jejunal loop
   c) for proximal staple line leaks, total gastrectomy and esophagojeujunostomy

3. Stenosis and Stricture

Patients can present with this immediately following surgery, after a few weeks or years later.

Following gastric banding, dysphagia in the immediate postoperative period is the result of stomal obstruction from postopertaive oedema or improper placement of band. Dysphagia at a later stage is due to either to an over-tightened band or band slippage.

In the operative procedure for sleeve gastrectomy, the use of too small a calibration tube, creation of a narrow acute angle at the incisura and ischaemia of the gastric tube can result in structuring (Fig. 2). Should watchful treatment with proton pump inhibitors, intravenous fluids and antiemetic fail, an endoscopic balloon dilatation with or without the placement of a retrievable stent can be helpful. The exact number of dilatation episodes and duration of stent placement have to be tailored. There are reports of segmental resection, stricturoplasty and of long seromyotomies

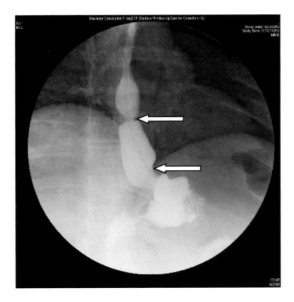

Figure 2.

Gastrografin meal with arrow head showing areas of structuring after sleeve gastrectomy.

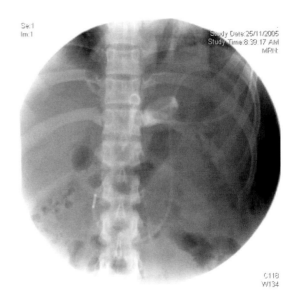

Figure 3.

Abdominal X-ray of normal orientation of gastric band.

with good results. If all the above mentioned options fail, then conversion to gastric bypass is an alternative.

The early strictures of GJ after gastric bypass are generally amiable to balloon dilatation. The aim of dilation is to have a GJ opening of around 1.5 cm. One should avoid the use of rigid dilator and too aggressive dilatation as this increases the risk of perforation.

4. Gastric Band Slippage and Intestinal Obstruction

The aetiology of intestinal obstruction include internal hernias, adhesions, jejunojejunostomy angulations, stenosis at anastomosis, incarcerated ventral or trocar hernia, intussusceptions, bezoars and the procedure-specific problems.

In gastric banding, band slippage and adhesions with a twist around the tubing can result in obstruction. Band slippage was a major concern with the bursa omentalis approach (Fig. 3). Now with the perigastric (pars flaccida) approach, the incidence has dropped to below 5%. The consequence of a slippage, be it anterior, posterior or complete, is a stricture or complete closure of the stoma through the band. The diagnosis is

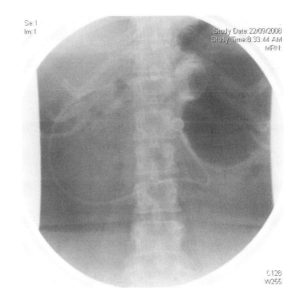

Figure 4.

Plain abdominal X-ray of slipped band.

established by a plain abdominal X-ray that would show an abnormal band position and further confirmation can be done with a UGI series or a CT scan (Figs. 4 and 5). Band slippage with obstruction is an acute emergency and would require deflating the band, nasogastric decompression followed by surgery to remove or reposition the band.

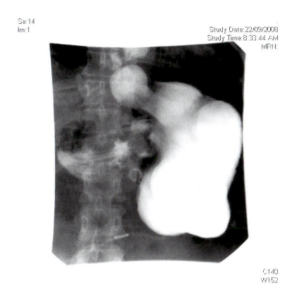

Figure 5.

Gastrografin meal showing gastric outlet obstruction due to band slippage.

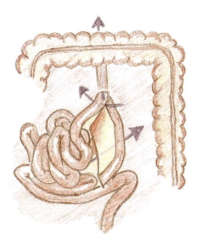

Figure 6.

Mesenteric defects through which internal hernia can potentially occur after gastric bypass.

In patients who undergo an antecolic gastric bypass, the space between the mesentery of the Roux limb and transverse mesocolon called the Petersen's defect and jejunojenunostomy defect are common sites of herniation (Fig. 6). An added defect through the transverse mesocolon is a potential site for internal hernias with the retrocolic technique. Antecolic Roux limb, routine closure of mesenteric defects, anti-obstruction suturing at JJ site, and use of dilating trocars can reduce the incidence of small bowel obstruction in patients undergoing gastric bypass. Patients can present with vague abdominal pain an hour or so after meals or with overt signs of intestinal obstruction, including vomiting, abdominal distention and failure to open bowels and pass flatus. A plain abdominal X-ray will show signs of intestinal obstruction. CT scan aids in confirming the diagnosis: it would show dilated loops of small bowel, mesenteric congestion or twisting call "swirl sign" or free gas if there is a perforation (Fig. 7).

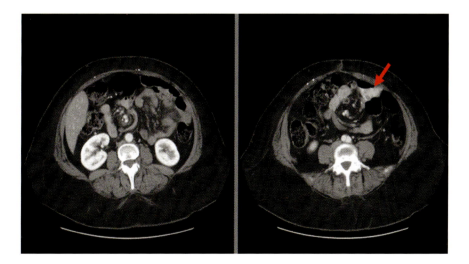

Figure 7.

Swirl sign on CT scan.

The principles of management of internal hernia obstruction include nasogastric decompression, fluid resuscitation, early confirmation of diagnosis to prevent gangrene, and surgical exploration. At surgery, a careful adhesiolysis is done followed by identifying the gastrojejunostomy, the duodenojejunal flexure and running the bowel to ileocaecal junction. Any mesenteric defect that is detected is closed with a non-absorbable suture.

5. Other Complications

Gastric banding

Band erosion

A better understanding of band erosion has led to the development of low pressure bands and improved surgical technique of placing band. Failure on the part of patients to comply with dietary advice to loose weight and over-enthusiastic filling of band to achieve weight loss goals in a patient who eats against the advice of the bariatric team are key to erosion. At erosion, patients note that they eat easily and are regaining their weight. Others may present with infected port site from a eroded band. Diagnoses can be established by a gastroscopy and further confirmed by a CT scan if necessary (Figs. 8 and 9). If the patient is asymptomatic, then allowing the band to completely erode through and then retrieving

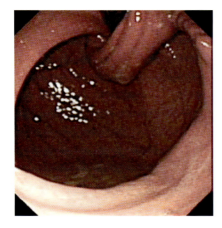

Figure 8.

Retroflexed view on gastroscopy of a normally placed band.

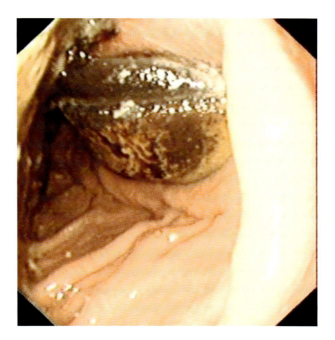

Figure 9.

Retroflexed view on gastroscopy of an eroded band.

it endoscopically is an option. If the patient has sepsis, then surgery is imminent during which removal of the band, drainage and a feeding mechanism is established.

Gastric bypass

Marginal ulcers

These occur in patients with a gastric bypass in whom the pouch size is larger and there is higher parietal cell load. Factors that promote or prevent healing of ulcers by either increasing acidity or mucosal damage, e.g. smoking, NSAID use, poor pouch blood supply of anastomosis and gastro-gastric fistula contribute to such ulcers. Patients generally complain of abdominal pain mainly in the epigastrium related to meals. They can also present to the emergency with signs of peritonitis if there is a perforation.

Upon recognition of an ulcer, a thorough investigation into what the inciting cause is needs to be made. This is accompanied by the use proton pump inhibitors along with avoidance of the inciting agent. In severe cases where surgical intervention is required for a non-healing symptomatic ulcer, or one that has perforated or is bleeding, surgical revision of the anastomosis would need to be done, along with correction of problems like large pouch or fistula.

Pouch dilatation

The aetiology of dilatation of gastric pouch after RYGB still remains controversial. Is it a natural phenomenon or the patients overeat causing dilatation? Whatever the case may be, it is definitely one of the many causes of weight regain. Diagnosis can be established by endoscopy and upper GI contrast study. The classical treatment is revising the pouch to 15–30 mL size, or using other procedures like biliopancreatic diversion. Newer endoscopic treatment options that have been published include circumferential injection of sodium morrhuate to induce scarring resulting in stenosis, and the use of endoscopic suturing or plication devices, but their long-term safety and efficacy remain to be determined.

Nutritional problems

After bariatric surgery till weight loss is stable, increased lipolysis and decreased intake contribute to macro- and micro nutritional deficiencies. For the restrictive procedures, namely gastric banding and sleeve gastrectomy, these changes are seen largely during the weight loss phase and patients need to be supported with multivitamins, minerals and trace elements. However, patients who undergo malabasorptive procedures like gastric bypass and biliopancreatic diversion, in order to absorb suffice macro- and micro nutrients, need to have a diet rich in proteins, supplements of iron, calcium, other trace elements and various vitamins for life. Failure to comply with the dietary supplement intake can result in deficiencies and their syndromes. At follow-up, patients are clinically screened for protein, vitamin and trace element deficiencies and their blood levels checked in order to adjust intake in an effort to prevent deficiency and toxicity.

Chapter 9

Surgery for Appendicitis

Tan Tse Kuang Charles*

1. Indications

Acute appendicitis may be the most common surgically correctable cause of abdominal pain. The diagnosis remains difficult in many instances. The classic presentation is an initial vague periumbilical pain, followed by migration of the pain to the right lower quadrant. It is often associated with nausea and vomiting, and a fever. These patients often have anorexia. On examination, the patients may look ill, with maximal tenderness of the abdomen at McBurney's point.

Patients often do not have this classic presentation, commonly having none or one of the few symptoms described. It is often understood that the natural history of appendicitis is a progressive inflammation of the appendix till perforation, thus presentation of the patient varies with the time at which the encounter with the patient and doctor occurs. Another reason for the variation of presentation is the position of the inflamed appendix.

What initially was a solely a clinical diagnosis has progressed to have radiological confirmation with an ultrasound or a computed tomographic scan.

Operative Strategy of Acute Appendicitis

The primary aim of surgery is to identify the inflamed appendix and resect it without any stump leak. This can be performed via the open or laparoscopic method.

2. Preoperative Preparation

1. Ensure adequate fluid resuscitation. May need a urinary catheter to monitor adequate volume status.
2. Intravenous antibiotics.

3. Surgery

Open Appendectomy

Exposure. The surgeon must decide on the location and type of incision. The patient should be re-examined after the induction of general anaesthesia, which allows deep palpation of the abdomen to determine where the mass of inflamed appendix is. The incision should be centred at that location. A skin crease incision is performed, followed by a muscle-splitting dissection down to the peritoneum. Too medial an incision is avoided as it would lead to injury to the anterior rectus sheath.

Locating the appendix. If it is an early appendicitis, the appendix is enlarged and free floating and thus palpable. Its location can vary from different individuals (Fig. 9.1). If it has been more than 24 hours, the appendix is frequently adhered to the adjacent structures. The adhesions can often be dissected by finger. Firmer adhesions necessitate formal dissection under direct vision. If the appendix is not found, locate the caecum. The appendix is invariably at the base of the caecum.

---

*Charles T. K. Tan, MBChB (UK), FRCSEd (Gen), FAMS, Consultant, Department of surgery, National University Hospital, Singapore.

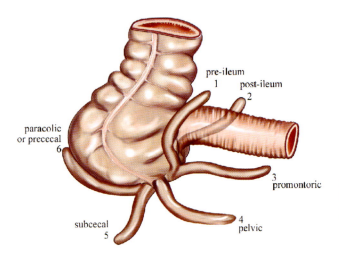

Figure 9.1.

Different positions of the appendix.

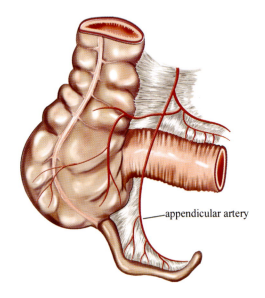

Figure 9.2.

Arterial supply of the appendix.

Excision of appendix. Extend the incision if needed. It is inadvisable to perform the next few steps in an inadequately large incision. Dissection of the appendix can be performed antegrade or retrograde depending on the location of the appendix. Ensure that the appendicular artery is secured before dividing it (Figs. 9.2 and 9.3). The stump should then be securely secured before dividing it. This is a crucial step to prevent a stump blowout. The decision to bury the stump is controversial and shown to have no added advantage. In certain cases, when the appendiceal

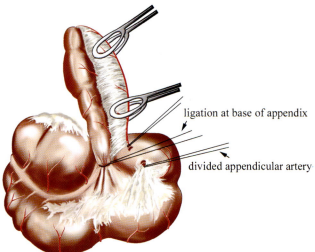

Figure 9.3.

Ligation of the appendicular artery.

inflammation extends to the caecum, resection of the inflamed appendix and inflamed caecum is performed with suturing up the un-inflammed caecum. This would prevent potential leakage. If the inflammation extends to the ileocaecal junction, an ileocaecotomy with primary anastomosis may be necessary.

Laparoscopic Appendectomy

Laparoscopic appendectomy is appropriate in virtually all patients as it provides the benefit of minimally invasive surgery; smaller incisions, less post-operative pain and quicker recovery. It is particularly useful in women, and there are other gynaecological pathologies that potentially mimic appendicitis. A comprehensive evaluation of the intra-peritoneal organs may be achieved with the laparoscope.

A three-port technique is used: a sub-umbilical optical port, one in the subra-pubic and one in the left lower quadrant. The patient is strapped so that the table and patient might be inclined at various angles to allow the bowel to "move" with gravity, away from the appendix. This allows better visualisation of the appendix. Dissection of the appendix is performed with the same principles as the open method. Division of the appendix and artery may be performed with a stapler (Fig. 9.4) or with endoloops.

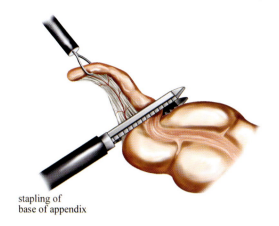

stapling of
base of appendix

Figure 9.4.

Transection of the appendix.

4. Postoperative care

Postoperative care for open and laparoscopic approaches is similar. Liquid diet may be commenced when ileus is resolved and patients discharged when normal diet is tolerated, and fever has settled.

If the fever persists, investigation may have to be carried out for a possible infected collection in the abdomen.

Special Situations

Perforated appendicitis

If the patient has generalised peritonism, free perforation is suspected. A right lower quadrant may not allow a good washout of the contamination. In this scenario, a midline laparotomy is advisable to prevent post-operative abscess formation. When frank pus is encountered, wound infection rates range from 30–50% with primary closure. It is thus advocated to perform delayed primary or secondary closure in such cases.

Appendiceal abscess

If there is an associated abscess, direct attention to drainage of all purulent material, elimination of any loculations, debridement of all necrotic tissue and placement of drains.

Post-operatively, these drains should be removed when output is minimal and non-purulent. Antibiotics should be continued.

Normal appendix

Obtaining an accurate diagnosis of appendicitis is difficult, thus surgeons are often caught in a situation where the intra-operative finding of a normal appendix is present. The surgeon must then decide on whether it is necessary to remove the appendix. The advantage of an appendectomy is that if pain recurs, the diagnosis of appendicitis is not re-entertained. The search for another pathology causing abdominal pain must not be ignored.

Neoplasm

Neoplasms of the appendix are rare. Variations include adenocarcinoma, carcinoid, mucoceles, lymphoma and cystic neoplasm. If encountered intra-operatively, a right hemicolectomy is performed. Laparoscopic approach is not recommended due to the possibility of spillage tumour cells throughout the abdomen.

Chapter 10

Emergency Surgery for Perforative Sigmoid Colonic Diverticulitis

Cheong Wai Kit*, Bettina Lieske† and Frances Sheau Huei Lim‡

Introduction

Colonic diverticula are false (acquired) diverticula consisting of only mucosa and submucosa layers. They are postulated to be formed as a result of high intra-luminal pressure predisposing to herniation of mucosa through the muscular defects that exist where vasa recta brevia penetrate to reach the submucosa and mucosa. These nutrient vessels are most commonly found on the anti-mesenteric border of the large bowel. The most frequent site for the development of colonic diverticula is the sigmoid colon.

Acute colonic diverticulitis occurs when there is infection and micro perforation through the wall of the diverticulum into the peri-colonic tissue. This perforation might be minute and form a micro abscess, sealed off by phlegmon (Hinchey stage I[a]) or form into a large abscess (Hinchey stage II[a]). Occasionally, rupture of this non-communicating abscess may lead to purulent peritonitis (Hinchey stage III[a]). However,

rarely, the communication with the bowel lumen fails to be obliterated by the inflammatory process and may lead to a free communication between the bowel and the peritoneal cavity, resulting in feculant peritonitis (Hinchey stage IV[a]).

The extent of the disease involvement at the time of presentation is one of the major factors in the decision making process on the best option of surgical treatment. This is complemented by the patient's hemodynamic status coupled with the status of the patient's co-morbidities.

Diverticular disease is increasingly common and its occurrence increases with age. Only approximately 10–20% of people with colonic diverticulosis suffer from symptoms of diverticulitis and from these, only 10–20% will require hospitalisation. Out of this 10–20% hospitalised patients, only 20–50% will eventually undergo operative intervention. The majority of patients with colonic diverticulitis follow an indolent clinical course. Overall, less than 1% of all patients with colonic diverticulosis will eventually require surgical management.[1]

*W. K. Cheong, MBBS, FRCS (Ed), FRCS (Glasg), FAMS, Head & Senior Consultant Surgeon, Division of Colorectal Surgery, Department of Surgery, National University Hospital, Singapore.

†B. Lieske, MD (Germany), FRCS (Eng), MA ClinEd (UK), Consultant, Division of Colorectal Surgery, University Surgical Cluster, National University Hospital, Singapore.

‡Frances S. H. Lim, Adv Dip Med Sci (1MU), MD (Canada), Associate Fellow ACS (USA), Consultant, Division of Colorectal Surgery, Department of Surgery, National University Hospital, Singapore.

[a]A common classification system used to stage complicated acute colonic diverticulitis with perforation was proposed by Hinchey et al.[2] in 1978 which takes into account the extent of spread of the inflammatory process.

Management of Acute Sigmoid Colonic Diverticulitis

A. Preoperative Management

Patients with clinical signs of more advanced disease, including marked leukocytosis, high fever, tachycardia, hypotension and physical signs demonstrating more advanced intra-abdominal pathology will definitely require urgent admission for resuscitation, administration of intravenous antibiotic therapy and bowel rest.

It is important to ensure adequate resuscitation with appropriate intravenous fluids, correction and normalisation of haematological and biochemical abnormalities and treatment with appropriate antibiotics before surgery.

As the group of patients who are affected with this condition is usually older and are associated with higher concomitant medical problems, particular attention must be paid to ensure preservation of homeostatic functions to reduce the possibilities of mortality and morbidity.

The choice of antibiotics to be administered must include coverage of Gram negative and anaerobic bacteria. The most predominant bacteria cultured include the aerobic and facultative bacteria *Escherichia coli* and *Streptococcus* spp. The most commonly isolated anaerobes include *Bacteroides* spp. (*B. fragilis* group), *Peptostreptoccus*, *Clostridium*, and *Fusobacterium* spp.[3]

All these patients will usually undergo a baseline computed tomography scan of the abdomen and pelvis to confirm the diagnosis, rule out potential alternative diagnoses (especially complicated colonic malignancy), and evaluate for complicated disease (peri-colic and pelvic abscesses and peritonitis) that would require a change in the initial management.[4]

Barium enema as an adjunctive or primary investigation is rarely used nowadays and should be avoided because of the risk of perforation, which can result in barium peritonitis. If a radiological contrast needed to be used, a water-soluble material (gastrograffin) should be used.

However, in cases in which treatment was successful in converting the surgery to an elective setting, if possible, a colonic evaluation should be carried out to rule out the all-important differential diagnosis of colonic adenocarcinoma. This is especially in elderly patients with low haemoglobin level where the haematological indices are suggestive of chronic blood loss type (hypochromic microcytic morphology on haematological indices and peripheral blood film examination).

B. Indications for Surgery

The indications for surgery of acute sigmoid colonic diverticulitis with perforation are:

1. Free perforation with peritonitis (purulent or feculent)
2. Failure to respond to nonoperative management including a persistent phlegmon, failure of percutaneous or trans-rectal drainage of an abscess, increasing fever, leucocytosis, tachycardia, hypotension, signs of sepsis or worsening clinical examination
3. Intestinal obstruction which does not resolve with conservative therapy (semi-emergency)

C. Options of Surgical Procedure

The management of acute perforative sigmoid colonic diverticulitis is based on the working principle of initial management of patients with complicated disease medically/conservatively, with the aim to convert (and avoid if possible) emergency surgery in favour of an elective resection later.

There are varied options and combinations in the surgical management armamentarium of complicated acute perforative sigmoid colonic diverticulitis. Deciding on the best surgical option requires a thorough knowledge of the options available and its indications. The choices of surgical procedure are:

Three-stage approach (rarely performed nowadays except in the most extreme cases of medical instability — described here for historical interest only)

1. Proximal diversion and drainage (occasionally modified using over-sewing of a visible perforation site with an omental patch[5])
2. Resection of the diseased bowel segment and primary anastomosis
3. Reversal of the proximal diverting stoma

Two-stage approach

1. Resection with proximal colostomy and over-sewing of the rectal stump (Hartmann's procedure) or exteriorisation of the distal stump as a mucous fistula (Mikulicz operation)
2. Re-establishment of bowel continuity

or

1. Primary resection with primary anastomosis and proximal diversion
2. Reversal of the proximal diverting stoma

Single-stage approach

1. Primary resection (segmental or subtotal/total colectomy) without proximal diversion.

   Intraoperative on-table colonic lavage is required when primary colonic anastomosis is performed.

The present day surgical approaches mainly concentrate on the single-stage and two-stage approaches in acute cases requiring urgent or emergent surgery.

In general

1. Most Hinchey stage I and some stage II disease can be managed with a single-stage operation (primary resection and primary anastomosis without proximal diversion) provided the patient fulfills the following conditions:

   — haemodynamically stable without inotropic support
   — extent of peritoneal contamination is limited
   — adequate bowel preparation is possible[6]

2. Most cases of Hinchey class III and IV disease will require a two-stage approach (especially Hartmann's procedure)

Hartmann's procedure has been the standard treatment in emergency setting with satisfactory results and a mortality rate between 2.6% and 7.3%.[7] The setback of this two-stage operation is that 35% to 45% of patients will never have their stoma reversed due to advanced age and severe co-morbidities.[8,9] However, in patients with pre-existing faecal incontinence, a Hartmann's procedure might be the procedure of choice. Reversal of the end colostomy created after a Hartmann's procedure is a technically challenging surgery[10] and is associated with significant morbidity and mortality (as high as 25% and 14%, respectively).[11,12]

Role of laparoscopic surgery in acute perforative sigmoid colonic diverticulitis

In the recent years, the role of laparoscopic approach for treating acute complicated sigmoid colonic diverticulitis has been explored and the evidence shows that this modality is still not adequately evaluated.

Firstly, the role of laparoscopic resectional surgery in perforative colonic diverticulitis is still limited. The result after laparoscopic resection with primary anastomosis is still lacking in the literature. Laparoscopic Hartmann's procedure appears to be a technically feasible operation with reasonable outcomes.[13]

Secondly, non-resectional laparoscopic surgery for perforative colonic diverticulitis, first described by Faranda *et al.*[14] in 1996, appears to be a promising alternative in the treatment of this acute condition. This technique of laparoscopic peritoneal lavage, inspection of the colon and the placement of abdominal drains in patients with peritonitis without gross faecal contamination appear to reduce morbidity and improve surgical outcome.[14, 15, 16] Myers *et al.* showed excellent results (morbidity and mortality rates <5%) after laparoscopic lavage and drainage of the peritoneal cavity in his series of 100 patients with perforative colonic diverticulitis.[17]

In short, laparoscopic damage control surgery seems to reduce the rate of more radical operations.[16,18] The advantage of this approach is that acute resection can still be performed in patients who fail to improve after lavage[18]. Karoui *et al.*[19] have shown no differences in the post operative morbidity and mortality rates in a comparative study between laparoscopic peritoneal lavage and open resection with primary anastomosis and diversion ileostomy. Laparoscopic peritoneal lavage reduced the duration of hospitalisation and the avoidance of stoma creation.

In summary, the choice of the surgical procedures performed depends not only on the extent of the disease but also on the experience of the surgeon, the clinical condition of the patient before and during the operation and the severity of the co-existing condition.

D. Important Considerations in the Techniques for Appropriate Resection

The practice parameters of the American Society of Colon and Rectal Surgeons set out some general recommendations regarding resection of colonic diverticular disease.[20]

1. In elective resection, it is not necessary to resect the entire proximal diverticula-bearing colon but it is important to remove all thickened and diseased colon. It may be acceptable to retain compliant proximal diverticula-bearing colon provided the colon is not hypertrophied.
2. The entire length of the sigmoid colon should be removed. The identification of the rectosigmoid colonic junction is crucial to ensure adequacy of the sigmoid colonic resection, i.e. termination of the taenia coli (flaring of the taenia coli to envelop the entire circumference of the colon), absence of diverticulae and appendices epiploicae and the level of resection just below the level of sacral promontory after rectosigmoid colonic mobilisations).
3. The colorectal anastomosis, when decided, should be made to normal rectum and must be fashioned to be tension-free and well-vascularised. The single most crucial predictor of recurrence after sigmoid colonic resection for uncomplicated sigmoid colonic diverticulitis is retention of the distal sigmoid colon.[21]

E. Position of Patient for Surgery

The patient is positioned on the operating table in the Lloyd Davis position (Trendelenburg position

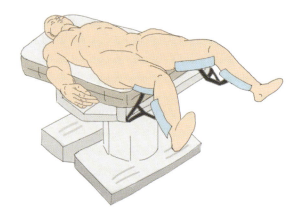

Figure 1.

Lloyd-Davis position.

with legs apart — 30° Trendelenburg and hips flexed at 150° as the basic angle which is adjustable with leg supports), using Allen Yellowfins Stirrups (Allen Medical System) (Fig. 1).

This position permits more effective retraction by the second assistant positioned between the patient's legs, insertion of vaginal probes which may assist in difficult anterior dissection (particularly after hysterectomy), irrigation of the rectum, occasional cystoscopy for ureteric stenting, and absolutely necessary for the insertion of the intraluminal stapling device.

F. Perioperative Precautions and Preparation

Prior to surgery, the patient is catheterised for perioperative urine output monitoring. A nasogastric tube is inserted to facilitate gastric decompression due to the high possibility of splenic flexure mobilisation and likely development of gastroparesis and paralytic ileus after surgery.

For patients with high cardiovascular and renal risks, a central venous line is required to assist in the adjustment of fluid management especially in patients with pre-existing fluid and electrolyte derangement and subsequently in anticipation of postoperative poor urine output issues. Occasionally, postoperatively, this central venous access can be used for temporary parenteral nutrition infusion. Preferentially, an intra-arterial line is inserted for intraoperative monitoring and to facilitate arterial blood taking for arterial blood gas assessment.

It is important to advocate thromboprophylactic measures such as perioperative application of TED stockings, usage of intermittent pneumatic calf compression device and administration of prophylactic anti-coagulation therapy as these surgeries are usually prolonged, located in the pelvis and the position of the lower limbs in the Lloyd-Davis position.

I cannot stress more on the importance of taking adequate measures to keep the patient warm during surgery. Besides ambient operating room temperature control, warming blanket and Bair Hugger warmer should be used. It is also important to keep the patient dry during surgery and one good way is the use of barrier drapes to divert fluid away from the patient's body, coupled with lining the patient with absorbable dressings. It is also useful to ensure all intravenous infusion fluid and operative irrigation fluid to be warmed to body temperature to ensure homeostasis and to reduce adverse consequences of hypothermia.

Intra-Operative Surgical Techniques

A. Incision and Laparotomy

A midline incision from the symphysis pubis inferiorly (to as far superior as necessary) to above the umbilicus to gain adequate exposure for thorough laparotomy and colonic mobilisation. The landmark for the mobilisation of the left colon is usually from the mid transverse colon to upper rectum with mobilisation of the splenic flexure to ensure adequacy of colonic length for an optimal tension-free colorectal anastomosis.

It is important to examine the entire colon and rectum to assess the extent of the diverticular disease involvement. Practically, identification of colonic diverticula can be difficult and sometimes can be confused with appendices epiploicae. It is also important to identify the presence and the extent of inflammatory changes on the colon and its demarcation. An experienced surgeon utilises the presence of muscular hypertrophic changes associated with colonic

diverticular disease to determine the optimal resection margin selection for anastomosis.

In some cases, the exact diagnosis is not firmly determined despite thorough preoperative investigations and assessment. Intra-operatively, perforated colonic adenocarcinoma can mimic perforated colonic diverticulitis unless the patient has overt signs of disseminated malignant disease. Sometimes, intra-operative flexible colonoscopic examination by a second surgeon can be carried out (if available), assisted by the abdominal surgeon, to confirm the diagnosis. Moreover, in situation of doubt, it is better to be cautious and it is advisable to perform the colonic resection according to oncological principles.

In the event of possible contamination, it is good to protect the laparotomy wound using wound protector or lining it with surgical packs and practise good containment methods. All septic adhesions should be broken using gentle finger dissection to ensure all potential collections are drained. The peritoneal pus or fluid in the septic peritoneal cavity should be collected for bacteriological culture and sensitivity testing. In the findings of colorectal malignancy, ascitic fluid should be sent for malignant cytology testing. It is prudent to explore all potential septic collection sites such as subphrenic, paracolic, subhepatic, pelvic and inter-loop spaces.

Copious amount of fluid should be used to ensure a thorough peritoneal lavage for washing and for its dilution effect. This should be carried out after this step before performing the definitive surgery.

B. Mobilisation of the Sigmoid and Descending Colon

The lateral to medial approach in the mobilisation of the left colon (sigmoid and descending colon) (using electrocautery) is the usual preferred technique in open surgery (Fig. 2). With proper medial traction of the left colon and its mesentery by the assistant standing on the right side of the patient (traction and counter-traction technique), the lateral peritoneal reflection (known as the white line of Toldt, the line of fusion of the colonic mesentery to the posterior parietal peritoneum) is incised. Dissection along this plane is usually relatively bloodless.

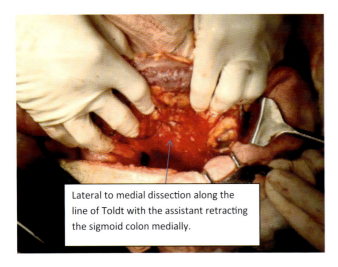

Lateral to medial dissection along the line of Toldt with the assistant retracting the sigmoid colon medially.

Figure 2.

Lateral to medial mobilisation of the left colon.

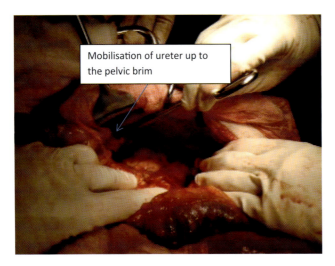

Mobilisation of ureter up to the pelvic brim

Figure 3.

Extent of left colon mobilisation.

After incision of the peritoneal lining, further mobilisation medially by using sharp dissection through the avascular loose areolar tissue plane beneath the peritoneum, will expose the left gonadal vessels and subsequently, the left ureter. It is important not to damage the branches of the gonadal vessels here to prevent haemorrhage, which can hamper easy identification of the left ureter.

The left gonadal vessels and left ureter should be mobilised from the renal level to the pelvic brim level (where the left ureter crosses over the bifurcation of the left common iliac artery) (Fig. 3). This is

to prevent injury to them especially to the left ureter during the high ligation of the inferior mesenteric artery and during the posterior mobilisation of the rectosigmoid colonic junction.

C. Identification of the Left Ureter

The standard surgical approaches to locate the left ureter are:

1. Lateral to medial approach by incising along the line of Toldt (as described above — commonly used by general surgeons and colorectal surgeons) (Fig. 4)
2. Entering the retroperitoneal space after division of the round ligament (commonly used by gynaecological surgeons)
3. Medial to lateral approach commonly used during laparoscopic mobilisation of the left colon.

Subsequently, the parietal peritoneal leaf on the right side of the rectosigmoid junction at the level of the sacral promontory is incised longitudinally to enter the retroperitoneal space. The left gonadal vessels and left ureter are easily identified and preserved upon widening of this retroperitoneal space.

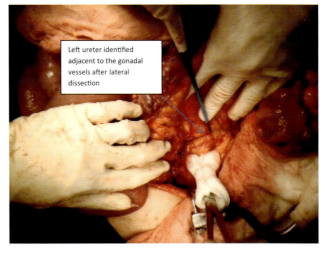

Left ureter identified adjacent to the gonadal vessels after lateral dissection

Figure 4.

Localisation of the left ureter.

Tips and tricks to help locate the 'difficult' left ureter

Every now and then, we will encounter difficulty in identifying the left ureter, usually due to obliteration of the left retroperitoneal space by locally advanced cancer, inflammation or prior surgery.

The principles to fall back on during these circumstances are:

1. Be familiar with the different approaches to identify the left ureter, as you may need to use either one or combination of these techniques to find it.
2. Always start your approach from normal anatomy/disease-free side first and then develop from this plane to the affected area.
3. The gonadal vessels almost always accompany the ureter and are usually located anterior to the ureter. Identification of the gonadal vessels would signal the proximity of the ureter and hence care should be exercised from hereon.
4. Be familiar with the macroscopic features of the ureter (vermiculating whitish muscular tube with superficial longitudinal capiliaries).
5. Preoperative insertion of ureteric stent in cases of anticipated "difficult" ureter, may facilitate palpation of the stent to aid localisation of the ureter and can also facilitate identification of ureteric injury and repair. However, the literature so far does not demonstrate that stents prevent ureteric injuries.

6. Goods surgical techniques to adhere to — always dissect along the longitudinal plane and not the transverse plane, do not transect any tubular structures transversely unless you are certain of its anatomy; sharp dissection using right angle forceps and diathermy is advisable; and judicious and careful application of diathermy to prevent thermal damage to the ureter is also advisable.
7. Be aware of suspicious signs of ureteric injury (either partial or complete) — might not just be as simple as a defect in the muscular tubular structure with fluid exiting through it. Subtle signs to take note are persistent pooling of heamoserous fluid in the vicinity of the ureter and mild haematuria. You must be aware of the possibility of thermal damage and must avoid overzealous mobilisation and devascularisation of segmental blood supply to the ureter (blood supply to the ureter is segmental in distribution and has limited transmural extension).

Common sites of left ureteric injury during anterior resection

Ureteric injuries typically involve one of the following three specific sites (Fig. 5):

1. During high inferior mesenteric artery (IMA) ligation, where this vessel lies in close proximity to the junction of the upper and middle thirds of

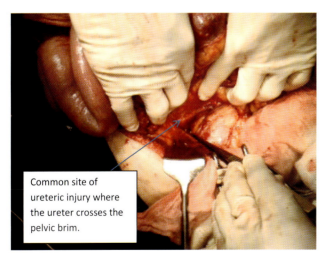

Common site of ureteric injury where the ureter crosses the pelvic brim.

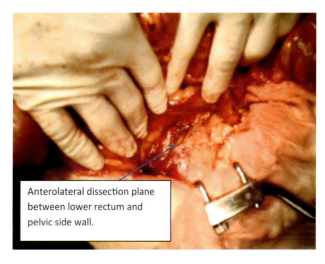

Anterolateral dissection plane between lower rectum and pelvic side wall.

Figure 5.

Common sites of ureteric injury.

the left ureter. Therefore, it is important to completely mobilise the ureter laterally before IMA ligation to prevent its inclusion during clamping and division of the IMA vascular pedicle.

2. During upper mesorectal mobilisation near the level of the sacral promontory, where the ureter crosses over the bifurcation of the iliac artery and courses medially to enter the pelvis. The left ureter may be closely associated to the sigmoid colon or even adherent to it as a result of prior inflammatory processes.

3. During pelvic dissection of the rectum in the anterolateral dissection plane between the lower rectum and the pelvic sidewall and bladder, including division of the lateral pedicle.

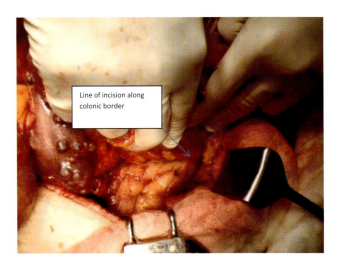

Line of incision along colonic border

Figure 6.

Mobilisation of the splenic flexure.

D. Splenic Flexure Take Down

Patients with colonic diverticular disease sometimes have a shortened colon (due to muscular hypertrophy) and therefore require mobilisation of the splenic flexure, to ensure adequate colon length to restore bowel continuity after sigmoid colon resection. This is to allow a tension-free well-vascularised proximal colonic stump to anastomose to the distal rectal stump.

Principles in splenic flexure take down:

1. It is most intuitive to approach mobilisation of the splenic flexure from both directions — proximally, antegrade direction from the transverse colon and distally, retrograde direction from the descending colon (which is the continuation from the descending colonic mobilisation).

2. Personally, I prefer to approach the splenic flexure first from the descending colon as the plane of dissection is already defined. The incision along the line of Toldt used for the descending colon mobilisation is extended proximally and then curve along the splenic flexure to mobilise it from the retroperitoneal Gerota's fascia and perinephric fat. The trick here is to keep the line of incision as close as possible to the colonic border and with gentle traction on the colon in the direction towards the right iliac fossa. Try to take this incision as proximally as possible and then leave the

remainder mobilisation from the direction of the distal transverse colon (Fig. 6).

3. To facilitate splenic flexure take down from the transverse colonic end, the posterior omental leaf is first released from the transverse colon to enter the lesser sac. From experience, the best spot to enter the lesser sac is at the mid transverse colon and the correct plane to follow is to keep as close as possible to the avascular plane adjacent to the colonic border. This plane is exposed by the assistant holding and maintaining traction on the greater omentum and the operating surgeon maintaining counter traction on the transverse colon.

4. The greater omental attachment to the distal half of the transverse colon and splenic flexure must be completely released. During this process, it is important that care be taken not to pull too hard on the greater omentum as occasionally, part of the greater ometum or its adhesions are adherent to the splenic capsule. This can cause splenic capsule avulsion injury resulting in troublesome haemorrhage.

5. After release of the greater omentum, the splenic flexure is fully exposed. It is important to identify the inferior border of the pancreas at this juncture as a reminder not to make the peritoneal releasing incision too close to it. With this in mind, the incision on the peritoneal reflection is then extended following the curve of the splenic flexure and

subsequently along the distal transverse colon, the incision being kept close to the colonic edge.

6. Another anatomical structure that must always be protected at this point of the surgery is the duodenojejunal flexure on the other side of the descending colonic mesentery.

7. It is also prudent not to create defects in the left colonic mesentery to avoid injuring the all-important marginal artery, which will be the main blood supply to the proximal colonic stump after ligation of the inferior mesenteric vessels.

Tips and tricks to tackle difficult splenic flexure

1. Ensure optimal exposure especially for difficult high splenic flexure. To ascertain the adequacy of the superior extent of the midline incision, a good indication is when part of the transverse colon and stomach are seen. Inadequate exposure increases the risk of splenic injury due to the need for excessive traction on the anatomical structures.

2. It is also important to straighten out the splenic flexure, especially if they are fused together by the greater omentum or congenital adhesions forming a hairpin loop.

3. Keeping the peritoneal reflection releasing incision close to the colonic edge and completely mobilise it from the retroperitoneal Gerota's fascia and perinephric fat till the inferior border of the pancreas is exposed.

E. Vascular Control

Ligation of the inferior mesenteric artery (IMA)

The inferior mesenteric artery can be ligated at two locations. These two locations are divided according to the origin of the left colic artery from the IMA.

1. High IMA ligation refers to ligation of the IMA proximal to the origin of the left colic artery. High IMA ligation is preferred if extra colonic length is required to ensure a tension-free anastomosis. However, with IMA ligation at this level, there is a

possibility of compromising the blood supply to the proximal colonic stump; therefore, it is important to scrutinise the blood supply carefully before deciding on the resection margin for anastomosis.

2. Low IMA ligation refers to ligation of the IMA distal to the origin of the left colic artery. The advantage of this ligation is that the blood supply to the descending colon is preserved. However, there will be a compromise on the length of the proximal colon available for low anterior resection.

Precautions to take when performing IMA ligation:

— Preserve adequate vascular stump length to ensure secure knotting and to avoid slippage (Fig. 7).

— Preserve and prevent injury to the para-aortic sympathetic nerves.

— Ensure that the left ureter is away from the site of vascular division and ligation.

How to identify the IMA?

With the mobilised sigmoid colon and mesentery held taut by the operating surgeon standing on the left side of the patient, the parietal peritoneum covering the rectosigmoid colonic junction at the sacral promontory level is incised on both sides of the gutter. The loose areolar tissue between the sigmoid mesocolon and retroperitoneum is separated to create a window. It is important not to dissect too deep into the

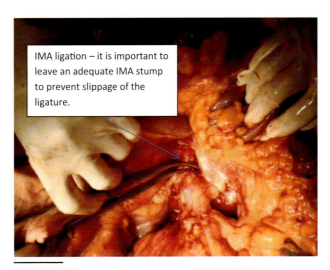

IMA ligation – it is important to leave an adequate IMA stump to prevent slippage of the ligature.

IMA ligation.

retroperitoneum to prevent injury to the branches of the superior hypogastric plexus (sympathetic plexus) and both the hypogastric nerves.

The IMA is located along the free edge of the sigmoid mesocolon and can be traced to the aorta superiorly. It is crucial then to isolate the root of the IMA by creating a mesenteric window superior to it. There is almost always an avascular mesenteric window at this site.

The root of the IMA is then skeletonised to enable optimal clamping and ligation. Care must be taken here to avoid damage to the para-aortic sympathetic nerves and the accidental injury of the left ureter and the left gonadal vessels (especially when these two structures are not completely lateralised).

Ligation of the inferior mesenteric vein (IMV)

After ligation of the IMA, the IMV can be identified as it enters posteriorly to the inferior border of the body of the pancreas to join the splenic vein. It is prudent to release the peritoneal attachments of the duodenojejunal flexure to allow easy isolation, ligation and division of the vein. It is also important to ligate at this point to ensure an adequate colonic mesenteric length for a tension-free anastomosis (Fig. 8).

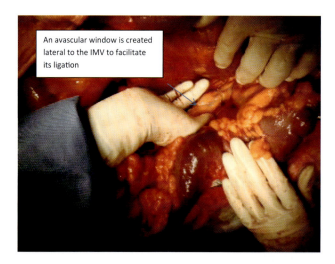

An avascular window is created lateral to the IMV to facilitate its ligation

Figure 8.

IMV ligation.

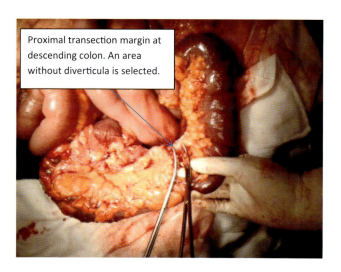

Proximal transection margin at descending colon. An area without diverticula is selected.

Figure 9.

Proximal transection margin.

F. Determination of the Proximal Transection Margin

The proximal transection margin should be in the distal descending colon approximately 5 cm from the involved diseased colonic point (Fig. 9). This margin should also be devoid of any diverticula to ensure an optimal anastomosis. The reason why the anastomotic margin must not incorporate any diverticulum is because the diverticulum does not have the all-important strength providing submucosa layer.

It is also important to ensure that the proximal stump has adequate blood supply, at this juncture provided only by the marginal vessels fed by the middle colic artery, a branch of the superior mesenteric artery. Brisk bleeding from the cut marginal artery must be present together with bright red arterial blood oozing from the cut edge of the colon must also be observed.

How to ensure adequate proximal bowel length for tension-free anastomosis

The following are some important steps to follow to achieve adequate proximal bowel length:

1. Complete medial mobilisation of the left colon.
2. Total splenic flexure mobilisation.

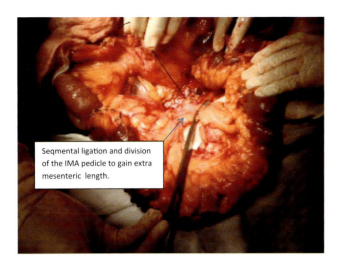

Seqmental ligation and division of the IMA pedicle to gain extra mesenteric length.

Figure 10.

"Segmental" ligation and division of the IMA pedicle.

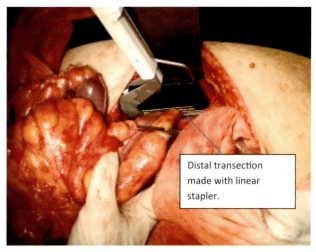

Distal transection made with linear stapler.

Figure 11.

Rectosigmoid junction.

3. Release of the greater omentum from the transverse colon beyond the right side of the midline of the transverse colon.
4. High ligation of the IMA and IMV.
5. "Segmental" ligation and division of the IMA pedicle distal to the left colic artery (in cases of high IMA tie) (Fig. 10).
6. Division of mesocolon up to the marginal artery.
7. Transverse scoring of the mesocolic peritoneum.

G. Determination of the Distal Transection Margin

From the oncological standpoint, it is adequate to have a 5 cm distal surgical margin. However, in surgical resection for complicated sigmoid colonic diverticulitis, the determination of the distal transection margin is more important because the entire sigmoid colon must be resected in order to reduce the possibility of recurrence of sigmoid colonic diverticulitis.

How to ensure that all the sigmoid colon is resected?

It has been shown that resection of the entire sigmoid colon is important to reduce the possibility

of recurrence of sigmoid colonic diverticulitis. The most crucial step here is to identify the distal resection margin which is the rectosigmoid junction (Fig. 11).

Where is this rectosigmoid junction?

1. The segment of the large bowel with confluence of the three bands of *tenae coli* (the *taenia coli* have fanned out to envelope the entire circumference of the bowel).
2. There is absence of appendices epiploicae.
3. Technically, the rectosigmoid junction is at the level of the sacral promontory when the mobilised sigmoid colon is pulled gently towards the cephalic direction.

H. Preparation for Colorectal Anastomosis

On-table colonic lavage

On-table colonic lavage is usually necessary to prepare the colon for colorectal anastomosis because bowel preparation is commonly not performed in emergency or semi-emergency operations and contraindicated in peritonitis.

The steps to perform on-table colonic lavage is described in the next chapter.

I. Construction of the Colorectal Anastomosis

Colorectal anastomosis is commonly achieved using either hand-sewn or stapling technique. Following high anterior resection, the proximal descending colon can be connected to the upper rectum using either a single-stapling technique or a double stapling technique.

The configuration of the colorectal anastomosis can either be a straight end-to-end colorectal anastomosis or a side-to-end colorectal anastomosis.

How to ensure an optimal and safe colorectal anastomosis?

Principles of good intestinal anastomosis:

1. **Tension-free** anastomosis with adequate proximal colonic stump length provided by optimal mobilisation of the left colon and splenic flexure.
2. **Optimal blood supply** of the transected colonic and rectal stumps as demonstrated by the healthy cut mucosa edges, fresh blood oozing at the cut edges and brisk fresh bleeding of the marginal vessel before ligation.
3. The intestinal ends used for anastomosis are **free of disease.**
4. There must be **no obstruction distal to the anastomosis.**
5. Ensure **good surgical and anastomotic techniques.**

When is it not safe to anastomose?

1. When the patient is in haemodynamic instability (from septic and cardiogenic shock) requiring inotropic support.
2. When the patient has signs of multiple organ failure (acute tubular necrosis, coagulopathy, etc.).

The safest and quickest surgical procedure to perform in an unstable patient is a Hartmann's procedure (end colostomy with over-sewing of the rectal stump), followed by peritoneal lavage and adequate drainage.

However, when the circumstance is equivocal for "optimal" anastomosis, primary anastomosis with creation of a proximal diverting ileostomy can be performed.

J. Completion of Surgery

The anastomotic line must be checked for viability and absence of tension of the bowel and its mesentery. In addition, air leak test should also be performed. If everything is satisfactory, rectal tube per rectally is usually inserted for decompression.

Thorough peritoneal lavage with heated saline solution must be advocated judiciously to cleanse the peritoneal cavity, especially in both the subphrenic fossae, Morrison's pouch, both paracolic gutters and pelvic cavity. The number of surgical drains required and the position of insertions are determined by the degree of peritoneal contamination.

K. Postoperation Care

Postoperatively, the patient is usually managed and monitored in the surgical intensive or high dependency care unit, depending on the patient's haemodynamic stability, co-morbidity status and extent of the artificial support required.

During the early postoperative period, it is vital to manage the following to promote recovery and to ensure healing of the anastomosis:

1. Optimal oxygen delivery to vital organs (maintain and support optimal mean arterial pressure, tissue oxygenation level and urinary output).
2. Correction of the patient's oxygen carrying capacity, intravascular volume, coagulopathy and electrolyte abnormalities.
3. Provision of early and appropriate nutritional support.
4. Support and maintenance of organ function.
5. Early detection of septic focus and anastomotic leakage to facilitate early and appropriate intervention.

References

1. Roberts PL, Veidenheimer MC. (1994) Current management of diverticulits. *Adv Surg* **27**: 189–208.

2. Hinchey EJ, Schaal PG, Richards GK. (1978) Treatment of perforated diverticular disease of the colon. *Adv Surg* **12**: 85–109.

3. Brook I, Frazier EH. (2000) Aerobic and anaerobic microbiology in intra-abdominal infections associated with diverticulitis. *J Med Microbiol* **49**: 827–30.

4. Hachigian MP, Honickman S, Eisentat TE, *et al.* (1992) Computed tomography in the initial management of acute left-sided diverticulitis. *Dis Colon Rectum* **35**: 1123–9.

5. Kronborg O. (1993) Treatment of perforated sigmoid diverticulitis: a prospective randomized trial; *Br J Surg* **80**: 505–7.

6. Maggard MA, Chandher CF, Schmit PJ, *et al.* Surgical diverticulitis: treatment options; *Am Surg* **67**: 1185–9

7. Fleming FJ, Gillen P. (2009) Reversal of Hartmann's procedure following acute diverticulitis: Is timing everything? *Int J Colorectal Dis* **24**: 1219–25.

8. Maggard MA, Zingmond D, O'Connell JB, Ko CY. (2004) What proportion of patients with an ostomy (for diverticulitis) gets reversed? *Am Surg* **70**: 928–31.

9. Vermeulen J, Coene PP, Van Hout NM, *et al.* (2009) Restoration of bowel continuity after surgery for acute perforated diverticulitis. Should Hartmann's procedure be considered a one-stage procedure? *Colorectal Dis* **11**: 619–24.

10. Banerjee S, Leather AJM, REnnie JA, *et al.* (2005) Feasibility and morbidity of reversal of Hartmann's. *Colorectal Dis* **7**: 454–9

11. Vermeulen J, Gosselink MP, Hop WCJ, *et al.* (2009) Hospital mortality after emergency surgery for perforated diverticulitis. *Ned Tijdschr Geneesk* **153**: 1209–14.

12. Salem L, Flum DR. (2004) Primary anastomosis or Hartmann's procedure for patients with diverticular peritonitis? A systematic review. *Dis Colon Rectum* **47**: 1953–64.

13. Agaba EA, Zaidi RM, Ramzy P, *et al.* (2009) Laparoscopic Hartmann's procedure: A viable option for treatment of acutely perforated diverticulitis. *Surg Endosc* **23**: 1483–86.

14. Faranda C, Barrat C, Catherine JM, Champault GG. (2000) Two-stage laparoscopic management of generalized peritonitis due to perforated sigmoid diverticula: Eighteen cases. *Surg Laparosc Endosc Percutan Tech* **10**: 135–38.

15. Franklin ME Jr, Portillo G, Trevino JM, *et al.* (2008) Long-term experience with the laparoscopic approach to perforated diverticulitis plus generalized peritonitis. *World J Surg* **32**: 1507–11.

16. Bretagnol F, Pautrat K, Mor C, *et al.* (2008) Emergency laparoscopic management of perforated sigmoid diverticulitis : a promising alternative to more radical procedures. *J Am Coll Surg* **206**: 654–57.

17. Myers E, Hurley M, O'Sullivan GC, *et al.* (2008) Laparoscopic peritoneal lavage for generalized peritonitis due to perforated diverticulitis. *Br J Surg* **95**: 97–101.

18. Taylor CJ, Layani L, Ghusn MA, White SI. (2006) Perforated diverticulitis managed by laparoscopic lavage. *ANZ J Surg* **76** (11): 962–65.

19. Karoui M, Champault A, Pautrat K, *et al.* (2009) Laparoscopic peritoneal lavage or primary anastomosis with defunctioning stoma for Hinchey 3 complicated diverticulitis: Results of a comparative study. *Dis Colon Rectum* **52**: 609–15.

20. Wong WD, Wexner SD, Lowry A, *et al.* (2000) Practice parameters for the treatment of sigmoid diverticulitis: Supporting documentation. The Standards Task Force. The American Society of Colon and Rectal Surgeons. *Dis Colon Rectum* **43**: 290–7.

21. Thaler K, Baig MK, Berho M, *et al.* (2003) Determinants of recurrence after sigmoid resection for uncomplicated diverticulitis. *Dis Colon Rectum* **46**: 385–8.

Chapter 11

Surgical Management of Obstructive Colorectal Malignancy

Bettina Lieske[*], Cheong Wai Kit[†], and Frances Lim Sheau Huei[‡]

Introduction

Colorectal cancer is the third most common cancer worldwide, with an estimated 1.24 million people diagnosed in 2008.[1] There is wide geographical variation with up to 10-fold differences in incidence across the world. Incidence rates of colorectal cancer are increasing in countries where the rates were previously low (especially in Asian countries), whereas in Europe the incidence is stabilising and in North America the trend is declining.

Colorectal cancer is now the most common cancer in Singapore.[2] The age-standardised incidence rates of colorectal cancer have steadily risen over the past 35 years, and is highest in Singapore Chinese, followed by the Malays and Indians.

The average age at diagnosis is 67 years for both males and females. Approximately 90% of colorectal cancer cases are diagnosed in patients at the age of 50 years and above. The current screening guidelines recommend annual screening for adults beginning from the age of 50. Despite this, the uptake of screening remains low, with only 14.2% of Singaporeans between the age of 50 and 69 years reporting to have

undergone screening in 2010.[3] As a result of the low uptake, the majority of colorectal cancer cases are diagnosed in symptomatic individuals at a later stage, leading to poorer prognosis.

A recent audit from the United Kingdom showed that the proportion of colorectal cancer patients admitted to hospital as emergency cases remained static over the past four years at 21%. One in seven patients undergoing emergency surgery did not survive 90 days after the operation,[4] highlighting the high risk of surgery in this group and the need for earlier diagnosis.

One of the emergency presentations of colorectal cancer is large bowel obstruction, which we will discuss in further detail in this chapter.

I. Preoperative Management

Patients with clinical signs of large bowel obstruction will usually require urgent admission for administration of intravenous fluid replacement and an attempt to decompress the bowel via a nasogastric tube. It is important to ensure adequate resuscitation with appropriate intravenous fluids, correction and

[*] B. Lieske, MD (Germany), FRCS (Eng), MA ClinEd (UK), Consultant, Division of Colorectal Surgery, University Surgical Cluster, National University Hospital, Singapore.

[†] W. K. Cheong, MBBS, FRCS (Ed), FRCS (Glasg), FAMS, Head & Senior Consultant Surgeon, Division of Colorectal Surgery, Department of Surgery, National University Hospital, Singapore.

[‡] Frances S. H. Lim, Adv Dip Med Sci (1MU), MD (Canada), Associate Fellow ACS (USA), Consultant, Division of Colorectal Surgery, Department of Surgery, National University Hospital, Singapore.

normalisation of haematological and biochemical abnormalities before any intervention.

As the group of patients who are affected with this condition is usually older, many will have concomitant medical problems, so particular attention must be paid to ensure preservation of homeostatic functions to reduce the possibilities of mortality and morbidity.

Initial abdominal radiograph should raise suspicion of large bowel obstruction if there is colonic dilatation with a distinct "cut off" or paucity of gas in the rectum (Fig. 1).

Small bowel dilatation indicates an incompetent ileocaecal valve, allowing the colon to decompress proximally (Fig. 2). A competent ileocaecal valve leads to

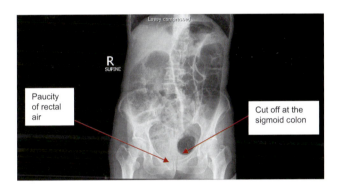

Figure 1.

Abdominal X-ray showing colonic dilatation with paucity of rectal air and "cut off" at the sigmoid colonic suggesting complete colonic obstruction.

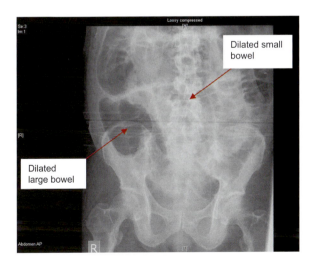

Figure 2.

Abdominal X-ray showing dilated small and large bowels suggesting large bowel obstruction in the presence of an incompetent ileocaecal valve.

closed loop obstruction, necessitating a more expedited course of action to decompress the obstructed colon.

Once the diagnosis of large bowel obstruction has been made, patients will usually undergo a baseline computed tomography (CT) scan of the abdomen and pelvis to confirm the diagnosis and assess the nature of the obstructing malignancy, particularly its location within the colon and rectum.

The CT scan should be carried out with intravenous and rectal contrast where possible, and serves as a staging scan to assess the local resectability of the malignancy as well as the liver for potential metastatic spread. As such, the thorax can either be included in the CT scan or the patient should undergo a chest radiograph.

II. Management Options

The management of acute malignant colonic obstruction can be divided into emergent resectional procedures with or without primary anastomosis, and procedures to decompress the colon and prepare for an elective resection later.

We will be discussing the management of left-sided colonic obstruction, as right-sided obstruction will easily be dealt with by a right hemicolectomy even in the emergency setting, thereby not conferring any advantage of deferring the surgery.

The practice parameters of the American Society of Colon and Rectal Surgeons[5] set out the following general recommendations regarding patients presenting with obstructing colonic malignancies:

1. Patients with an obstructing right or transverse colon cancer should undergo a right or extended right colectomy. A primary ileo-colic anastomosis can be performed in the appropriate clinical setting.
2. For the patient with a left-sided colonic obstruction, the procedure selected should be individualised from a variety of appropriate operative approaches.
3. Options for treatment may include resection with or without anastomosis (e.g. Hartmann resection), resection of the distended bowel (e.g. subtotal/total colectomy), or temporary relief of obstruction and faecal load (e.g. preoperative stenting as a bridge to resection).

The management of left-sided colonic malignant obstruction, including the rectum offers three main options:

1. Endoscopic colonic stenting
2. Proximal defunctioning loop colostomy or ileostomy
3. Resectional surgery with or without primary anastomosis

Each of these options has advantages and disadvantages and the ultimate decision must be made with the best interest of the patient and the individual scenario in mind.

III. Endoscopic Colonic Stenting

Indications

1. Patients with disseminated metastatic disease
2. Patients suitable for laparoscopic resectional surgery

Although randomised clinical trial data are lacking, the role for preoperative stenting in the emergent management of acute malignant colonic obstruction has been supported by cost-effectiveness analysis studies and several pooled analyses that demonstrate efficacy and safety.[7]

Endoscopic stenting serves the dual purpose of avoiding a major operation in patients with disseminated malignancy, thus allowing them to proceed to palliative chemotherapy faster, and secondly in patients who are suitable for curative resection of their obstructing malignancy, allowing a less extensive elective surgery as opposed to an emergency procedure, which is especially important in patients who might be able to undergo laparoscopic resection.

Its availability depends on local expertise and the availability of fluoroscopy, as well as the specialised endoscopic equipment for the stent placement.

After initial trials, there were some concerns regarding the safety of colonic stenting; however, more recently colonic stenting has become an accepted treatment approach for obstructing left-sided colon

malignancy,[8–10] particularly as a bridge to palliative therapy[8] as well as a bridge to surgery.[11–13]

The suitability for stenting is evaluated on CT scan and includes anatomical considerations, tumour location, as well as tumour characteristics and length of the stricture. Acute angulation of the bowel distal to the tumour or at the tumour site itself, possibly due to invasion of underlying structures, will make colonic stenting more challenging and occasionally impossible. Long segment obstruction might require placement of more than one stent to bridge the obstruction, and can lead to inadequate expansion of the stent subsequently.

A tumour in the lower rectum cannot be stented as the distal end of the stent will cause tenesmus and will give the patient poor quality of life.

Risks of stenting that need to be discussed with the patient prior to the procedure are:

— Unsuccessful stenting attempt with subsequent need for operative procedure. This includes the inability to cannulate the tumour and pass the guide wire through, and unsuccessful stent deployment and failure of stent to relieve the obstruction, often due to inadequate expansion of the stent. The radiological success rate (successful stent deployment) reported in systematic reviews is 92% and the clinical success rate (colonic decompression without need for surgical intervention) is around 80%[10,14]
— Stent migration occurs in around 10%[10,14] of the patients
— Stent perforation occurs in around 4%[10,14] of the patients
— Re-obstruction when tumour continues to grow into the stent occurs in 7–10%[10,14] of the patients

It is advisable to obtain consent of the patient for possible surgical intervention in the event that the stenting is not successful, as the abdominal distension can deteriorate during the endoscopic procedure due to gas insufflation, or an inadvertent perforation can occur, necessitating immediate transfer to the operating theatre.

The procedure is carried out endoscopically under image intensifier guidance. This can either be done in the endoscopy suite (usually the procedure room used for ERCP), the fluoroscopy room at the department of diagnostic imaging using portable endoscopic equipment, or the operating theatre (especially if there is a hybrid theatre for endovascular procedures).

Ensure that the patient receives an enema for clearance of the bowel distal to the obstruction before stenting.

The initial colonoscopic procedure is carried out in the usual fashion with the patient in the left lateral position and under conscious sedation. A double-lumen colonoscope is preferred as it facilitates simultaneous suction and irrigation via one channel whilst advancing the guide wire in the other channel. If available, CO_2 insufflation should be used in preference to room air.

Identify which area of the tumour is most likely to allow passage of the guide wire into the proximal bowel (sometimes there is still a pinpoint hole visible) (Fig. 3), and advance the guide wire under fluoroscopy. More often than not multiple attempts of passing the guide wire are necessary, and sometimes turning the patient into the supine position can help.

Once the guide wire is passed through the obstructing lesion, its position is confirmed with fluoroscopy and then the guide wire is advanced into the proximal bowel (Fig. 4).

The cannula is then inserted over the guide wire using the Seldinger technique into the proximal bowel

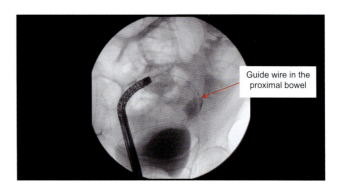

Figure 4.

Fluoroscopic picture confirming the successful cannulation of the tumour with the guide wire well placed proximal to the tumour.

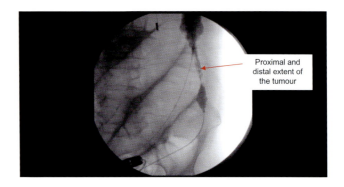

Figure 5.

Fluoroscopic picture showing the length of tumour obstruction after injection of contrast.

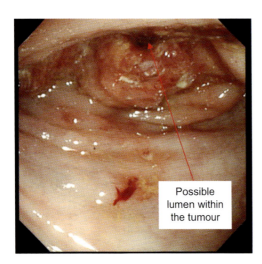

Figure 3.

Colonoscopic picture showing a stenotic cancer with a pinpoint hole.

to allow injection of water soluble radiological contrast (gastrograffin) to establish the proximal and distal extent of the tumour using fluoroscopy.

The length of the tumour is measured to decide on the optimal length of stent to be used to bridge the tumour with enough overhanging ends to prevent migration of the stent after its full expansion (Fig. 5).

The cannula is then exchanged for the stent in its deploying device, whilst the guide wire is kept in position (Fig. 6). Frequent confirmation with fluoroscopy during this process is necessary.

The stent deploying device is advanced under direct fluoroscopic and endoscopic visualisation until the entire stent is optimally straddling the tumour.

The stent is deployed once its position is confirmed by fluoroscopy. The stent on expansion will have a tendency to draw into the proximal bowel, which requires counter traction on the device during the deployment process (Fig. 7). Simultaneous monitoring with fluoroscopy as well endoscopy is mandatory.

Once the stent is fully expanded, the distal end should be visible beyond the malignant lesion, and there is often a gush of liquid faeculent material, confirming successful deployment and expansion (Fig. 8).

The patient is monitored overnight and an abdominal X-ray is taken on the following day to confirm the position and expansion of the stent (Fig. 9) and to look out for possible complications (Fig. 10).

Oral intake can be restarted once the abdominal distension eases. We routinely prescribe for the patient stool softener (e.g. Lactulose) and a low residue diet.

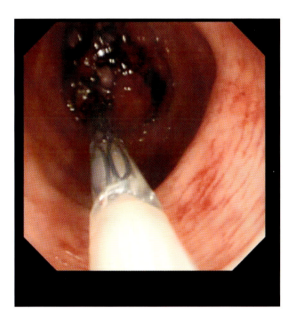

Figure 6.

Colonoscopic view of the self-expanding metallic stent (SEM) in its deploying device transversing the stenotic tumour.

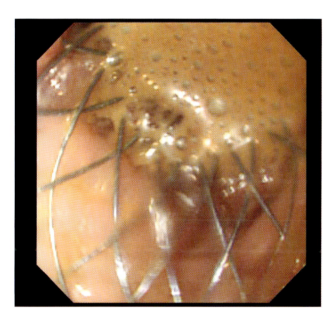

Figure 8.

Colonoscopic view of gush of faeculent material confirmation of successful stent deployment and stent expansion.

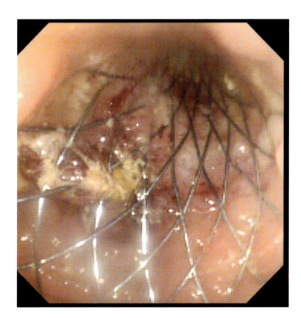

Figure 7.

Colonoscopic view showing optimal distal stent position.

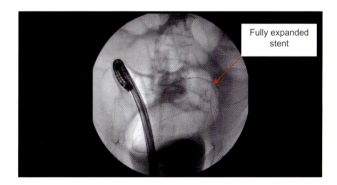

Fully expanded stent

Figure 9.

Fluoroscopic view showing a fully expanded stent in good position.

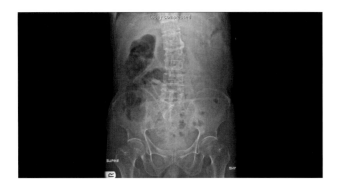

Figure 10.

Abdominal X-ray post stenting showing the stent in its optimal position and expansion.

Most conventional colonic stents expand to a diameter of 25 mm, and high dietary fibre can theoretically and potentially cause obstruction of the stent.

Patients planned for palliative therapy should be referred to medical oncology after discharge from hospital.

For patients proceeding to elective resectional surgery, there is currently no evidence to suggest an ideal interval period from insertion of the stent to definitive surgery. Considerations are adequate nutritional state, especially if the patient has been subacutely obstructed for some time prior to presentation and stenting, resolution of colonic distension and oedema of the colonic wall to facilitate primary anastomosis. The timing must take into consideration the safety and potential success of surgery and balance it against the risk and possible complications, including stent migration and re-obstruction when planning for the elective resection. In the pooled analysis by Sebastian *et al.*,[10] the mean time to resection was 8.9 days (range 2–115 days).

IV. Defunctioning Stoma

Indications

1. Patients unfit to undergo major resectional surgery
2. Patients with disseminated metastatic disease
3. Patients declining major resectional surgery
4. Patients unsuitable for stenting but suitable for elective resection later

A defunctioning stoma can be lifesaving in the event of an obstructing colonic tumour in the setting of a competent ileocaecal valve leading to closed loop obstruction. The siting of the stoma is dependent on the location of the tumour.

The most common sites are the left iliac fossa for a sigmoid colostomy, left upper quadrant for a distal transverse colostomy, right upper quadrant for a proximal transverse colostomy and right iliac fossa for an ileostomy. The guiding principle is to place the defunctioning stoma as distal as possible, allowing the patient as much functional bowel as possible, especially if the stoma is the only surgical intervention planned for the patient, with the aim to facilitate palliation, which may include chemotherapy.

For patients planned to undergo restorative resection later, the stoma should be sited to avoid interference with the blood supply to the anticipated anastomosis. On that note it is not advisable to injure the marginal artery during stoma creation. For a rectal cancer, the stoma can be a sigmoid loop colostomy, with the aim to include the stoma site in the resection specimen, or a defunctioning loop ileostomy, which can then serve to divert after the anastomosis following definitive resection. This, however, can only be carried out if the ileocaecal valve is incompetent and allows venting of the colon via the distal limb.

A sigmoid colon cancer might benefit from a defunctioning transverse colostomy, depending on the location of the tumour and the length of proximal colon available to reach the anterior abdominal wall. A descending colon tumour requires a transverse colostomy.

Preoperative marking of the stoma site is essential. However, if this is not possible, the following principles should be followed:

- The ideal stoma site should be easily accessible for the patient and must be away from bony prominences and not within skin creases, as well as away from the belt line (often located at the level of the umbilicus), whilst allowing the bowel to traverse the rectus sheath.
- A trephine incision is made, and after incising the skin, subcutaneous fat, and anterior rectus sheath, the rectus muscles is gently retracted to either side

to allow incision through the posterior sheath. Be careful to avoid injury to the inferior or superior epigastric artery.

Once inside the peritoneal cavity, identify the loop of bowel chosen for the anastomosis. The colon should be distended with gas and therefore close to the anterior abdominal wall, but identification of the correct part of the bowel is paramount.

- Sigmoid colon is characterised by the presence of taenia coli and appendices epiploicae. Transverse colon, in addition to the taenia coli and appendices epiploicae, has got the greater omentum attached to it. The terminal ileum is characterised by the fat pad as it joins to the caecum.
- The loop of bowel identified is gently eased out of the abdominal cavity through the incision. The width of the incision must be adequate to accommodate the bowel loop. Once the loop of the bowel is prolapsed out of the abdominal cavity, a small window is made at the mesentery close to the bowel wall to allow insertion of the stoma rod (stoma bridge) through it. The purpose of the stoma rod is to prevent retraction of the bowel loop back into the abdominal cavity.
- A transverse incision is made on the bowel loop (half of the circumference of the bowel) to allow decompression of gas and faeces. The abdominal distension should immediately ease with the decompression of the distended bowels. Be prepared to aspirate considerable amounts of faeces.

After the bowel is decompressed, the stoma opening is matured by anchoring the everted bowel wall to the wound skin edge using interrupted absorbable suture (e.g. Vicryl).

Postoperative Considerations

Patients who are planned for palliative therapy should be referred to medical oncology after discharge from hospital.

V. Resectional Surgery With or Without Primary Anastomosis

For this section, we refer the reader to the previous chapter 10 on advice for patient position and technical aspects of the surgery.

General considerations in the setting of an obstructive colonic malignancy include the adequacy of the oncological resection, the extent of the colonic resection, which will be determined by the viability of the colon when encountered at laparotomy, as well as the suitability of the proximal colon for primary anastomosis or the need for a Hartmann's procedure.

When entry into the abdominal cavity is achieved, the entire colon should be assessed for viability. Due to the obstruction, the colon will be distended, and if there is an incompetent ileocaecal valve, then the small bowel will be distended, too. Handling of these thin walled and fluid filled intestines must be carried out with great care, as they tend to slip over the edge of the incision laterally and then often drag to the side of the patient with significant pull on the mesentery, potentially leading to impaired perfusion and impending ischaemia.

Inspection should start at the caecum, as its state will determine the further proceedings of the surgery. Significant distension with serosal tears and impending perforation, as well as ischaemia determine the need for resection of the caecum, and in these cases, a subtotal colectomy will be indicated. Evacuation of the gaseous distension via a needle colotomy can make the surgery much easier at this stage. Choose a large bore needle, insert it tangentially through the bowel wall at a taenia coli and connect to the suction to deflate the colon. On withdrawal of the needle, close the defect suture to avoid spillage of faecal content during the surgery.

A subtotal colectomy requires mobilisation of the entire colon from the obstructing lesion distally to the caecum proximally. This can be carried out in a clockwise or anti-clockwise fashion. Proceed from lateral to medial, leaving the division of vascular structures till last.

Upon completion of the mobilisation and vascular division, including the pedicle supplying the part of the bowel containing the malignancy, the bowel should be divided distal to the malignancy. Proximal division is carried out at the terminal ileum, followed by an ileocolic or ileorectal anastomosis. The anastomosis can be hand-sewn or stapled.

For a stapled anastomosis, the choice is between side-to-side and end-to-end/side-to-end via the anus. We recommend a side-to-side or hand-sewn approach for an anastomosis well above the peritoneal reflection, whereas an end-to-end/side-to-end approach is feasible for an anastomosis at the peritoneal reflection and below.

If the caecum is found viable, then the usual oncological resection can be carried out. After removal of the specimen, the decision for primary anastomosis with or without defunctioning ileostomy versus Hartmann's procedure has to be made.

Hartmann's procedure has long been considered the gold standard for obstructive colonic malignancies,[15,16] however, a benefit in mortality has not been demonstrated in various non-randomised studies.[17–19] There is to date no randomised controlled trial.

The principles of safe colonic anastomosis have been described in the previous chapter, and should be adhered to in the setting of obstructive colonic malignancy as well. In addition, a significant size discrepancy of the distended proximal colon to the distal colon or rectum might make a primary anastomosis more challenging.

Secondly, the proximal bowel should be decompressed and faecal material evacuated prior to anastomosis. Colonic lavage has previously been advocated; however, following recent trials showing that bowel preparation in the elective setting is not necessary, it has been demonstrated that intraoperative colonic irrigation or lavage confers no benefit over manual decompression of the proximal bowel.[20]

If colonic lavage is deemed necessary, then the entire colon should be mobilised, to control the flow of the lavage fluid, and ensure that it is evacuated safely. The easiest entry is gained at the appendix, which acts as a natural entry tube into the colon. Use a Foley catheter or similar soft tubing and ensure that it is fixed securely within the appendix, and that the fluid used to irrigate the colon is warmed to body temperature.

The distal bowel needs to be mobile enough to be moved out of the operative field towards the left side, and a big basin placed securely between the patient's side and the operating surgeon's abdomen to steady it can be used to collect the effluent. Manual compression along the colon to move fluid and faeces distally is necessary to achieve good clearance of the bowel contents. Once the effluent is clear and all bowel content evacuated, remove the tubing from the appendix and perform a formal appendicectomy, securely tying the appendicular stump to prevent a stump blow-out.

The distal end of the bowel can then be prepared for the anastomosis.

VI. Clinical Consideration after Surgery

For this section, we refer the reader to the previous chapter 10 on advice for patient's post operative care.

References

1. Ferlay J, Shin HR, Bray F, *et al*. GLOBOCAN 2008, International Agency for Research on Cancer. http://globocan.iarc.fr/factsheet.asp. Accessed July 2013.
2. Trends of Colorectal Cancer in Singapore, 2007–2011. Health fact sheet. National Registry of Diseases Office. February 27, 2013, INP-13-1.
3. National Health Survey 2010. Epidemiology & Disease Control Division, Ministry of Health, Singapore.
4. *BMJ* 2013; **347**: f4266.
5. Wolff BG, Fleshman JW, Beck DE, *et al*. (eds.) (2010) The ASCRS *Textbook of Colon and Rectal Surgery*. Springer.
6. Chang GJ, Kaiser AM, Mills S, *et al*. (on behalf of the Standards Practice Task Force of the American Society of Colon and Rectal Surgeons). (2012) Practice Parameters for the Management of Colon Cancer. *Dis Colon Rectum* **55**: 831–843.
7. Farrell JJ. (2007) Preoperative colonic stenting: How, when and why? *Curr Opin Gastroenterol* **23** (05): 544–549.
8. Stefanidis D, Brown K, Nazario H, *et al*. (2005) Safety and efficacy of metallic stents in the management of colorectal obstruction. *JSLS* **9**: 454–459.

9. Khot UP, Lang AW, Murali K, Parker MC. (2002) Systematic review of the efficacy and safety of colorectal stents. *Br J Surg* **89**: 1096–1102.

10. Sebastian S, Johnston S, Geoghegan T, *et al.* (2004) Pooled analysis of the efficacy and safety of self-expanding metal stenting in malignant colorectal obstruction. *Am J Gastroenterol* **99**: 2051–2057.

11. Balague C, Targarona EM, Sainz S, *et al.* (2004) Minimally invasive treatment for obstructive tumors of the left colon: Endoluminal self-expanding metal stent and laparoscopic colectomy. Preliminary results. *Dig Surg* **21**: 282–286.

12. Dulucq JL, Wintringer P, Beyssac R, *et al.* (2006) One-stage laparoscopic colorectal resection after placement of self-expanding metallic stents for colorectal obstruction: A prospective study. *Dig Dis Sci* **51**: 2365–2371. Large series looking at a laparoscopic resection of colon cancer after colonic stenting.

13. Ng KC, Law WL, Lee YM, *et al.* (2006) Self-expanding metallic stent as a bridge to surgery versus emergency resection for obstructing left-sided colorectal cancer: A case-matched study. *J Gastrointest Surg* **10**: 798–803.

14. Morino M, Bertello A, Garbarini A, *et al.* (2002) Malignant colonic obstruction managed by endoscopic stent decompression followed by laparoscopic resections. *Surg Endosc* **16**: 1483–1487.

15. Desai DC, Brennan EJ, Reilly JF, Smink RD. (1998) The utility of the Hartmann procedure. *Am J Surg* **175**: 152–4.

16. Meyer F, Marusch F, Coch A, Kockerling F *et al.*, and the German Study Group 'Colorectal Carcinoma (Primary Tumor)'. (2004) Emergency operation in carcinomas of the left colon: value of Hartmann's procedure. *Tech Coloproctol* **8**: S226–9.

17. Zorcolo L, Covotta L, Carlomagno N, Bartolo DC. (2003) Safety of primary anastomosis in emergency colo-rectal surgery. *Colorectal Dis* **5**: 262–9.

18. Villar JM, Martinez AP, Villegas MT, *et al.* Surgical options for malignant left-sided colonic obstruction. *Surg Today* **35**: 275–81.

19. Biondo S, Pares D, Frago R, *et al.* (2004) Large bowel obstruction: predictive factors for postoperative mortality. *Dis Colon Rectum* **47**: 1889–97.

20. Lim JF, Tang CL, Seow-Choen F, Heah SM. (2005) Prospective, randomized trial comparing intraoperative colonic irrigation with manual decompression only for obstructed left-sided colorectal cancer. *Dis Colon Rectum* **48**: 205–9.

Chapter 12

Surgical Management of Acute Cholecystitis

Davide Lomanto* and Iyer Shridhar Ganpathi**

- Acute cholecystitis accounts for 3–9% of hospital admissions for acute abdominal pain.[1,2]
- The majority of patients with upper abdominal complaints are subsequently found to have a relatively benign cause of pain or non-specific abdominal pains,[2] but the possibility of acute cholecystitis must be ruled out with a comprehensive diagnostic evaluation.
- Laparoscopic cholecystectomy is now advocated by clinicians based on lower complication rates, reduced costs, and shortened hospital stay.

Definition

Cholecystitis is a syndrome encompassing a continuum of clinicopathologic states; at one end of the spectrum with acute attacks of pain that resolve, at the other end an obtunded patient presenting with septic shock. Typically, cholecystitis means upper abdominal pain accompanied by fever, Murphy's sign or abdominal tenderness in right upper quadrant and laboratory markers of inflammation.

One of the proposed standardised definitions for acute cholecystitis is the presence of[3]:

a) **Local signs of inflammation**

- Murphy's sign
- RUQ pain/tenderness

b) **Systemic signs of inflammation, etc.**

- Fever
- Elevated WBC Count

c) **Imaging findings**

- Double-ring sign on ultrasound
- Pericholecystic fluid
- Thickened gallbladder wall

Risk Factors for Difficult Laparoscopic Cholecystectomy in Acute Cholecystitis

a) **Acute acalculous cholecystitis:** Gallbladder inflammation without gallstones (i.e. acalculous cholecystitis) typically occurs in critically ill patients and is consequently associated with a high mortality rate.[4] In such patients, percutaneous transhepatic cholecystostomy should be considered, and if patient improves, subsequent laparoscopic cholecystectomy should be performed. Acalculous cholecystitis may occasionally occur in a non-ICU setting, and these patients should be treated just as for any patient with cholecystitis with early laparoscopic cholecystectomy if feasible.[5]

b) **Recurrent acute cholecystitis.** One of the most significant factors and independent predictors of

D. Lamanto, MD, Phd, FAMS (Surg), *Department of Surgery, National University of Singapore and Khoo Teck Puat Advanced Surgery Training Centre, National University Hospital, Singapore.
**Division of Hepatobiliary and Pancreatic Surgery, National University Hospital, Singapore.

conversion is the presence of or a previous attack of acute cholecystitis.[6] Previous repeated attacks of inflammation cause repeated healing by fibrosis leading to obliteration of dissection planes.

c) **Timing of cholecystectomy** has been a subject of considerable debate. Several studies report increased risk of conversion with increasing delay from time of admission to surgery, while there are other studies which fail to show timing as a factor.[7] This may be due to variable progression of inflammation, adhesion formation, severity of acute cholecystitis, and the immune responses. It may be too simplistic to attribute the conversion risk to delay in timing of surgery.

d) **Previous abdominal surgery** could lead to an increase in conversion rates.[8] Surgery of the stomach and duodenum may make laparoscopic biliary surgery more difficult, particularly with dense adhesion in the triangle of Calot. The patient should be advised on increased risk of conversion.

e) **Liver cirrhosis and portal hypertension.** The elevated portal venous pressure and extensive collateral portosystemic shunts may cause troublesome bleeding. Although technically difficult, laparoscopy has become the preferred method of treatment in recent years.[9] It is feasible in most child's A and B patients with an acceptable conversion rate. Some modification of technique and subtotal cholecystectomy are required. Dealing with inflamed gallbladders in cirrhotic patients also poses higher risks for conversion and intraoperative bleeding.

f) **Thickened gallbladder wall** seems to contribute to conversion to open surgery in acute cholecystitis.[10] Thickened gallbladder makes grasping by laparoscopic instrumentation and manipulation of gallbladder difficult.

Preoperative preparation

a) **Routine measures**
  - A thorough review of patient with history, clinical examination, investigations, liver function tests, and ultrasound/CT scan of abdomen must be done.

  - Prior to surgery, dehydration or electrolyte imbalance must be corrected by intravenous fluid administration, and broad-spectrum antibiotic treatment (e.g. second-generation cephalosporin and metronidazole) is given.
  - A naso-gastric tube should be placed prior to the surgery to decompress the stomach and to optimise exposure.

b) **Special measures**
  - Ultrasound scan pictures may be useful in pre-operative planning. If the gallbladder wall is thicker than 5 mm, a different set of instrumentation may be required, such as toothed grasper, needle aspiration, endoloop, etc.

Surgical Treatment

Laparoscopic approach

a) **Standard procedure**
  - LC is performed under **general anaesthesia** with endotracheal intubation.
  - The **surgeon** stands on the left side of the patient with the video-monitor positioned at the patient's upper right side (Fig. 12.1), so that if any conversion is required, patients don't require repositioning.

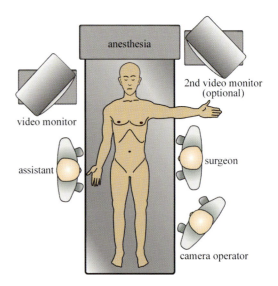

Figure 12.1.

Patient positioning.

- A high-definition **telescope** angled at 30° to 45° camera is used.
- To create the **pneumoperitoneum**, different techniques can be utilised such as Veress needle, open insertion of Hasson's trocar or optical trocar. Special precaution must be exercised in obese patients. Three further 5 mm trocars are inserted under direct vision: 1st, subcostally in the epigatrium; 2nd, the subcostal midaxillary line; and 3rd, four finger-breadths from the costal margin on the right anterior axillary line.
- A diagnostic laparoscopy must be performed. The patient is tilted in an anti-Trendelenburg (20–25°) position and turned to the left side as needed to optimise exposure. Adhesions between the gallbladder, liver, duodenum and the omentum are divided by blunt dissection or with scissors.
- **Dense adhesions** are dissected with a hook electrode taking precaution to avoid diathermy injury by transmitted heat. An alternative or the latest energy device (Ligasure, harmonic scalpel, thunderbeat, etc.) can be useful. Once the adhesions are peeled off, we can determine the grade of inflammation to choose the better surgical strategy.
- If it is **difficult for the surgeon to hold the gallbladder**, a decompression is indicated. Decompression can be established with either an aspiration needle or with a small opening in the fundus to suction out the thick pus and the stones (Fig. 12.2). After decompression, the surgeon can seal the puncture site by grasping the empty gallbladder opening with toothed graspers. The gallbladder is pulled cephaled and laterally, in order to put under tension the Calot's triangle and its structures (i.e. cystic duct, cystic artery, inferior border of the liver and CBD). If there is any adhesion to the liver, they are released to avoid tearing the liver capsule. Tension on the gallbladder must be "elastic" to avoid changing the "natural course" of the CBD.
- **Dissection** of the peritoneal layer starts near the Hartmann's pouch of the gallbladder and

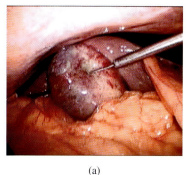

(a)

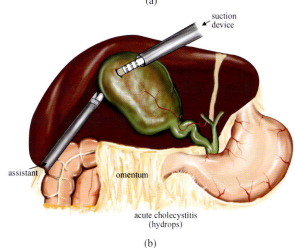

(b)

Figure 12.2.

Aspiration of gallbladder.

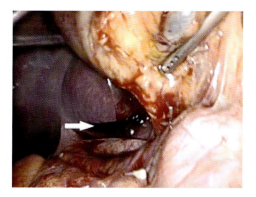

Figure 12.3.

Rouviere's sulcus, which marks the lower limit of dissection (solid arrow).

proceeds upwards to the liver. The dissection is kept above the level of the Rouviere's sulcus if it can be identified (Fig. 12.3). The Rouviere's sulcus is sometimes not clear due to adhesions and obliteration. The dissection is continued close to the gallbladder wall by blunt dissection or using the hook dissector. After identifying the transition of the gallbladder into the cystic duct at the area of the lymph node of Lundh/Mascagni (landmark transition mascagni gallbladder/cystic duct), the surgeon retracts the gallbladder in a slightly ventral position and exposes the cystic duct, using mainly blunt dissection. Calot's triangle is now completely exposed by blunt dissection. No structure presumed to be ductal or vascular should be divided until all the anatomical features have been identified and the triangle of safety is clearly demonstrated (Fig. 12.4).

- If any **cystic duct stones** are present, a clip is applied to the cystic duct at the neck of the gallbladder. Then, the cystic duct is incised proximal to the clip, with scissors, and then "milked" towards the gallbladder with a traumatic forceps.
- If there is any doubt regarding the anatomy, an **intraoperative cholangiogram (IOC) is performed**. The 4fr catheter is inserted through the midclavicular port via the cholangiography clamp and the cystic duct cannulated. Absence of leak from site of cannulation is confirmed with injection of saline initially. Subsequently, the contrast is gently injected and monitored with fluoroscopy. The patient

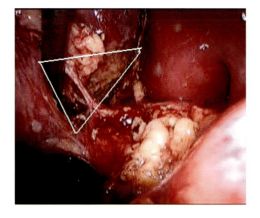

Figure 12.4.

Demonstration of "triangle of safety".

is then tilted in a Trendelenburg position and further contrast dye is injected to visualise the intrahepatic bile ducts. Care must be taken not to inject any air bubbles, which can mimic CBD stones. After IOC has been completed, the cystic duct is routinely sealed and divided using two clips. The cystic artery is then clipped and divided.

- **If there is difficulty in identifying the structures in the Calot's triangle to the extent that even a cholangiogram cannot be performed, a retrograde cholecystectomy** or fundus-first cholecystectomy may be performed. The dissection between the gallbladder and liver bed is performed using monopolar cautery hook and/or hydrodissection. A careful dissection in the right plane is important to avoid gallbladder perforation or severe bleeding from the liver parenchyma. Care must be taken to avoid getting a bleed from the terminal portion of the middle hepatic vein. Bleeding from the gallbladder bed should be controlled immediately with diathermy in spray fulgurate mode, irrigation and suction devices. However if difficulty is encountered, it is advisable to apply pressure by pressing the gallbladder against the liver bed. It gives time for surgeon to take stock of situation, the anaesthetist to prepare for blood loss, the nursing staff to arrange for additional instrumentation and to prepare to open if necessary. Another important aspect of performing a fundus-first cholecystectomy is to avoid carrying the dissection inadvertently above the cystic plate and then above the hilar plate. This may lead to damage to right hepatic artery and right hepatic duct. Keeping close to gallbladder at all times helps in avoiding complications. Once the cholecystectomy is completed, the gallbladder is extracted using an endobag. The abdomen is carefully inspected and irrigated thoroughly with saline (2–3 L). The operating field is checked for bleeding or bile leaks from the liver bed or the cystic stump.

- **Drainage** of gallbladder bed is not routinely performed. However, if it is used, a closed suction drain is preferred for 24–48 hr.

- Next, the **trocar sleeves are removed** under direct vision to detect abdominal wall bleeding and, if necessary, to perform haemostasis by diathermy or transfascial sutures. The fascia at the 10 mm port site is closed with a resorbable suture while the other incisions require only skin closure.

b) **Tricks and tips in challenging cases**

1. In case of **difficulty in exposure despite a steep Trendelenburg position**, a fan blade retractor may be used to push the colon and duodenum down.

2. In rare occasions if the **Calot's anatomy is not clear**, a subtotal cholecystectomy can be performed by leaving the posterior wall of the gallbladder intact. The cystic duct, if accessible, is controlled by intra-corporeal suturing or with endo-loop. If subtotal cholecystectomy is performed, consider closed suction drainage of Morrison's pouch.

3. Often, acute cholecystitis is due to **occlusion of the cystic duct, and** performing an IOC can be difficult. The cystic duct is "milked" with a blunt grasper and then attempts can be made to introduce the catheter. In difficult circumstances, an intraoperative ultrasound can be used to identify the common bile duct and the anatomy or an IOC can be performed by puncturing the bile duct under vision using a spinal needle.

4. Grasping a **thick-walled gallbladder** may require additional toothed forceps or 10 mm trocar to introduce a "crocodile" grasper to hold and manipulate the gallbladder.

5. **"Hydrodissection"** either with a water jet dissector or simply with a suction irrigation cannula is an extremely useful maneuver that can be used in acutely inflamed gallbladder (Fig. 12.5). The water helps separate out natural planes allowing further dissection.

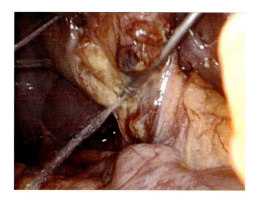

Figure 12.5.

Hydrodissection with suction-irrigation cannula.

Furthermore the blood and blood clots can be constantly washed away for clearer vision. This is very useful in the early stage of the inflammation before fibrosis sets in.

6. In the case of thick or **scarred cystic duct**, the occlusion by titanium clips might be difficult. As an alternative option, larger clips such as 10 mm clips (through the umbilical port and a 5 mm camera through the epigastric port), Röder loops or an endo-GIA can be used (all these devices can only be used when anatomy is clearly identified with performance of IOC if necessary).

7. **Bleeding from deeper vessels in liver bed**, in most cases, is managed with a laparoscopic argon-beam coagulator, higher powered monopolar ball-tipped diathermy. As a final alternative, an attempt to control liver-bed bleeding can be made by the laparoscopic suturing.

8. In **cirrhotic liver** with many collaterals along the liver bed, the ultrasonic dissectors may be used to dissect the gallbladder off the liver bed, and eventually hemostasis can be secured after cholecystectomy and lavage with the use of fibrin glue sealant.

c) **Contraindications: When to convert to open procedure**

Conversion to open surgery is at times perceived as a "failure" of the laparoscopic procedure, and surgeon's enthusiasm to keep the conversion rate low may lead to unwanted biliary tract injuries and complications.

Conversion is appropriate when there is uncertainty about the patient's anatomy, identification of the Calot's triangle and the triangle of safety, or if concerns of injury exists. There is no clear-cut guideline as to the extent to which a surgeon should struggle to complete the procedure laparoscopically and when to convert to open procedure. When operating on a high-risk patient, the surgeon has to make an early decision to convert if dissection seems to be very difficult; early conversion shortens the operation time and decreases morbidity.[11] A policy of converting if there is no progress in dissection of Calot's triangle within 15–30 min may be adopted for high-risk patients. In low-risk patients, in general, if no progress is made in identifying the biliary anatomy within an hour, the procedure is converted to open, and if the structures are seen and the feasibility of dissection is there, the procedure is continued.

Conversions can be decreased if

- The cholecystectomies are performed early after admission.
- Surgical instrumentation is modified (grasping instruments, hydro-dissection, fan blade retractors).
- Use of IOCs is liberal.
- Performed by dedicated surgical units.

d) **Management of unexpected pathology**

Preoperatively undiagnosed common bile duct stones (CBDS) are found in only 2.3–3.5% intraoperatively.[12] The optimal management of CBD stones in the laparoscopic area is controversial. The major treatment options are intraoperative laparoscopic bile duct exploration (trans-cystic or choledochotomy) and intraoperative or post-operative ERCP. Duct clearance and morbidity and mortality rates for these three procedures are similar, except that laparoscopic CBD exploration results in a significantly shorter hospital stay. Intraoperatively identified CBDS can initially be treated laparoscopically by the transcystic or transcholedochal approach, if possible. If this procedure fails, intraoperative or postoperative

endoscopic retrograde cholangio-pancreatography (ERCP) are alternative options. If intraoperatively a biliary stent can be placed and post-operative ERCP can be delayed. Large stones, amenable neither to the trans-cystic approach nor to ERCP, might be treated by open bile duct exploration. Always keep a watch for the "Moynihan's Hump", or the right hepatic artery cruising close to the gallbladder, which may be occasionally mistaken for the cystic artery.

e) **Postoperative care**

- **Standard care**

  o Post-operatively antibiotics may be continued as clinically indicated.

  o Feeding may be resumed in the early post-operative period as tolerated.

  o Analgesics and intravenous fluids administered post-operatively as necessary.

  o Drains if placed are removed in 1–2 days post-operatively.

- **Special care for complicated case**

  CBD injuries during LC remain the most serious complication encountered with this procedure. At present it is accepted that the incidence of CBD injuries during LC is only approximately double the rate for OC, reaching 0.4–0.7%, as reported in larger trials.[12] Strict adherence to the principles of surgical dissection is obviously of utmost importance for the prevention of CBD injuries. Whether the routine use of IOC decreases the incidence of CBD injuries remains controversial. If the anatomical features are unclear during surgical dissection, IOC must be performed to give a surgical "road map". CBD injury must be suspected in the presence of contrast material extravasation or lack of opacification of the right posterior intrahepatic bile duct. Hospital mortality rates, post-operative biliary complications and re-interventions can be reduced in patients with early intraoperative CBD injury detection during IOC.[13]

- **Management of complications**

  Bile leak: Bile leaks may be detected through drains if placed or clinically if a scan is performed which may show a biloma. Principles of management of bile leaks include: adequate resuscitation, drainage of collections, antibiotics based on cultures, and early ERCP and stenting of bile duct. This may suffice for treatment of minor bile leaks from gallbladder bed, from minor sectoral ducts or cystic duct. However if bile duct injury is suspected then immediate surgical repair by specialist hepatobiliary surgeon is mandated. Post-operative peritonism and sepsis should raise suspicion of subphenic abscesses, collections and bile leaks. Early imaging and radiological drainage along with ERCP is indicated.

References

1. Powers RD, Guertler AT. (1995) Abdominal pain in the ED. *Am J Emerg Med* **13**: 301–303.
2. Irvin TT. (1989) Abdominal pain. *Br J Surg* **76**: 121–1125.
3. Kimura Y, Takada T, Kawarada Y, *et al.* (2007) Definitions, pathophysiology, and epidemiology of acute cholangitis and cholecystitis: Tokyo Guidelines. *J Hepatobiliary Pancreat Surg* **14(1)**: 15–26.
4. Cornwall EA, Rodriguez A, Mirvis SE, Shorr RM. (1989) Acute acalculous cholecystitis in critically injured patients. *Ann Surg* **210**: 52–55.
5. Shridhar Ganpathi I, Diddapur RK, Eugene H, Karim M. (2007) Acute acalculous cholecystitis: challenging the myths. *HPB (Oxford)* **9(2)**: 131–34.
6. Alponat A, Kum CK, Koh BC, *et al.* (1997) Predictive factors for conversion of laparoscopy cholecystectomy. *World J Surg* **21**: 629–33.
7. Soffer D, Blackbourne LH, Schulman CI, *et al.* (2007) Is there an optimal time for laparoscopic cholecystectomy in acute cholecystitis? *Surg Endosc* **21**: 805–09.
8. Schrenk P, Woisetschläger R, Wayand W. (1995) Laparoscopic Cholecystectomy — Cause of conversion in 1,300 patients and analysis of risk factors. *Surg Endosc* **9**: 25–28.
9. Yeh CN, Chen MF, Jan YY. (2002) Laparoscopic Cholecystectomy in 226 cirrhotic patients. Experience of a single center in Taiwan. *Surg Endosc* **16(11)**: 1583–87.
10. Low SW, Iyer SG, Chang SK, *et al.* (2009) Laparoscopic cholecystectomy for acute cholecystitis: safe implementation of successful strategies to reduce conversion rates. *Surg Endosc* **23(11)**: 2424–29.
11. Lo CM, Fan ST, Li CL, *et al.* (1997) Early decision for conversion of laparoscopic to open cholecystectomy for treatment of acute Cholecystitis. *Am J Surg* **173**: 513–17.
12. Z'graggen K, Wehrli H, Metzger A, *et al.* (1998) Complications of laparoscopic cholecystectomy in Switzerland. A prospective 3-year study of 10,174 patients. Swiss Association of Laparoscopic and Thoracoscopic Surgery. *Surg Endosc* **12**: 1303–10.
13. Gigot J, Etienne J, Aerts R, *et al.* (1997) The dramatic reality of biliary tract injury during laparoscopic cholecystectomy. An anonymous multicenter Belgian survey of 65 patients. *Surg Endosc* **11**: 1171–78.

Chapter 13

ERCP in the Management of Cholangitis and Bile Duct Injuries

Lim Lee Guan* and Ho Khek Yu**

Biliary obstruction presenting with symptoms of cholangitis can occur as a result of choledocholithiasis, malignancy, or injury to the bile duct. Sepsis from biliary obstruction is life threatening. ERCP plays a central role in the diagnosis of biliary pathology, immediate relief of obstruction and helps healing of bile duct injuries.

Pre-ERCP Preparation

The management of sepsis should include sending blood for culture and sensitivity, administration of broad-spectrum antibiotics, correction of circulatory volume and ensuring adequate urine output. Associated coagulopathy would also require correction before performance of ERCP.

ERCP for Choledocholithiasis

EUS is more accurate than transabdominal US for detecting choledocholithiasis. Radial array echoendoscopes are preferred by many endosonographers for biliary imaging because elongated views of the bile

duct can be obtained easily. The CBD stone appears as a hyperechoic proximal edge with distal shadowing (Fig. 13.1).

Guidelines recommend that ERCP be reserved for patients in whom therapeutic intervention will most likely be needed. ERCP is not recommended for use

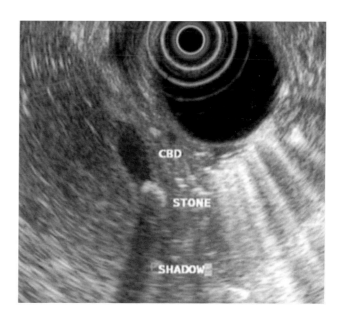

Figure 13.1.

EUS image of stone in the common bile duct.

*L.G. Lim, MBBS, MRCP(UK), Consultant, Department of Gastroenterology & Hepatology, National University Health System, Singapore.
**K.Y. Ho MBBS, MD, FRACP, FAMS, FRCP (Glasgow), Head, Department of Medicine, Department of Gastroenterology & Hepatology and Endoscopic Centre, National University Health System, Singapore.

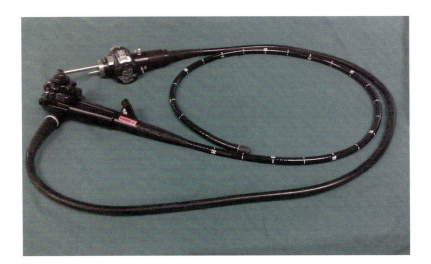

Figure 13.2.

Duodenoscope.

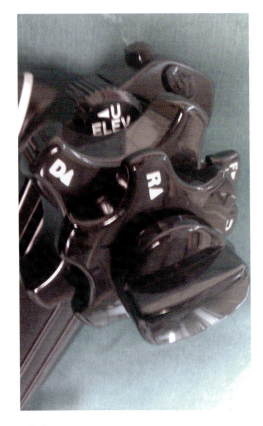

Figure 13.3.

Elevator lever on the duodenoscope.

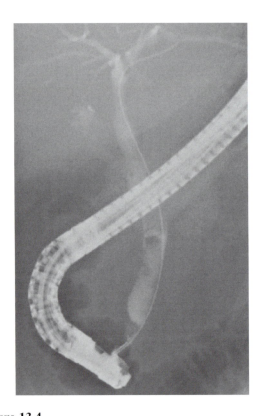

Figure 13.4.

Cholangiogram showing filling defect in the common bile duct.

solely as a diagnostic test in patients with suspected CBD stone.[1,2]

ERCP involves inserting a duodenoscope (Figs. 13.2 and 13.3) perorally till the ampulla. Following cannulation of the ampulla, radio-opaque contrast medium is injected into the CBD to obtain a cholangiogram.

The presence of CBD stone, as evidenced by a filling defect on cholangiography (Fig. 13.4), necessitates stone removal. Enlargement of the biliary sphincter is most commonly performed with electrocautery sphincterotomy, after which 90% of CBD stones can be retrieved by a basket or balloon catheter. Although balloon sphincteroplasty is associated with lower rates of bleeding compared to sphincterotomy, balloon sphincteroplasty is less commonly used in routine clinical practice because it is associated with increased short-term morbidity rates and death due to pancreatitis compared to sphincterotomy.

Large CBD stones need to be broken into smaller fragments before extraction, using either intracorporeal or extracorporeal lithotripsy. Intracorporeal means include mechanical lithotripsy, electrohydraulic lithotripsy and laser lithotripsy. Mechanical lithotripsy is performed by entrapping the stone in a strong wire basket and breaking the stone into several pieces as the basket filaments cut through the stone (Fig. 13.5).

Electrohydraulic lithotripsy[3] involves the use of a probe which is connected to an electrohydraulic shockwave generator. Charges transmitted across the electrodes at the tip of the probe create sparks that result in expansion of the surrounding fluid which creates oscillating spherical shock waves that fragment the stone. The procedure is usually performed under direct choledochoscopic guidance so that the probe can be aimed directly at the stone. This decreases ductal trauma and perforation risk. A new solid-state laser lithotripter, the frequency-doubled double-pulse neodymium YAG laser ("FREDDY") system,[3,4] is less likely than electrohydraulic lithotripsy to cause mucosal damage because of its stone/tissue discrimination system. Extracorporeal shock wave lithotripsy (ESWL) generates a shock wave originating outside the body using piezoelectric crystals, underwater spark gap (electrohydraulic), or electromagnetic membrane technologies.

In a feasibility study, the newly developed single operator peroral cholangioscope, the SpyGlass Direct Visualization System (Boston Scientific, Natick, Mass), is performed successfully and safely in the vast majority of patients. In patients with biliary stones, complete stone clearance was achieved in 92.3%.[5] Direct peroral cholangioscopy using an ultra-slim upper endoscope GIF-XP260N and GIF-N260 (Olympus, Tokyo, Japan) by a single endoscopist yielded an overall success rate of 89% for bile duct clearance by lithotripsy.[6] A retrospective study of a prospectively maintained database of 3475 ERCPs and 402 ERCPs with cholangioscopy using either conventional cholangioscope (Olympus) or catheter-based cholangioscope (SpyGlass Direct Visualization System) reported complications in 7.0% in the ERCP with cholangioscopy group and 2.9% in the ERCP-only group (odds ratio [OR], 2.50; 95% CI, 1.56–3.89). There was a significantly higher rate of cholangitis in the cholangioscopy group vs. ERCP group (1.0% vs. 0.2%; OR, 4.98; 95% CI, 1.06–19.67) but identical rates of pancreatitis (2.2% vs. 1.3%; OR, 1.75; 95% CI, 0.74–3.65) and perforation (1.0% vs. 0.3%; OR, 3.16; 95% CI, 0.73–10.75).[7]

Biliary stent placement for choledocholithiasis may be performed as a temporising measure for CBD stones which are hard to remove, or in frail and or old patients who may not tolerate prolonged attempts at stone removal (Fig. 13.6).

ERCP in Malignancy Involving the Biliary Tract

ERCP allows the localisation of bile duct strictures. The presence of asymmetric, irregular strictures suggests malignancy. However, cholangiography alone cannot be relied upon to differentiate between malignant and benign lesions. During ERCP, tissue sampling can be done with brush cytology and tissue biopsies. A study comparing these two modalities

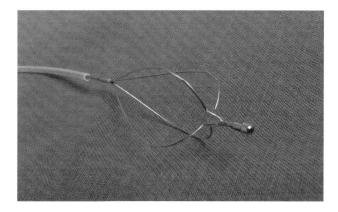

Figure 13.5.

Dormia basket.

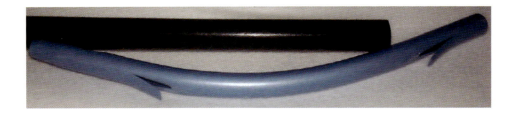

Figure 13.6.

Biliary stent.

showed diagnostic yield for malignancy of 41% by brush cytology, 53% by forceps biopsy, and 60% by the combination of both techniques.[8] Cholangioscopy is a useful diagnostic tool for biliary lesions.[9] Probe-based confocal laser endomicroscopy has also been reported to aid in the diagnosis of biliary malignancy.[10,11] Intraductal ultrasound can aid in the local staging of cholangiocarcinoma. EUS-fine needle aspiration may also be used to obtain a diagnosis, although the diagnostic accuracy varies in different studies.

In a meta-analysis of 21 trials involving 1,454 patients undergoing palliative biliary stenting for obstructing pancreatic carcinoma, endoscopic stenting with plastic stents had a reduced risk of complications, but higher risk of recurrent biliary obstruction prior to death when compared with surgery. There was no difference in technical or therapeutic success. Metal biliary stents were associated with lower risk of recurrent biliary obstruction than plastic stents. One single eligible trial which studied types of metal stents reported higher patency with covered stents, but at higher risk of complications. It appears that endoscopic metal stents are the intervention of choice in patients with malignant distal biliary obstruction due to pancreatic carcinoma. In patients with short predicted survival, their patency benefits over plastic stents may not be evident.[12]

A study which compared self-expandable metal stents made from nitinol versus conventional stainless steel stents for malignant biliary strictures showed similar outcomes regarding efficacy, duration of stent patency, occlusion rates, and complications between the two types of stents. The role of pre-surgical biliary stenting prior to pancreaticoduodenectomy for patients with malignant pancreatico-biliary stricture is less clear. In a Cochrane review of two randomised trials involving 125 patients undergoing pancreaticoduodenectomy, 62 patients underwent ERCP with biliary stenting and 63 had ERCP without biliary stenting prior to surgery. Stenting had no significant effect on the pre-surgical and post-surgical mortality. Overall mortality and complications were similar in the two groups.[13]

When biliary drainage by ERCP is unsuccessful, EUS-guided biliary drainage may be attempted. This can be achieved by the rendezvous technique, EUS-guided choledochoduodenostomy, or EUS-guided hepaticogastrostomy. The EUS-rendezvous technique involves puncturing the obstructed bile duct under EUS guidance and passing a guide wire antegradely through the papilla to aid subsequent ERCP.[14] In EUS-guided choledochoduodenostomy, puncturing the bile duct under EUS guidance is followed by stenting through the choledochoduodenostomy site into the extrahepatic bile duct.[15] EUS-guided hepaticogastrostomy involves puncturing a dilated peripheral branch of the left intra-hepatic system via the transgastric route and stenting via the hepaticogastrostomy site into intrahepatic bile ducts.

ERCP in Bile Duct Injuries

Most bile duct injuries are not recognised intraoperatively. The gold standard for evaluating bile duct injuries is cholangiography, which includes ERCP, percutaneous transhepatic cholangiography and magnetic resonance cholangiopancreatography. ERCP allows the exact location of the bile leak to be determined and treated simultaneously. Endoscopic biliary stenting creates a path of least resistance which allows the biliary flow away from the site of the leak and bridges the defect, consequently allowing time for healing as well as preventing stricture formation.[16] In a multi-centre study of patients with CBD post-cholecystectomy stricture treated with stenting for a median of 12 months and a mean follow-up of six years, the overall success rate was 67% after one period of stenting and 82% after additional treatments.[17] In patients with biliary fistulas after complex liver resection, fistulas dried up completely in 96.1% of patients after ERCP therapy.[18] In a French multi-centre study, patients with anastomotic biliary strictures after liver transplantation had partially covered self-expandable metal stents placed across the stricture for two months and then removed. Stents were placed and removed successfully in all patients. Short-term stricture resolution was seen in 86%, and sustained stricture resolution was achieved in 46%.[19] In a study of patients who had multiple endoscopic stenting of post-operative biliary strictures, 11% of patients had postoperative biliary stricture recurrence which was retreated endoscopically with placement of stents, and 9% had CBD stones which were extracted. There was no stricture or CBD stone recurrence post-retreatment after a further mean follow-up of seven years.[20]

Difficult Biliary Cannulation

Various methods have been described to aid in difficult biliary cannulation. Selective biliary cannulation using pancreatic guide-wire placement has been described.[21] A guide wire is inserted into the pancreatic duct and is left *in situ* after withdrawal of the catheter. A second catheter is then advanced via the same endoscope channel.

While pushing the pancreatic duct with the guidewire, biliary cannulation is attempted in the 11 o'clock direction. In the initial pilot trial,[19] this method yielded a significantly higher success rate compared with the conventional method (93% vs. 58%), with no pancreatitis occurring in either group. However, a recent multi-centre randomised trial showed that biliary cannulation using pancreatic guide-wire placement was not superior to the standard technique, and it was associated with a higher incidence of post-ERCP pancreatitis (17% vs. 8%).[22]

Another reported technique is physician-controlled wire-guided cannulation over a pancreatic duct stent,[23] in which pancreatic duct cannulation is followed by insertion of a guide wire to the level of the mid-pancreatic body to allow placement of a soft polyethylene stent. When the stent is in its desired position, the wire is pulled back into the sphincterotome and attempts at biliary cannulation resume. Physician-controlled wire-guided cannulation of the bile duct is then attempted over the pancreatic duct stent. This technique facilitates biliary cannulation while maintaining a low rate of pre-cut sphincterotomy.

Needle-knife pre-cut papillotomy may be used if biliary cannulation fails despite a number of attempts with a pancreatic guide wire placement, with or without a stent *in situ*, or as an alternative to the pancreatic guide wire placement if performed by experienced endoscopists. Several pre-cut techniques have been described.[24] Early implementation of precut papillotomy results in similar overall cannulation rate and reduces post-ERCP pancreatitis risk but not the overall complication rate compared to persistent cannulation attempts.[25]

Post-ERCP Care

Complications of ERCP include pancreatitis (1–7%), cholangitis (0.5–1.1%), bleeding (0.6–4%) and perforation (0.3–0.6%). In order to minimise the infective complications of ERCP, antibiotics are recommended for patients with ongoing cholangitis or sepsis elsewhere (patients should already have been established on antibiotics) and in biliary obstruction. Current evidence shows that pancreatic stent placement decreases the risk of post-ERCP pancreatitis and hyperamylasemia in high-risk patients.

References

1. ASGE Standards of Practice Committee, Maple JT, Ben-Menachem T, Anderson MA, *et al.* (2010) The role of endoscopy in the evaluation of suspected choledocholithiasis. *Gastrointest Endosc* **71(1)**: 1–9.

2. Arya N, Nelles SE, Haber GB, *et al.* (2004) Electrohydraulic lithotripsy in 111 patients: a safe and effective therapy for difficult bile duct stones. *Am J Gastroenterol* **99**: 2330–34.

3. Maiss J, Tex S, Bayer J, *et al.* (2001) First clinical data on laser lithotripsy of common bile duct stones with a new frequency-doubled double-pulse Nd:YAG laser (FREDDY) in 22 patients. *Endoscopy* **33**: AB2726.

4. Cho YD, Cheon YK, Moon JH, *et al.* (2009) Clinical role of frequency-doubled double-pulsed yttrium aluminum garnet laser technology for removing difficult bile duct stones (with videos). *Gastrointest Endosc* **70**: 684–89.

5. Draganov PV, Lin T, Chauhan S, *et al.* (2011) Prospective evaluation of the clinical utility of ERCP-guided cholangio-pancreatoscopy with a new direct visualization system. *Gastrointest Endosc* **73(5)**: 971–79.

6. Moon JH, Ko BM, Choi HJ, *et al.* (2009) Direct peroral cholangioscopy using an ultra-slim upper endoscope for the treatment of retained bile duct stones. *Am J Gastroenterol* **104(11)**: 2729–33.

7. Sethi A, Chen YK, Austin GL, *et al.* (2011) ERCP with cholangiopancreatoscopy may be associated with higher rates of complications than ERCP alone: a single-center experience. *Gastrointest Endosc* **73(2)**: 251–56.

8. Garrow D, Miller S, Sinha D, *et al.* (2007) Endoscopic ultrasound: a metaanalysis of test performance in suspected biliary obstruction. *Clin Gastroenterol Hepatol* **5**: 616–23.

9. Itoi T, Osanai M, Igarashi Y, *et al.* (2010) Diagnostic peroral video cholangioscopy is an accurate diagnostic tool for patients with bile duct lesions. *Clin Gastroenterol Hepatol* **8(11)**: 934–38.

10. Giovannini M, Bories E, Monges G, *et al.* (2011) Results of a phase I-II study on intraductal confocal microscopy (IDCM) in patients with common bile duct (CBD) stenosis. *Surg Endosc* **2011 Mar 18**. [Epub ahead of print].

11. Lim LG, von Delius S, Meining A. (2011) Cholangioscopy and probe-based confocal laser endomicroscopy in the diagnosis of an unusual liver cyst. *Gastroenterology* **141(4)**: e5–6.

12. Moss AC, Morris E, Mac Mathuna P. (2006) Palliative biliary stents for obstructing pancreatic carcinoma. *Cochrane Database Syst Rev* **2006 Apr 19;(2)**: CD004200.

13. Mumtaz K, Hamid S, Jafri W. (2007) Endoscopic retrograde cholangiopancreaticography with or without stenting in patients with pancreaticobiliary malignancy, prior to surgery. *Cochrane Database Syst Rev* **2007 Jul 18;(3)**: CD006001.

14. Kim YS, Gupta K, Mallery S, *et al.* (2010) Endoscopic ultrasound rendezvous for bile duct access using a transduodenal approach: cumulative experience at a single center. A case series. *Endoscopy* **42**: 496–502.

15. Giovannini M, Moutardier V, Pesenti C, *et al.* (2001) Endoscopic ultrasound-guided bilioduodenal anastomosis: a new technique for biliary drainage. *Endoscopy* **33**: 898–900.

16. Weber A, Feussner H, Winkelmann F, *et al.* (2009) Long-term outcome of endoscopic therapy in patients with bile duct injury after cholecystectomy. *J Gastroenterol Hepatol* **24(5)**: 762–69.

17. Tuvignon N, Liguory C, Ponchon T, *et al.* (2011) Long-term follow-up after biliary stent placement for postcholecystectomy bile duct strictures: a multicenter study. *Endoscopy* **43(3)**: 208–16.

18. Farhat S, Bourrier A, Gaudric M, *et al.* (2011) Endoscopic treatment of biliary fistulas after complex liver resection. *Ann Surg* **253(1)**: 88–93.

19. Chaput U, Scatton O, Bichard P, *et al.* (2010) Temporary placement of partially covered self-expandable metal stents for anastomotic biliary strictures after liver transplantation: a prospective, multicenter study. *Gastrointest Endosc* **72(6)**: 1167–74.

20. Costamagna G, Tringali A, Mutignani M, *et al.* (2010) Endotherapy of postoperative biliary strictures with multiple stents: results after more than 10 years of follow-up. *Gastrointest Endosc* **72(3)**: 551–57.

21. Maeda S, Hayashi H, Hosokawa O, *et al.* (2003) Prospective randomized pilot trial of selective biliary cannulation using pancreatic guide-wire placement. *Endoscopy* **35**: 721–24.

22. Herreros de Tejada A, Calleja JL, Diaz G, *et al.* (2009) Double-guidewire technique for difficult bile duct cannulation: a multicenter randomized, controlled trial. *Gastrointest Endosc* **70**: 700–09.

23. Coté GA, Ansstas M, Pawa R, *et al.* (2010) Difficult biliary cannulation: use of physician-controlled wire-guided cannulation over a pancreatic duct stent to reduce the rate of precut sphincterotomy (with video). *Gastrointest Endosc* **71(2)**: 275–79.

24. Deng DH, Zuo HM, Wang JF, *et al.* (2007) New precut sphincterotomy for endoscopic retrograde cholangio-pancreatography in difficult biliary cannulation. *World J Gastroenterol* **13**: 4385–90.

25. Cennamo V, Fuccio L, Zagari RM, *et al.* (2010) Can early precut implementation reduce endoscopic retrograde cholangiopancreatography-related complication risk? Meta-analysis of randomized controlled trials. *Endoscopy* **42(5)**: 381–88.

Chapter 14

Surgical Management of Bile Duct & Pancreatic Emergencies

Alfred Kow Wei Chieh* and Krishnakumar Madhavan**

Common surgical emergencies of the bile duct and pancreas include:

A. Acute cholangitis
B. Acute pancreatitis with or without necrosis
C. Bile duct injuries during surgery
D. Pancreatic trauma
E. ERCP perforation

A) Acute Cholangitis

○ Cholangitis is one of the most common causes of severe hepatobiliary sepsis leading to septic shock and multi-organ dysfunction.

Common causes of cholangitis include:

- Choledocholithiasis with Mirizzi's syndrome
- Malignant ductal obstruction
- Benign ductal stricture (secondary to inflammation or post-anastomosis)
- Parasitic infection of biliary tree by liver flukes, ruptured hydatid cysts and ascariasis, and
- Foreign bodies such as a blocked stent

○ Cholangitis typically presents as Charcot's triad (Fever, RHC pain and jaundice).
○ Reynold's pentad describes additional symptoms of hypotension and altered mental status (secondary to septic encephalopathy and poor cerebral perfusion).
○ Investigations:

- FBC — Raised TW suggests infective process. However, the patient can become neutropenic in severe sepsis.
- Renal function — patient may develop pre-renal dysfunction in sepsis due to hypotension and dehydration.
- LFT — Conjugated hyperbilirubinaemia with elevated alkaline phosphatase (ALP) is usually suggestive of cholangitis. However, prolonged and severe biliary obstruction can also lead to moderate transaminitis in certain situations.
- Coagulation profile — Deranged PT, especially with significant biliary obstruction, leads to deficiency of vitamin K-dependent clotting factors.
- Ultrasound HBS — To detect the presence of bile duct dilatation, with or without aerobilia. It is also useful to ascertain the underlying

*Alfred K. W. Chieh, MBBS, MMed (Surg), MRCS (Ed), MRCS (Ire), FRCS Ed (Gen Surg), Consultant, Division of Hepatobillary and Pancreatic Surgery and Liver Transplantation, Department of Surgery, National University Hospital, Singapore.
**K. Madhavan, MBBS, MS (Gen Surg), FRCS (Ed), FRCS (Gen), Head and Senior Consultant, Division of Hepatobiliary & Pancreatic Surgery, Director of Liver Transplant Program, Department of Surgery, National University Hospital, Singapore.

aetiology, e.g. stone vs. non-stone diseases. The presence of concomitant liver abscess in cholangitis can also be seen on US.

- Contrast CT scan — Especially useful to evaluate conditions related to malignancy, such as head of pancreas tumor. It is also useful in studying the relationship of biliary tree with Hartmann's pouch such as that in Mirizzi's syndrome.
- MRCP — Useful only in diagnostic situation when other imaging modalities are inconclusive.
- EUS — Another modality to evaluate the bile duct to look for small CBD stones in selected patients.
- ERCP — Rarely used solely for diagnosis nowadays. However, it is very useful as a therapeutic tool. In fact, one of the most important aspects of initial management of acute cholangitis is decompression of the obstructed biliary tree. ERCP with stenting is an ideal option in many situations.

○ Treatment

- Appropriate resuscitation with IV fluid.
- Initiate appropriate empirical IV antibiotics (after blood culture) to cover for common gram-negative organisms and anaerobes.
- Correct coagulopathy in preparation of possible intervention (coagulopathy secondary to prolonged biliary obstruction or sepsis).
- Early biliary decompression either via ERCP (Figs. 1A and 1B) and stenting or PTC decompression (Fig. 2). Decompression of the infected & obstructed biliary system is one of the most important steps of managing acute cholangitis. Such early decompression is done in the hope of reversing the triggering factors for SIRS and MODS.
- Monitor in high-dependency or ICU if patient shows signs of haemodynamic compromise (with the necessary monitoring devices such as CVP line and IA line).
- Start inotropic support if patient is hypotensive from septic shock.
- Plan for elective surgery to relieve biliary obstruction at later date.

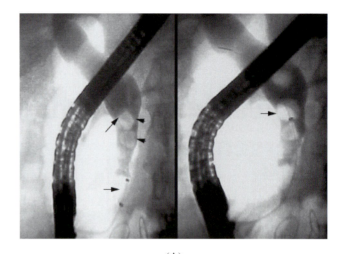

(A)

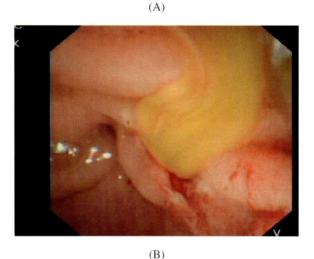

(B)

Figure 1A and 1B.

Common bite duct stone.

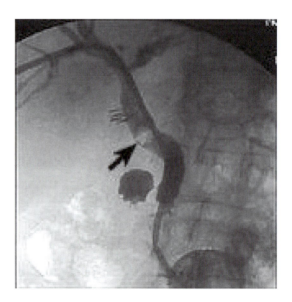

Figure 2.

Stone with bite duct obstruction with stent inserted.

○ Surgery for stone in the common bile duct/common hepatic duct:

- Definitive surgery might be required after successful treatment of acute cholangitis with ERCP/PTC decompression. In the situation of CBD stone(s), repeat ERCP can be performed to try to remove the stones in the bile duct. PTC with rendezvous ERCP can also be performed with the same intent. Failure of removal of stones via ERCP would necessitate exploration of the CBD and removal of stones operatively.
- In cases where the stone(s) in the CBD is too large and endoscopic removal is unlikely to be successful (>1.5cm), surgical removal of the stone(s) might be required.
- Exploration of the bile duct can be performed in various ways:

1. Open/Laparoscopic CBD exploration and T-tube insertion.
2. Open/Laparoscopic CBD exploration with insertion of internal CBD stent and primary closure of the bile duct (using on-table OGD to guide the position of the internal stent in the duodenum, stent inserted using Seldinger technique with guide wire inserted into CBD through ampulla of Vater to the duodenum).
3. Open/Laparoscopic transcystic CBD exploration with primary closure of the cystic duct.
4. Open/Laparoscopic CBD exploration with bilioenteric bypass.

- The steps to perform open CBD exploration and T-tube insertion are shown in Fig. 3.

○ Identification of the CBD is the key for CBD exploration.

- Careful dissection of the hepatoduodenal ligament in inflamed/post-inflammation tissue around the region is important to avoid unnecessary injury to the structures such as hepatic artery and, rarely, the portal vein posterior to the bile duct. It is important to be aware of anatomical anomalies such as displaced or accessory right hepatic artery within the vicinity of the bile duct.
- Needle aspiration of the CBD (using butterfly needle/catheter) may be helpful in certain situations.
- Intra-operative cholangiogram can also provide essential information regarding biliary anatomy, location and number of stones to be removed.

○ Upon identification of the CBD, two stay sutures are placed along the longitudinal axis on the anterior surface of the CBD (Fig. 3A).

○ Choledochotomy is performed using a sharp size 11 blade and extension of the opening using Potts scissors to about 2cm long (if IOC was performed

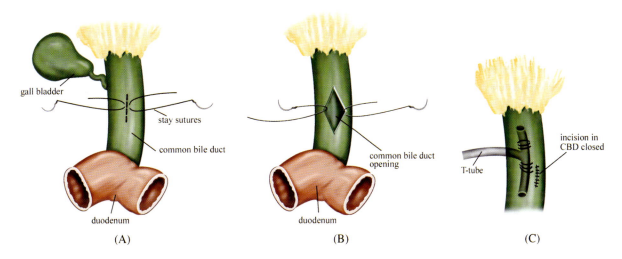

(A)   (B)   (C)

Figure 3.

Exploration of common bile duct.

prior to this, we can inject saline into the catheter that is within the biliary system to further distend the bile duct prior to puncturing it) (Fig. 3B). Usually a gush of biliary content will be seen upon entering the biliary system. Oftentimes, dislodged stones will flow out together with the fluids.

o Exploration of CBD can be performed with stone forceps and flushing with Nelaton's catheter.

o Further exploration can be achieved using choledochoscopy and remnant stones can be removed using Dormia baskets or flushed down into the duodenum.

o T-tube is inserted and choledochotomy closed primarily using 4/0 to 5/0 PDS sutures in an interrupted manner, with care not to narrow the lumen of the CBD excessively (Fig. 3C).

B) Acute Pancreatitis with or without Necrosis

o Acute pancreatitis is commonly encountered in surgical practice. Patients with severe acute pancreatitis (necrotising and/or haemorrhagic) can present to the emergency department, in a variety of presentations.

o The common aetiologies of acute pancreatitis include:

- Gallstones
- Alcohol
- Post-procedure (e.g. ERCP, post-surgery)
- Others (drug-induced, e.g. thiazides; toxin, e.g. snake venom; scorpion bite; hypercalcemia; hypertriglyceridemia; neoplasm, trauma; autoimmune, etc.)

o Clinical presentation of patients with acute pancreatitis includes:

- Epigastric pain with radiation to the back, maybe relieved by leaning forward
- Nausea and vomiting
- Fever (usually when associated with cholangitis)
- In severe episodes, haemodynamic compromise with hypotension, tachycardia or even circulatory collapse may occur.
- Physical signs include Grey-Turner's, Cullen's or Fox's sign.

o The management of patients with acute pancreatitis can be outlined as follows:

- Diagnosing acute pancreatitis
- Assessing severity of pancreatitis
- Looking for aetiology of acute pancreatitis
- Evaluation of need for surgical intervention

o Diagnosis of acute pancreatitis

- Acute pancreatitis can be diagnosed based on clinical presentation that is suggestive with supportive evidence from biochemical markers or imaging studies.
- Raised serum amylase of >3–5 X upper limit of normal (or >1000 U/L) is consistent with acute pancreatitis (bearing in mind other causes of raised serum amylase).
- In the event that serum amylase level is not diagnostic, serum lipase level may be helpful in making the diagnosis (half-life of serum lipase is much longer, and it peaks later compared to serum amylase).
- Other tests include urine diastase (amylase).
- Ultrasound of the abdomen is not efficient at diagnosing acute pancreatitis, but CT scan can confirm the diagnosis — showing oedematous and inflamed pancreas with peripancreatic stranding.

o Looking for aetiology of acute pancreatitis

- The reason for looking for aetiology of acute pancreatitis is to differentiate acute severe gallstone pancreatitis from non-gallstone pancreatitis.
- It has an impact on early intervention using ERCP in acute severe gallstone pancreatitis, especially when concomitant acute cholangitis is present as a result of stones in the CBD.
- The first line of radiological investigation is usually US HBS. Ultrasonic evidence of gallstones or bile sludge in the GB would suggest gallstone pancreatitis. Concomitant dilated biliary tree (especially with raised bilirubin level and ALP) would suggest presence of CBD stone as well. Early ERCP with decompression of obstructed bile duct might help to turn the process of SIRS around

(removing another potential offending agent in the inflammatory pathway, i.e. cholangitis).

○ Assessing severity of pancreatitis

• It is crucial to assess the severity of acute pancreatitis as patients with severe acute pancreatitis might require closer monitoring, haemodynamic support, respiratory support and other organ supports in event of deteriorating MODS. In fact, a small number of patients with mild acute pancreatitis may progress to severe conditions while in the hospital.

• Assessing severity of acute pancreatitis includes:

1. Clinical evaluation — Patients who present at initial stage to ED with hypotension, respiratory distress, tachycardia, discolouration of abdomen suggestive of haemorrhagic pancreatitis usually have severe acute pancreatitis

2. Composite scoring system

a. Many scoring systems have been used in an attempt to differentiate between mild and severe forms of acute pancreatitis.

b. Scoring systems that employ clinical and biochemical markers in the scores include Ranson's score, Imrie score (modified Glasgow), APACHE II scoring etc.

c. Other parameters include CRP level (at 48 hours), pepsinogen-activating enzyme level, etc.

d. The scoring system helps to streamline the right-siting of patients for proper monitoring and treatment of patients with acute severe pancreatitis.

3. Radiological evaluation

a. Balthazar's score — CT severity index based on Balthazar score of combining CT grade score (extent of pancreatic tissue involvement) and necrosis score (based on percentage of pancreatic necrosis).

○ Treatment of acute pancreatitis

• In most situations, acute pancreatitis will resolve spontaneously with appropriate supportive therapy.

• In the event of gallstone pancreatitis, definitive cholecystectomy would be required to reduce risk of future pancreatitis (although bile sludge in the biliary system might still be able to precipitate pancreatitis).

• Early ERCP (within the initial 72 hours) might be necessary in cases of concomitant obstructive jaundice and/or acute cholangitis.

• IV antibiotics in selected cases (especially in severe cases — those with associated cholangitis).

• The role of surgery is limited in acute pancreatitis (other than cholecystectomy for gallstone pancreatitis). However, in selected patients with necrotising pancreatitis (esp. in proven infected necrosis), necrosectomy might be necessary.

• Indications of pancreatic necrosectomy include:

1. Proven infected necrosis of pancreatitis.
2. Especially in event of continuing downward spiral of clinical conditions despite maximal supportive measures.

• There is a trend towards delayed operation to allow better demarcation between viable and nonviable pancreatic tissues. There is also a need for multiple-staged operation to evaluate the area of necrosis in this situation.

• Types of operation for necrosectomy include:

1. Conventional open necrosectomy with or without tube drainage (into the lesser sac) (See Figs. 4A and 4B for access to lesser sac in pancreatic necrosectomy).
2. Conventional open necrosectomy with temporary abdominal closure to facilitate relook laparotomy.
3. Percutaneous drainage and peritoneal lavage.
4. Minimally invasive retroperitoneal pancreatic necrosectomy (MIRP) (See Fig. 5). A nephroscope is used to access the retroperitoneal space on the left to gain access to the pancreas. Piecemeal debridement of necrotic pancreatic tissue can be performed using the nephroscope, drains can be inserted for continuous lavage, and drain tracts can be used for further approach to necrosectomy.

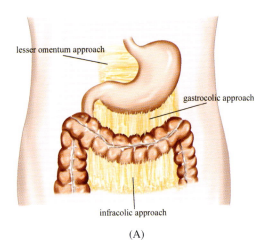

(A)

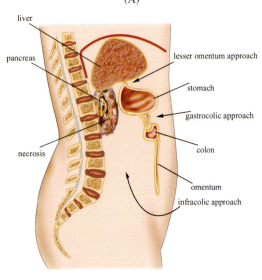

(B)

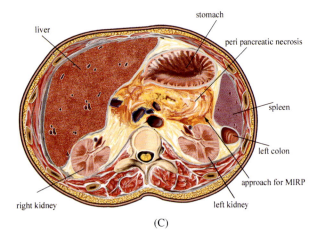

(C)

Figure 4.

Sections of abdomen showing position of pancreatic abscess and surgical approaches.

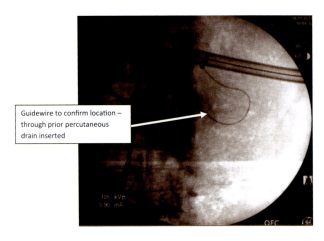

Figure 5A.

A position of the sheath for the retroperitoneoscope using guidewire under the guidance of image-intensifier.

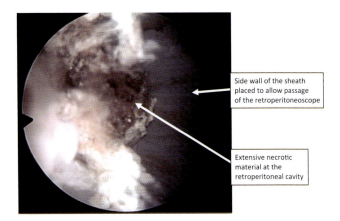

Figure 5B.

Appearance of necrotic (brownish black) retroperitoneal tissue during the first MIRP. The tissue was friable following the extensive necrosis and was amenable for piecemeal necrosectomy.

○ Approach to open necrosectomy is dependent on getting access to the necrotic pancreatic tissue.

○ In the *infracolic approach*, the transverse colon is lifted up to expose the inferior part of the pancreas, which is bounded by the mesentery of the transverse colon anteriorly and root of the small bowel mesentry inferiorly. If there is a pointing area at this region, it would suggest the collection of necrotic tissue, likely to be semi-liquefied, and thus amenable to necrosectomy.

○ Hydrodissection technique using saline spraying, gentle wiping of the necrotic pancreatic tissues

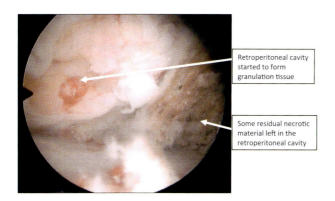

Figure 5C.

A cleaner retroperitoneal cavity after previous MIRP followed by continuous intraperitoneal lavage for a few days to flush out the remaining necrotic material. Only some residual brownish necrotic material was left as shown.

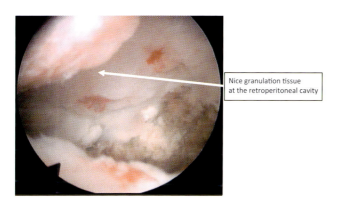

Figure 5D.

Nice granulation tissue at the retroperitoneal cavity. This cavity was then converted to passive drainage and the intraperitoneal lavage of the cavity was stopped.

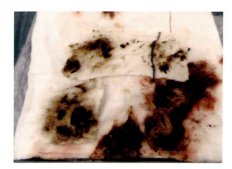

Figure 5E.

The tissue collected from the necrosectomy. The friable and easily removed tissue is typically described as 'dead-rat' tissue.

using wet gauzes or, in well demarcated pancreatic necrosis, piecemeal removal of the tissue using sponge forceps or sterile spoon are a few techniques to remove the necrotic tissue.

o *Gastrocolic approach* is another approach to perform this operation, especially if post-necrosectomy irrigation is required.

o Catheters can be inserted (total four, two on either side) for post-operative continuous lavage of the lesser sac.

o Lesser sac approach is usually not ideal for open necrosectomy as the lower extent of the pancreatic tissue may be obscured by stomach, colon and bowel, making the surgery difficult. In addition, this space is difficult to seal to facilitate catheter irrigation as the superior limit is the left lobe of the liver.

o Access to the retroperitoneum can be achieved in two ways: Progressive dilatation of percutaneous drain track or direct approach of the infected material with a retroperitoneoscope. Position of the track can be confirmed using image-intensifier on-table (Fig. 5a).

o Access is usually from the left flank (can be from the right flank if necrotic material has tracked to the right paranephric space).

o Piecemeal debridement of the necrotic material from the retroperitoneum is performed via the nephroscope/retroperitoneoscope (Figs. 5B, 5C and 5D showing progressive improvement of retroperitoneal cavity after repeated pancreatic necrosectomy via MIRP. Figure 5E shows the debrided material from the necrosectomy, classifically described as dead-rat tissue).

o Low-pressure water jet can be used to dislodge necrotic debris in the space.

o Drainage catheter can be placed in the space to facilitate post-operative lavage and drainage, at the same time, maintaining the tract for further surgery if necessary.

C) Bile Duct Injuries During Surgery

o One of the uncommon complications during gallbladder operation is bile duct injury (BDI).

o In various series quoted in the literature, the incidence of BDI in laparoscopic cholecystectomy was reported to be 0.3%–0.7%, while it was 0.13% in open cholecystectomy.

o The causes of BDI during cholecystectomy can be attributed to the following reasons:

- Previous severe inflammation around the porta hepatis region (such as pancreatitis, cholangitis, and cholecystitis), causing adhesion and scarring that obscure the anatomy of the region.
- Misinterpretation of the biliary anatomy.
- Partial injury to the bile duct due to thermal injury.
- Over vigorous traction on the cystic duct causing avulsion from the bile duct during cholecystectomy.

o Presentation of BDI:

- BDI may be recognised intra-operatively or may present later.
- The patient might present in the early post-operative period with complication of biliary leakage or biliary obstruction.
- Presence of bile fistula might cause bile peritonitis, intra-abdominal abscess and deranged LFT, while biliary obstruction would present with obstructive jaundice with or without cholangitis, stricture formation in the biliary tree, or in very late cases, secondary biliary cirrhosis.

o Management of BDI

- Intra-operative recognition

  1. If a BDI is identified during the surgery, it is important to call for the help of an experienced HPB surgeon. "A repair undertaken by the surgeon who has caused the injury is far less likely to be successful than one performed by a surgeon experienced in performing the repair."
  2. Effort can be made to insert a T-tube into the bile duct with closure of the small choledochotomy over the T-tube.
  3. If CBD is completely transected, a hepaticojejunostomy would be required after careful assessment of the injury.

- Post-operative presentation:

  1. In event of bile peritonitis/localised bile collection in the Morrison's pouch, percutaneous drainage to remove the infected material would be necessary at the beginning. After the sepsis is taken care of, anatomical study of the biliary tree can be performed either using MRCP or ERCP. ERCP can be therapeutic as stenting can be performed in minor CBD injury. PTC can be considered as an alternative to gain access to the biliary tree if ERCP fails.
  2. After resolution of the sepsis, reconstruction with bilioenteric anastomosis should be planned.
  3. Similarly, late post-operative biliary stricture would require bilioenteric reconstruction after careful study of the biliary anatomy using radiological modalities.
  4. An example of Roux-en-Y hepaticojejunostomy is shown in Fig. 6.
  5. The ideal option, especially in high injuries, is done to open up the left hepatic duct (Hepp-Couinaud procedure) to perform the anastomosis. This should be done by an experienced HPB surgeon (Fig. 7).

o Careful assessment of the extent of biliary injury is necessary to decide on the best modality for repair. Intra-operative cholangiogram is mandatory to provide this crucial information.

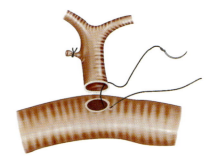

Figure 6.

Roux en- hepatico-jejunostomy.

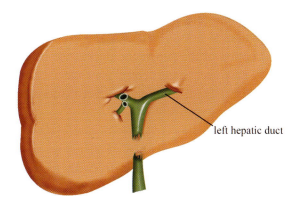

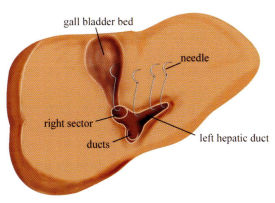

Figure 7.

Left hepatic duct used for anastomosis in high bile duct injuries.

○ BDI identified intra-operatively is usually associated with normal (non-dilated) biliary tree. Anastomosis is often associated with higher risk of stricture at later date.

○ Careful dissection at the hilum of the liver will help expose the area of bile duct injury and display the anatomy of the biliary tree. Care must be taken to avoid injury to surrounding structures (e.g. anomalous right hepatic artery).

○ In complete transection of the CBD, Roux-en-Y hepaticojejunostomy is the appropriate choice of reconstruction. A roux loop of jejunum is brought up via the retrocolic route (shortest route) without tension.

○ Stay sutures are placed at the corners of the anastomosis to mark the ends of the suturing margin. Full-thickness stitch on the bile duct side is accompanied by serosubmucosal layer stitching on the jejunum side.

○ Single-layer interrupted sutures are placed and tied for both anterior and posterior layers of the HJ anastomosis.

○ Mesenteric window of the colon is closed with interrupted sutures.

D) Pancreatic Trauma

○ Traumatic injuries to the pancreas and duodenum pose a major challenge due to the difficult exposure of these organs in the retroperitoneum.

○ Injury to the pancreas can be either blunt or penetrating in nature. As the pancreas is situated across the spine, blunt injury to the epigastric region can result in fracturing of the pancreas. The duodenum, being closely adherent to the pancreas, is usually traumatised as well.

○ Investigations of pancreatic injury

  • Serum amylase has little value in the initial evaluation of pancreatic injury.

  • Ultrasonography is not likely to yield important information due to the retroperitoneal location of the organ.

  • Contrast CT scan — Best modality to evaluate pancreatic injury.

  • ERCP — Might provide information on the ductal system in the pancreas. There might be a role in pancreatic stenting if the guide wire is able to bridge across the injured pancreatic duct.

○ Operative evaluation of pancreatic injury

  • It is necessary to have a complete exposure of the pancreatic gland.

  • A central retroperitoneal haematoma must be thoroughly evaluated and intra-abdominal bile staining necessitates proper evaluation of possible pancreatic and/or duodenal injury.

  • In case of trauma with haemodynamic instability, damage control surgery to achieve haemostasis will be the first priority. Placement of drains and packing are preferable.

  • Definitive surgery for pancreatic injury is dependent on the location of trauma.

- Injury to the distal part of the pancreas in the tail region necessitates distal pancreatectomy with closure of pancreatic stump and drainage of the area. Spleen preservation can be attempted if patient's condition allows.
- In ductal injuries, especially combined injuries of the head of pancreas and duodenum, integrity of the distal CBD and ampulla of Vater on cholangiogram will dictate the operative procedure. Intact duct and ampulla requires simple repair and drainage or repair and pyloric exclusion.
- Pyloric exclusion is widely adopted in the management of Grade III and IV combined pancreaticoduodenal injuries. The technique involves temporary diversion of enteric flow away from the injured duodenum by closure of the pylorus and creation of a gastroenterostomy.
- Closure of the injured area over a T-tube in combined injuries when D2 is involved has also been advocated.
- Injury to the body of the pancreas with disruption of the pancreatic duct may necessitate central pancreatectomy (See Fig. 8).

o Lesser sac is entered by opening the gastrocolic ligament.
o Careful assessment of the injured pancreatic tissue and surrounding structures such as the

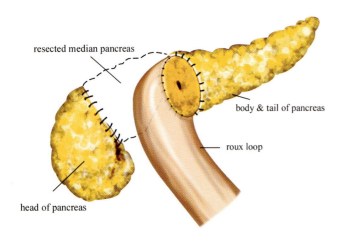

resected median pancreas

body & tail of pancreas

roux loop

head of pancreas

Figure 8.

Central pancreatectomy and reconstruction.

duodenum is essential to plan the next step of the operation.
o Disruption of the pancreatic duct at the neck and body may necessitate central pancreatectomy but, recently, PD disruption has been successfully treated conservatively.
o SMV-PV tunnel is created with careful dissection of the neck of pancreas. Pancreatic neck is transected using GIA stapler (with or without buttress material).
o Further dissection of the pancreatic body is performed from medial-to-lateral. Vessels connected to the pancreatic tissue are progressively ligated and divided.
o Pancreatic neck and part of the body are transected with cold-blade after adequate margin is achieved with all devitalised and unhealthy tissue removed.
o Bleeding from the cut surface of pancreas is secured with prolene 5/0 interrupted sutures.
o A roux loop of jejunum is brought up in retrocolic manner without tension to facilitate PJ anastomosis.
o Options of anastomosis are dependent on the surgeon's choice. Preferably, the surgeon should perform the type of pancreatico-enteric anastomosis that they are most familiar with at most times.
o In single-layer PJ, both anterior and posterior layer of anastomosis can be performed using PDS sutures. The sutures will be placed from the pancreatic side, parenchyma-to-capsule, to bowel side, seromuscular layer. Pancreatic stent is usually not required.
o In double-layer anastomosis, the outer posterior layer can be performed using prolene 4/0 suture in continuous manner while the inner posterior and anterior layer can be completed using PDS 5/0 sutures in interrupted manner. Pancreatic stent can be secured in the duct-to-seromucosa anastomosis if necessary. The outer anterior layer of the PJ can be completed with prolene 4/0 sutures.

- In fewer than 10% of cases, severe injury with unreconstructable injury to the duct or ampulla of Vater or duodenum would require pancreaticoduodenectomy (Whipple procedure).

- Some centres would advocate the use of somatostatin or its analogue (octreotides) in order to reduce pancreatic secretion. However, the evidence for administration of this pharmacological agent is controversial at the moment.

E)   ERCP Perforation

○   Incidence of ERCP-related perforation is rare (about 1%).

○   Types of ERCP injury can be classified as follows:

- Type I — Lateral duodenal wall injury (Or medial injury)
- Type II — Injury to the sphincter of Oddi
- Type III — Ductal injury
- Type IV — Retroperitoneal air only

○   Type I injuries tend to be large and remote from the ampulla of Vater. Persistent contrast leak in the retroperitoneal and/or intraperitoneal spaces may be evident on scans. Exploratory laparotomy and repair of the damaged structures is necessary.

○   Type II usually represents perivaterian injuries with varied severity, but usually the injury is discrete and less likely to require surgery.

○   Type III is usually due to distal bile duct injury related to wire of basket instrumentation near the obstructing entity (e.g. stones). The site of injury is usually small. Conservative management is often possible.

○   Type IV injuries are probably related to the use of compressed air to maintain patency of a lumen and are not true perforations. Surgical intervention is not required.

○   In short, the surgical indications after ERCP-related duodenal perforation are as follows:

- Large amount of contrast extravasation at the time of ERCP (defined as incomplete dissipation of contrast after one minute on follow-up plain film). If the contrast dissipated after one minute, it may represent small contrast extravasation and a repeat Gastrografin study should be performed four to six hours later. If contrast extravasation is noted, surgical exploration should be done.
- Any follow-up scans showing fluid collection in the retroperitoneal or peritoneum consistent with perforation, not pancreatitis.
- Documented ERCP perforation with cholelithiasis, choledocholithiasis or retained hardware.
- Massive subcutaneous emphysema after ERCP with what appears at endoscopy to be a large duodenal diverticulum.
- Failure of nonsurgical management.

Chapter 15

Laparoscopic Drainage of Liver Abscess

Stephen Chang Kin Yong* and Liza Tan Bee Kun†

I. Introduction

In the majority of cases, the aetiology of liver abscess remains unknown (cryptogenic). In patients with a known aetiology, ascending infection from choledocholithiasis is the most common source of liver abscess. In the West, malignancy of the head of pancreas or of bile ducts leading to biliary sepsis is a common cause of liver abscesses.

In the authors' institutional experience, *Klebsiella pneumoniae* and *Escherichia coli* were the most common organisms isolated; 9.2% were amoebic in origin. Diabetes mellitus was associated with 45.5% of these patients.

The majority of the abscesses are found in the right lobe of the liver. The segmental distribution based on the authors' institutional experience is shown in Fig. 15.1. 97.7% of abscesses are solitary.

II. Management Strategy for Liver Abscesses

Most liver abscesses can be treated by intravenous antibiotics and percutaneous drainage without general anaesthesia. Nevertheless, a proportion of patients with complicated abscess require surgical drainage.

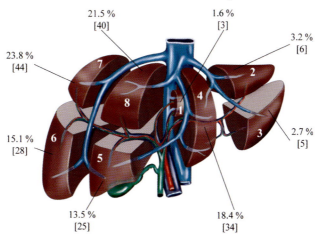

Figure 15.1.

Location of abscesses.

*K.Y. Chang, MBBS, MRCSED, MMed (Surg), FRCS (Gen Surg), FAMS, Associate Professor, YLL School of Medicine, National University of Singapore, Senior Consultant, Research Director, Division of Hepatobiliary and Pancreatic Surgery, Liver Transplant Program, National University Health System, Singapore.
†B. K. Tan, MBBCh, BAo (Nul), MRCS (lve), Department of Surgery, University Surgical Cluster, National University Hospital, Singapore.

In the authors' experience, surgical drainage can usually be achieved by a laparoscopic technique described as follows:

Preoperative Preparation

1. Ensure adequate infusion of fluids and blood components to restore and maintain blood volume and coagulation ability.
2. Broad-spectrum antibiotics with a view to streamlining it to targeted therapy based on culture results from blood or from the drained pus.
3. Ensure patient's condition is safe for general anaesthesia.
4. Informed consent with attention to the possible need of more than one intervention.

III. Operative Procedure Via Laparoscopic Approach

a. Position

The patient is prepared in the "French position" (Fig. 15.2), which is a supine position with both thighs abducted, knees straightened and soles supported. In such a position, the patient can be placed in a reverse Trendelenburg position to allow bowels to be displaced towards the pelvis and the patient prevented from sliding off the operating table.

The lower limbs must be abducted enough to permit the surgeon to position himself between them.

Port Siting

A 10-mm transumbilical incision is made for the camera port. Two 5-mm ports are placed along the midclavicular line cephalad to the camera port (Fig. 15.3).

b. Diagnostic laparoscopy

After a thorough inspection of the abdominal organs in a systemic fashion, the camera is focused onto the liver.

Note: The common primary diseases to look for include appendicitis, diverticulitis, cholecystitis and pelvic inflammatory diseases.

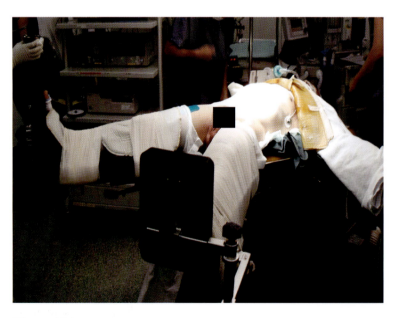

Figure 15.2.

Positioning of the patient.

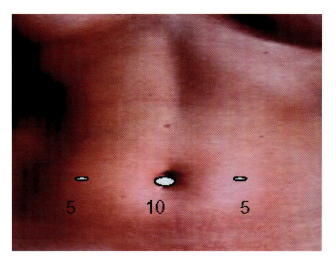

Figure 15.3.

Port sites.

c. Intra-operative ultrasound

The 10-mm telescope is exchanged for a 5-mm telescope and inserted through one of the 5-mm ports. A 10-mm laparoscopic ultrasound is introduced through the 10-mm port and a systematic examination of the liver is performed (Fig. 15.4).

The aims of performing the ultrasound are:

i. To confirm the position of the abscess.
ii. To identify the site on the liver closest to the abscess, i.e. the site where the abscess is "pointing", which usually serves as the site of initial parenchyma entry. The depth at this point is noted.

iii. To determine if the abscess is septated.
iv. To locate any other smaller abscesses that may not have been visible on preoperative scans.
v. To verify that no major vasculature crosses the path of drainage, i.e. from the site of parenchyma entry to the abscess cavity.
vi. To exclude Hydatid cyst, which is characterised by the presence of daughter cysts within the cavity. This is a relative contraindication to laparoscopic surgical drainage.

d. Drainage procedure

Having completed the ultrasound examination and determined the most suitable site of parenchyma entry, the surface of the liver at this site is scored with diathermy to serve as a marker. The laparoscopic ultrasound probe is then withdrawn and the 5-mm telescope is replaced by the 10-mm telescope. An aspirator is introduced through one of the 5-mm working ports and a hook with diathermy is introduced through the other. The site of parenchyma entry is further diathermised to coagulate a 1 cm diameter area of liver and induce sufficient "dimpling" of the liver. The power of the diathermy is then increased to 50, and the hook is advanced through the site of entry towards the abscess cavity keeping the power of the

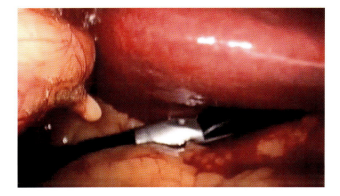

Figure 15.4.

Performing laparoscopic ultrasound.

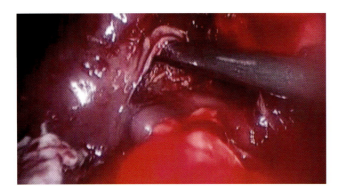

Figure 15.5.

Breaking down the septa using the aspiration catheter.

diathermy activated all the time. When the abscess cavity is reached, purulent material will be released. The pus is aspirated and sent for culture and sensitivity. The aspiration catheter is also used to gently break down the septa within the abscess if these were found during the ultrasound examination (Fig. 15.5). The cavity is then washed with saline.

Precautionary note

i. *It is important to coagulate a 1 cm diameter around the site of entry before attempting to enter the abscess cavity. This will reduce the likelihood of tearing the liver and induce bleeding at this site when the aspiration catheter is introduced later to break down the septa. The coagulated "capsule" at the surface will resist tearing of the liver at the point of entry and serves as point of pivoting for the instrument movements.*

ii. *Advancement of the hook with diathermy into the abscess cavity must be performed slowly in a controlled manner to allow the liver parenchyma with its microvasculature to coagulate sufficiently to reduce the amount of blood loss.*

iii. *The aspirator must be position close to the site of entry in anticipation of the exit of the pus to reduce contamination to the rest of the abdominal cavity. The prior knowledge obtained during the ultrasound step with regards to the depth of the abscess helps the surgeon to judge when the abscess wall is about to be breached.*

Special tricks!

Occasionally there may be bleeding encountered while trying to break down the septa within the abscess cavity. The important point then is to stop aspirating! This will allow the pneumo-peritoneal pressure to build up again, which will then serve as tamponade to further bleeding!

e. **Placement of drains**

A large-bore drain (14 fr) is introduced through the 5-mm port into the cavity. A second similar drain is placed into the sub-hepatic space near the abscess cavity. The ports are then removed.

Special tricks!

The placement of the first drain into the cavity may be guided by another grasper introduced via the other 5-mm port. But given that there are only two working ports, the placement of the second drain may be difficult. The trick is to use the port itself to direct the position of the drain towards the subhepatic space!

IV. Postoperative Management

i. Post-operatively, the patient is monitored for signs of intra-peritoneal bleeding such as tachycardia, hypotension, generalised abdominal pain and significant bloody drainage from the drains.

ii. The abscess catheter may be flushed daily with 10 mL of sterile saline to prevent it from being blocked.

iii. Appropriate antibiotics are started after obtaining the culture results.

iv. A CT scan may be repeated two weeks later to check that no other abscesses have developed and that the drains are still in appropriate position. It is possible to observe a reduction in size of the abscess cavity, but it is unlikely to contract fully.

v. The timing of drain removal varies. The authors' preference is that there must be absence of clinical signs of active infection, radiological evidence of contraction of the abscess cavity and absence of any partially necrotic liver tissue in the cavity.

Special situations

i. Abscesses in segments 7, 8

When the abscess is mainly in the superior segments of the right lobe, i.e. segments 7 and 8, it is often pointing towards the bare area of the liver. It is important to adequately mobilise the right lobe of the liver to allow access to this area (Fig. 15.6). The use of a snake retractor is useful in helping to mobilise the liver towards the left. Often both the falciform ligament and the right triangular ligament have to be divided to achieve this. This is a better way than to attempt to drain the abscess through a longer path via an entry point in the lower segment.

ii. Ruptured abscess

This is not a contraindication to laparoscopic approach. Certainly, percutaneous drainage will not be adequate. The key issue is adequate lavage of the peritoneal cavity, including the inter-loop areas of the small bowel. An additional drain may be placed in the pelvis to reduce the chance of pelvic abscess.

iii. Concurrent pathology

Occasionally the causative pathology for the liver abscess can be determined pre-operatively or during diagnostic laparoscopy. This may be addressed at the same time of the liver abscess drainage although additional ports may be placed to help in the dissection of the organs involved. Usually for an appendicectomy, an additional suprapubic port is placed while an additional right lateral port is placed for a cholecystectomy.

iv. Caudate lobe abscess

The drainage of a caudate lobe abscess is better done laparoscopically than percutaneously as the

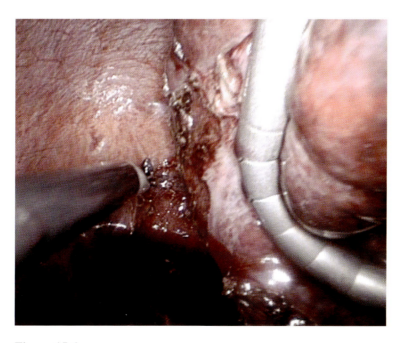

Figure 15.6.

Dividing the right triangular ligament to mobilise right lobe.

caudate lobe is "sandwiched" between the portal structures and the inferior vena cava, which may be at risk during percutaneous drainage. The laparoscopic approach will require opening the lesser omentum and lifting the left lobe towards the right. Occasionally the left triangular ligament may have to be divided before the left lobe can be lifted enough to expose the caudate lobe. More often with the caudate abscess, the lesser omentum lying on it becomes inflamed and adherent to the caudate lobe, but it can still be dissected from the caudate lobe. More often, an additional port may be necessary for the purpose of retraction.

v. **Deep-seated abscess**

In deep-seated abscesses in the right lobe of the liver where there is more than 2 cm of parenchyma tissue all around the abscess, it may be prudent to attempt drainage of the abscess percutaneously rather than surgically. If this fails, the patient can then be brought into the operating room for surgical drainage using the percutaneous drainage catheter as a guide to reach the abscess.

In the occasional situation where there is an obvious concurrent pathology that needs to be addressed in the first instance, the "percutaneous aspect" can be done intra-operatively under laparoscopic ultrasound guidance, and the surgical drainage can then be performed again using intra-operatively placed catheter (or guide wire) as a guide to reach the abscess cavity.

Final Note

As in all laparoscopic procedure, it is important that the surgeon is comfortable with the open approach in the event that the procedure has to be converted. This situation may arise when the patient cannot tolerate peritoneal insufflation and develops haemodynamic instability. The surgical principle remains the same as described above except for a larger incision placed usually at the right subcostal. In such situations, it is therefore unlikely that a posterior transpleural approach can be undertaken.

Chapter 16

Interventional Radiology in the Management of Intra-Abdominal Abscess

Anil Gopinathan,* Quek Swee Tian† and Lenny Tan‡

Introduction

Intra-abdominal abscess, when leading to septic shock, has a mortality of over 50%.[1] Until the late 1970s, surgical incision and drainage was the only practical way for achieving source control. Following the first report of percutaneous aspiration for abdominal abscess by McFadzean in 1953,[2] percutaneous drainage of abdominal abscesses has had to wait another two decades for the advent of cross-sectional imaging techniques to enable universal acceptance as a less invasive alternative or complement to surgery.

Advantages of Radiological Drainage

1) It can avoid a major surgical undertaking without precluding future surgery if indicated.
2) It permits multiple and repeated drain placements with relatively little patient morbidity. This is a major advantage as repeat laparotomies are often a nightmare for both the patient and the surgeon.
3) It allows precise drain placement into deep intra-abdominal locations that would otherwise warrant extensive organ mobilisation and tissue dissection to reach surgically, e.g. peripancreatic abscess.
4) It is almost always performed under local anaesthesia which is rarely feasible for most surgical drainages.
5) Bedside drain insertion may be possible when amenable to ultrasound guided drainage.
6) Direct procedural complications are uncommon with radiological drainage.
7) It may be the best and only rational approach in certain select situations, e.g. percutaneous transhepatic biliary drainage (PTBD) in the treatment of post-biliary enterostomy strictures.
8) Radiological drainage may be possible in certain situations when surgical intervention is relatively contraindicated, e.g. high surgical risk patients, postoperative abscess following recent major surgery.

*Anil Gopinathan, MBBS, MD, DNB, FRCR (Lond), FAMS, Consultant Radiologist, Department of Diagnostic Imaging, National University Hospital, Singapore.
†Quek Swee Tian, MBBS, FRCR, FAMS, Chief & Senior Consultant, Department of Diagnostic Imaging, National University Hospital, Singapore.
‡Lenny Tan, MD, FSIR, Emeritus Consultant, Department of Diagnostic Imaging, National University Hospital, and Professor, National University of Singapore, Singapore.

Disadvantages of Radiological Drainage

1) In multiloculated abscesses, radiologically placed drains may be less effective. Unlike surgical drainage, it is difficult to disrupt all the septae and drain every locule with percutaneous techniques.
2) Thick contents of an abscess may drain poorly in spite of wide bore drainage catheters.
3) Decortication of the wall of a chronic/thick walled abscess is not possible with radiological technique.
4) In rare instances, complications from a radiological drainage may expedite the need for surgical intervention.

Radiological Evaluation of the Abscess

An abscess is a collection of pus made up of microorganisms, tissue debris, fluid and neutrophils enclosed within a capsule of fibrin, surrounded by hyperaemic healthy tissue/granulation that walls off the infective process. A well formed abscess is drainable. However, abscess is the end stage of an inflammatory infective process and the earlier stages in its evolution are often not amenable to percutaneous drainage. Hence, it is important to remember the concept of "phlegmon," which is an inflamed tissue with the potential to form an abscess, but still receiving perfusion; phlegmon is not liquefied and not suitable for percutaneous drainage.

1) Diagnosis of Abscess

Plain radiograph has very little value in diagnosing an abscess. In the appropriate clinical setting, if mass effect is noted or abnormal extraluminal pocket of air is seen, one may raise the possibility of an abscess.

Sonography is a quick and useful modality in the diagnosis of intra-abdominal abscess. The typical sonographic description (Fig. 16.1A) of an abscess is, as an anechoic collection of fluid with good through transmission, low level internal echoes and often irregular margins. This appearance is indistinguishable from that of a cyst with debris/haemorrhage or lymphocele. The USG appearance can differ substantially, depending on the surrounding tissue and organ where it is located as well as on its composition. It may appear as a complex or solid mass when the abscess is poorly liquefied, has multiple septations or when it contains blood/blood products. Air within an abscess is seen as echogenic foci with dirty shadowing. The presence of ileus, deep location of an abscess or recent post-surgical status may limit the acoustic

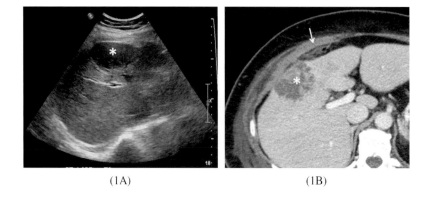

(1A) (1B)

Figure 16.1.

Typical ultrasound (**1A**) and contrast enhanced CT (**1B**) appearance of a liver abscess (*) is shown here. Note the anechoic appearance with increased through transmission and low level internal echoes on ultrasound. On CT scan it appears hypodense with few enhancing septae within. CT also shows the perilesional fat stranding (arrow) with a locule of air representing the inflammatory nature of the lesion.

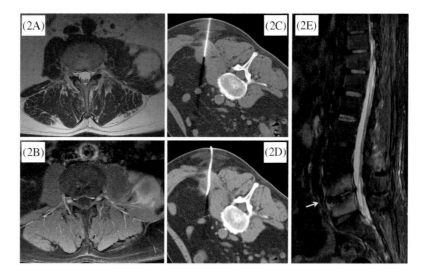

Figure 16.2.

MRI shows a bulky left psoas muscle with a hyperintense lesion (*) on T_2 weighted image (**2A**) that shows irregular, rind-like rim enhancement on post contrast T1W image (**2B**), that was diagnosed as psoas abscess. Percutaneous aspiration (**2C**) through a posterior approach (without contaminating the peritoneal/ anterior pararenal/ perinephric spaces) confirmed the diagnosis. Subsequently a drainage catheter was inserted (**2D**). Spondylodiscitis (arrow), the cause of this psoas abscess, is demonstrated in the sagittal MRI image of the spine (**2E**).

window and make USG an inadequate modality to evaluate an abscess.

Contrast enhanced CT is the recommended modality in the primary evaluation of an abscess. Just as with ultrasound, there is significant overlap between the appearances of a sterile collection and an abscess. At CT scan (Fig. 16.1B), an abscess is seen as a soft tissue mass with attenuation values in the range of 10–25 HU, with fat stranding in the vicinity and sometimes surrounded by a slightly hyperdense/ enhancing irregular rim. The contents of an abscess can show variable heterogeneity with uniform water density suggesting complete liquefaction. The presence of blood or thick debris can make the contents of an abscess look more hyperdense. The rim and internal septae may enhance on contrast administration. When the abscess is located within a solid organ, reactive hyperaemia or hypodensity from reactionary oedema may be seen beyond the enhancing rim. Fat stranding and reactionary slivers of fluid around an abscess is often seen on CT scan.

MRI is seldom employed for diagnosing an abscess. Generally, an abscess is seen as a mass lesion hypointense on T1W images and heteroneously hyperintense on T2W images with rim and septal enhancement (Fig. 16.2). Abscesses may appear bright on T1W image if it contains protein-rich contents or blood products.

The use of radionuclide scan is reserved for detecting occult abscesses or in certain cases when a diagnostic dilemma exists. Gallium 67 and Indium-111 labelled leukocytes can accumulate in an abscess and be seen as "hot spots". The latter is more specific and has higher accuracy in detecting an abscess.

2) Identify a Potential Cause for an Abscess

Definitive control of the cause of an infection is necessary to prevent continued or repeated episodes of sepsis and to restore optimal anatomic and physiologic function to the affected part. For example, if there is an abscess in the paracolic gutter secondary to perforated diverticulitis or a sub-hepatic abscess secondary to cholecystitis, it is essential to identify and treat the underlying cause in addition to draining the abscess. Likewise, a patient with psoas abscess

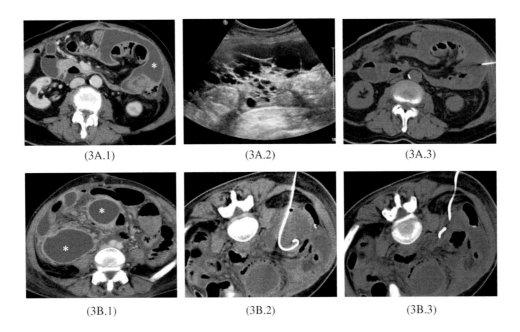

(3A.1)   (3A.2)   (3A.3)

(3B.1)   (3B.2)   (3B.3)

Figure 16.3.

Image series **3A** and **3B** demonstrate peritoneal collections (*) in two different patients; the former is a post surgical collection while the latter is complicated Crohn's disease.

On contrast enhanced CT, both are homogenously hypodense with enhancing rims (**3A.1** and **3B.1**). In spite of the similar appearance, on percutaneous aspiration, **3A** was sterile seroma while **3B** had frank pus within.

Ultrasonography (**3A.2**) shows multiple septae within the collection shown in **3A.1** that is not seen on CT. The higher spatial resolution of ultrasound permits better visualisation of the septae within a fluid collection compared to CT scan.

A direct safe access is the best approach to reach an abdominal collection as shown in **3A.3**. However, the abscess in **3B.1** does not have a direct safe access as it is surrounded by bowel loops; hence, a retroperitoneal approach (**3B.2** and **3B.3**) to a peritoneal abscess is justified here.

secondary to spondylodiscitis requires prompt identification and treatment of the underlying condition in addition to dealing with the abscess. Radiological imaging plays a vital role in identifying the root cause of an abscess (Fig. 16.2).

3) Determine Drainability of an Abscess

If the contents of an abscess is organised and not liquefied or if it is still a phlegmon, the infective focus may not be suitable for drainage. This can often be determined by imaging. In doubtful cases, this may need a diagnostic aspiration to confirm the same. The presence of multiple internal septa is a factor that can impact the effectiveness of percutaneous drainage. Broadly speaking, CT scan is superior to USG in evaluating an abscess but, when it comes to detecting these internal septa, ultrasound by virtue of its higher resolution is better than CT (Fig. 16.3).

Percutaneous drainage may not be the best option for all intra-abdominal abscesses, even if there is a safe window to drain it. Infected echinococcal cyst or suppuration in a necrotic tumour are classical examples of such abscesses; the former runs the risk of anaphylactic reaction while the latter may cause tumour seeding and fistula formation.

4) Identifying the Complications from an Abscess

For example, a pancreatic abscess causing splenic vein thrombosis or gastroduodenal artery aneurysm or a hepatic abscess causing hepatic vein thrombosis or rupture into the pleural abscess.

5) Aid Drainage Planning

CT scan is the preferred modality to identify the presence of a safe window and aid percutaneous drainage planning, especially for complex abscess locations. For example, interbowel abscesses are especially challenging to distinguish from dilated bowel loops. MDCT with multiplanar reconstruction and positive small/large bowel contrast administration is useful to make this differentiation.

Patient Preparation for Radiological Drainage

Appropriate patient selection for percutaneous drainage is vital to achieve the desired therapeutic results. This should be a multidisciplinary effort with good coordination between the surgeon, infectious disease specialist and interventional radiologist. Although one should strive to achieve 100% success, in practice this is not possible. With appropriate patient selection, successful diagnostic aspiration of intra-abdominal abscess should be possible in approximately 95% of cases and successful drainage in about 85% of cases.[3] Curative drainage, which means complete resolution of the abscess with no need for any further surgical intervention, can be achieved through radiological guidance in more than 80% of patients.

Radiological drainage has a low complication rate but is not entirely complication free (Table 16.1). While obtaining informed consent from the patient for abscess drainage, the primary clinician should explain to the patient the need for and role of the procedure in the overall management of the condition. However, the onus of explaining the possible outcome of the procedure and its complications, as described earlier, lies with the interventional radiologist.

Safe radiological drainage of abdominal abscess requires an intact coagulation pathway. However, when a patient is in sepsis it is not unusual for the

Table 16.1. Published Complication Rates and Suggested Thresholds

Specific Major Complication	Reported Rate (%)	Suggested Threshold (%)
Septic shock	1–2	4
Bacteraemia requiring significant new intervention	2–5	10
Haemorrhage requiring transfusion	1	2
Superinfection (includes infection of sterile fluid collection)	1	2
Bowel transgression requiring intervention	1	2
Pleural transgression requiring intervention (abdominal interventions)	1	2

(*The above table is adapted from the Society of Interventional Radiology Guidelines (Ref. 5)*)

coagulation function to be deranged. This has to be corrected before the drainage procedure is carried out.

We routinely obtain international normalised ratio (INR), activated partial thromboplastin time (aPTT) and platelet count for all patients who undergo abscess drainage. As most of the intra-abdominal drainage procedures carry moderate risk for haemorrhagic complication, we correct INR and aPTT when they are more than 1.5 times the normal. Platelet transfusion is recommended for counts less than 50 000/cu mm.

Aspirin is not considered as a contraindication while clopidogrel is preferably stopped for 5 days before the procedure. In emergency situations where there is insufficient time for 5 days of stoppage of thionepyridines (e.g. clopidogrel), platelets may be given 6–8 hours from the last dosage of the drug. In patients on low molecular weight heparin, one dose is omitted before the patient goes for the procedure or fresh frozen plasma supplementation is used.[4] There are anecdotal reports of delayed haemorrhage with fatal outcome occurring more than 24 hours from the drainage procedure, especially in patients with severe coagulapathy that was temporarily corrected for the procedure. This awareness can enable early recognition and treatment of complications.

Role of Radiological Intervention

1) To obtain fluid sample for diagnosis: An intra-abdominal fluid collection can be of varying a etiology. It is not always possible to determine by imaging alone that a collection is infected. A biloma, seroma, urinoma, resolving haematoma can have a similar appearance as an abscess (Fig. 16.3). Hence, the least invasive, confirmatory technique for ascertaining the nature of the fluid collection is through percutaneous aspiration. Microbiology can provide the organic cause of the infection. Even if an organism cannot be identified, high white cell count would suggest the infective nature of the fluid. In some cases, biochemical analysis of a specimen may reveal the cause of an abscess; for example, a high creatinine level helps confirm a diagnosis of a urinoma while a high bilirubin content would help confirm the diagnosis of a biloma or bile leak.

2) To completely drain the abscess: If infected appearing material is obtained or if the operator suspects the presence of an infection after a diagnostic aspirate, a drainage catheter may then be placed. Percutaneous drainage along with antibiotics may be adequate to treat the abscess in many cases. For smaller collections, a dry tap may suffice instead of placing a drain (Fig. 16.4).

3) To treat a recurrent collection by instilling sclerosing agent: The percutaneous drainage catheter may also be used as a conduit for infusing a sclerosing agent into a recurrent collection.

4) Temporising manoeuver to stabilise the patient's condition before definitive surgery, e.g. percutaneous cholecystostomy to be followed by interval cholecystectomy in a high surgical risk candidate presenting in acute sepsis (Fig. 16.5).

5) As an adjunct to facilitate further surgical intervention, e.g. a percutaneously placed drain into a pancreatic collection can be adequately upsized to provide a mature pathway for subsequent minimally invasive pancreatic necrosectomy (Fig. 16.6).

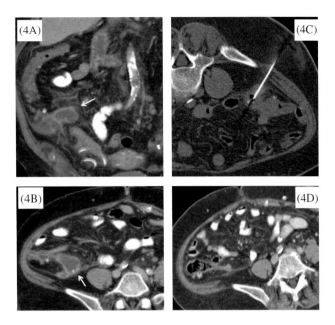

Figure 16.4.

The coronal (**4A**) and axial (**4B**) CT images show a rim enhancing fluid collection (arrow) with surrounding fat stranding and slivers of fluid in the right iliac fossa closely related to the ileocecal junction. In appropriate clinical settings, this is consistent with an appendicular abscess. Note the appendicolith (radio-opaque tiny density) within the collection on **4B**. Multiple comorbidities precluded surgery in this patient; hence, the collection was aspirated dry under CT guidance (**4C**). CT scan done 2 weeks post aspiration (**4D**) shows complete resolution of the abscess and the inflammatory changes.

Contraindications

Almost every fluid collection can be percutaneously drained. However, the risk associated with such a procedure has to be weighed against other surgical/alternative options available. Hence, most contraindications are relative, with the common ones being coagulopathy and necrotic tissue requiring surgical debridement. The absence of a safe percutaneous path is probably the only absolute contraindication to percutaneous abscess drainage. Although there are techniques of creating a safe pathway to a seemingly unreachable abscess, such as hydrodissection or artificial pneumoperitoneum, the magnitude of these efforts should be weighed against other therapeutic options. For certain complex abscesses, e.g. abscess related to

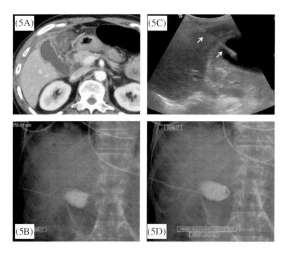

Figure 16.5.

CT scan shows acute cholecystitis (**5A**). As the patient was unfit for surgery, percutaneous cholecystostomy was performed. Under ultrasound guidance, a 22-G needle (*arrows* in **5B**) was inserted through the liver into the gall bladder. Through this needle, contrast was injected to opacify the gall bladder. A co-axially passed guidewire was secured in the gall bladder lumen (**5C**). Over this wire, a drainage catheter (**5D**) was inserted to complete the percutaneous transhepatic cholecystomy.

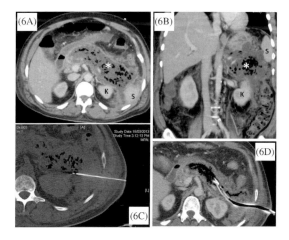

Figure 16.6.

Axial (**6A**) and Coronal (**6B**) images show a rim enhancing fluid collection (*) with several pockets of extraluminal air in the pancreas, consistent with pancreatic abscess. It was accessed percutaneously through a narrow window between the spleen (S), kidneys (K) and adjoining colon without going through the perinephric fat or peritoneal cavity under CT guidance (**6C**). This track was serially dilated over a few days and later necrosectomy was done and surgical drain inserted (**6D**).

Crohn's disease/tuberculosis, collections that need pleural transgression to drain, those with high risk of fistula formation, etc., percutaneous drainage may be a relative contraindication; such abscesses often need prolonged drainage, and have high risk of complications and failure of adequate source control. In such complex cases a thorough discussion between the surgeon and radiologist is essential before a percutaneous drain insertion is embarked on.

Technique

The procedure is usually done under local anaesthesia. In special circumstances, sedation with intravenous analgesia may be used. Rarely (usually in children) deep sedation or general anaesthesia may be required.

Imaging Guidance

The type of imaging guidance used for percutaneous drainage is determined by the location of the collection and the preference of the operator.

USG provides real-time guidance, involves no radiation and has lower procedure time; it is the method of choice for the relatively superficial abscesses, where there is little risk of transgressing a vascular structure, bowel, or pleural cavity.

CT guidance is essential for deep-seated abscesses when attempts at drainage carry a high risk of injuring structures in the vicinity. Large patient habitus, recent postoperative patients, the presence of air within the abscess are other scenarios where we routinely prefer CT guidance.

Combining CT/USG with fluoroscopy can increase both the safety and effectiveness of the procedure (Fig. 16.7). Here the abscess is opacified with contrast using CT or USG guidance, and under fluoroscopy guidance the drainage catheter is precisely positioned.

Insertion of the Drain

Various methods to catheterise an abscess have been described. Each method has its proponents, as well as its advantages and disadvantages. Usually it is

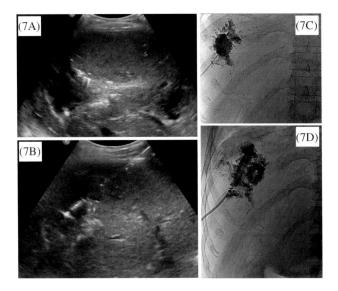

Figure 16.7.

This is an example of percutaneous drain placement with combined ultrasound and fluoroscopy guidance. Note the liver abscess (*) in segments 7 and 8 of the liver (**7A**). Under ultrasound guidance a needle is introduced into the abscess. The entire course of the needle from the surface of the skin to the abscess is well visualised (*arrows* in **7B**). This real time guidance is helpful in organs such as the liver that keeps moving with respiration. An abscessogram is performed with contrast injected through the access needle (**7C**). Now the abscess is visible to flouroscopy and once again under real time fluoroscopy guidance, a drainage catheter is placed within the abscess (**7D**).

an operator preference. In our practice, the "trocar technique" or the "Seldinger technique" is used.

Trocar technique: This involves direct introduction of a catheter mounted on a sharp trocar into the abscess. Once the assembly has entered the abscess, the trocar is held steady and the catheter is slid in further into the abscess. Usually such catheters are preshaped and once disengaged from the trocar they form a loop within the abscess. This loop provides greater surface area for drainage as well as prevents the catheter from getting easily dislodged.

Trocar technique is essentially a "one-step technique", hence, it is faster to perform, requires limited hardware and saves both time and cost. However, this technique is not suitable for abscesses in difficult locations such as (1) repositioning is often difficult; (2) the primary entry is with a wide bore

catheter-trocar assembly thereby limiting the manoeuverability. This technique also requires greater level of experience and skill from the operator, as minor digression from the expected path may cause the trocar to injure vital structures.

Seldinger technique: In this technique, a hollow needle is initially introduced into the abscess. Through this needle, a guide-wire is secured in the abscess cavity. Subsequently, the needle is removed, the track around the guide wire is dilated appropriate to the size of the drain to be inserted, and finally a catheter is introduced over the wire into the abscess. Once the catheter is placed in the desired location, the guide wire is removed. Over a 0.035 inch or 0.038 inch guide wire, drainage catheters in the size range of 8–14 Fr can be inserted. In patients with high risk of haemorrhagic complications and for abscesses with very limited window of entry, this technique can be performed using a minimal access system. Here, the initial entry into the collection is made with a skinny needle (22 or 21G) through which a microwire (usually 0.018 inch) is secured in the abscess. Using a dilator-sheath assembly, the microwire is replaced with a standard 0.035 inch or 0.038 inch guide wire, and the subsequent steps are as described earlier.

The Seldinger technique involves multiple steps and use of multiple items such as guide wires and dilators; this increases the time and cost of the drainage procedure. However, the index of safety is significantly higher with this technique. It increases the drainability of collections that otherwise would have been deemed inaccessible. It also permits precise localisation of the drain.

Drainage Catheter

Commercial drainage catheters come in a wide range of shapes and sizes, including non-sump catheters ranging from 6 to 12-Fr in diameter; sump drains with double lumen available in 12–18 Fr size; and Malecot catheters of various sizes. Although the largest size that can be safely placed is recommended for an effective drainage, Rothlin *et al.*[5] found no difference in the success rate, recurrence rate, incidence of surgical drainage, drainage time, complication rate, and post-drainage hospital stay between the percutaneous treatment of abdominal abscesses with a 7-Fr pigtail catheter and a 14-Fr sump drain. Through an *in vitro* analysis, Haaga's group[6] showed that for viscous fluid, larger catheters provide for more rapid drainage. However, at review of literature, the same group found similar clinical success with large and smaller caliber drainage catheters.

The authors routinely use an 8-Fr single lumen catheter for abscesses that are not so thick or a 10-Fr single lumen catheter for thick and viscid collections. If the contents of the abscess are too thick to drain through the indwelling catheter, we upsize the catheter in another session. We prefer using self-retaining pig tail catheters as they are more stable and the chance of accidental dislodgement is less.

Tips on Drain Insertion and Maintenance

1) Preferably take the shortest pathway with minimum angulation from the skin surface to the abscess.
2) Intervening bowel loops often preclude drainage catheter insertion into an abscess. In such cases, it is generally safe to transgress small bowel/stomach with a small caliber needle (19–22 G) and perform a one-time aspiration of the collection. However, transgression of the colon should be avoided, as the colonic flora will contaminate the specimen and may cause infection in the fluid collection.
3) Try to place the catheter at a position convenient to the patient, e.g. a drain entering from the lateral abdominal wall would be more convenient for the patient than one along the back.
4) When inserting drains over a guide wire, one should always watch out for kinking of the guide wire. This can lead to inadvertent perforation or placement of the drain in a wrong place.
5) If there is an intention to place a drainage catheter, the contents of a small to moderate size abscess should not be completely aspirated. Once the abscess cavity collapses, it would be difficult to place a drain.

6) Abrupt decompression of an abscess with thick and well vascularised wall may incite bleeding into the abscess. Hence, it is preferable to let it drain gradually through the drainage catheter rather than aspirating all the contents by forceful aspiration, immediately after inserting the drain.
7) Use of fibrinolytics like urokinase and irrigation through the drainage catheter often helps in clearing thick viscid collections.
8) Irrigation of the abscess must be performed with a lesser volume of fluid than that previously drained from the abscess, to avoid an increase in intracavitary pressure with resultant bacteraemia and sepsis.
9) After the catheter is secured in place in the decompressed abscess, the catheter should be flushed every 8–12 hours with 5–10 mL of saline solution to clear the tube of any adherent plugs or encrustations that might cause blockage.
10) Difficulty in flushing a catheter suggests a blocked catheter. If the abscess is not completely evacuated, such a blocked catheter needs to be exchanged for a new one, preferably under fluoroscopy guidance.
11) If the catheter is patent, yet the drain output is minimal, it may be due either to resolution of the abscess or a need for repositioning of the catheter. A CT scan or abscessogram may be done to evaluate this.
12) In spite of the abscess being empty at cross sectional imaging, if the drain output is light, an abscessogram to seek for a fistulous communication with some other epithelial surface should be done.

Site Specific Comments on Radiological Drainage of Intra-Abdominal Abscess

Liver Abscess

Untreated liver abscesses have a uniformly fatal outcome. Antibiotic therapy as the sole treatment is often inadequate, and drainage, either surgical or radiological is essential in most cases. Most of them are pyogenic in origin. Percutaneous aspiration as well as drainage can be done for liver abscess. Traditionally, catheter drainage is recommended for liver abscess, but some researchers have reported success rates up to 98% with needle aspiration alone with antibiotic therapy. There is no consensus on the best approach. The authors restrict the use of needle aspiration only for simple, small (usually less than 3 cm) abscesses. For large and complex abscesses, we prefer drain insertion. Needle aspiration may also be attempted when abscess is in a difficult to reach location, e.g. caudate lobe.

The authors use a combined approach with ultrasound and fluoroscopy for percutaneous drain insertion for liver abscess (Fig. 16.7). CT guidance is used if the abscess is not visible at ultrasound. It is always advisable for the drainage catheter to traverse some amount of normal liver parenchyma, before entering the abscess. This decreases the risk of procedure-related rupture of the abscess (and peritoneal contamination) as well as provides stability to the catheter.

Pyogenic liver abscesses are often multiloculated with several internal septations (Fig. 16.8). As the abscess matures, it tends to become more liquefied and can be more safely and completely drained. In a multiloculated abscess, a drain may be placed into the dominant locule and the smaller ones may be just aspirated. The septae are vascularised and it is not unusual for patent blood vessels to traverse an immature abscess. Hence, if there are too many septae and the locules are very small (Fig. 16.9), we generally avoid inserting a drain as there is potential increase in the risk for haemorrhagic complications. In such cases, we restrict the radiological intervention to diagnostic aspiration for microbiological purposes.

Once the drain output is negligible and imaging (contrast enhanced CT or abscessogram) show no drainable pus within the collection, the drain may be removed. The post-treatment changes in the liver parenchyma may take several months to clear in spite of complete clinical recovery (Fig. 16.8).

Haematoma, tumours and simple cysts may get infected and form secondary abscesses. Excluding the tumours, all of them can be treated like the pyogenic abscesses. A tumoural abscess can also be drained if the tumour is not resectable.[7] Amebic abscess are

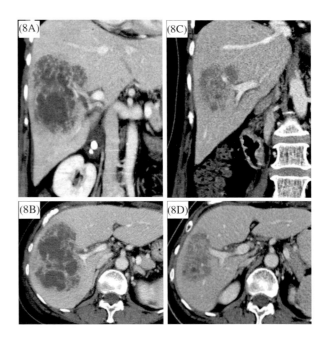

Figure 16.8.

Contrast enhanced CT scan of right lobe liver abscess is shown in coronal (**8A**) and axial (**8B**) planes. Note the ill defined mass with areas of fluid attenuation and multiloculated appearance. There is a large locule in the caudal half of the abscess into which we placed a percutaneous drain. Three weeks from drainage, the patient had clinically recovered; however, follow up scans (**8C** and **8D**) show ill defined hypodensity in the area corresponding to the previous abscess. This stigma of a healed liver abscess may be seen on imaging for several months after recovery.

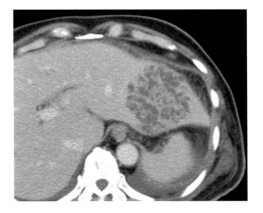

Figure 16.9.

A left lobe liver abscess with innumerable tiny loculations and enhancing septae is shown here. The central part of the abscess is almost solid. Such a poorly liquefied abscess is not a good candidate for percutaneous drain insertion.

treated in a different manner. They are highly responsive to antimicrobial treatment and drainage is only required in refractory cases, those at high risk of haemorrhage or for large abscesses (6–8 cm).

Subphrenic and Lesser Sac Abscess

Subphrenic and lesser sac abscesses are often post surgical or post traumatic. Lesser sac is also a common site for abscesses following complicated duodenal ulcer and pancreatitis. The preferred approach for a subphrenic abscess is to go subcostally or intercostally without injuring the liver/spleen and without pleural transgression. As the pleural recess is most shallow along the anterior aspect, it is often best to enter from here. The skin entry is much caudal to the location of the abscess and then the catheter has to be carefully navigated towards the abscess, at variable angles in all the three dimensions (Fig. 16.10). Hence, these are among the most technically difficult abscesses to drain percutaneously. Sometimes, hydrodissection to create a plane between the abdominal wall and liver/spleen may be required to place such drains. In select circumstances, a transhepatic or transdiaphragmatic drain insertion into a subphrenic abscess may be done. This should be avoided as far as possible; it should be performed only after the patient and the primary treating physician have been informed about the potential risk of hepatic abscess or emphyema.

The lesser sac is a fairly closed space and it can be impossible to get safe percutaneous access to an abscess in this region. If there is no response to medical management, the abscess often tracks out from the lesser sac, thereby giving a window to drain if percutaneously. If the patient is too sick for such an expectant management, transhepatic approach may be required for draining the lesser sac. The risk of secondary liver abscess exists with this approach.

Percutaneous Cholecystostomy

Percutaneous cholecystostomy involves placement of a needle into the gallbladder to aspirate bile. This is

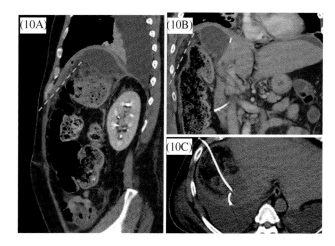

Figure 16.10.

A right subphrenic abscess following right hepatectomy is shown in the sagittal (**10A**) and coronal (**10B**) CT images. Note the peculiar location of this abscess interlocked between the lung and the colon along the anterior and right aspect, right kidney and lung posteriorly and residual liver anteromedially. There was no direct window to access this collection. Hence the drain was inserted from the anterior side with skin entry several centimetres caudal to the abscess, and then the needle was navigated cranially along a steep angle, obliquely oriented in both the sagittal and coronal planes. The dotted yellow line shows the plane through which the catheter was navigated to reach the final position (**10C**). This is an example of the frequently encountered technical difficulty in percutaneously draining a sub-phrenic abscess.

commonly followed by placement of a tube for external drainage. Such percutaneous decompression can be performed with the intent of definitive therapy in patients at high risk with medical comorbidities or as a temporising measure preceding subsequent elective cholecystectomy.

In patients with large ascites and bowel interposition, the transhepatic route is preferred (Fig. 16.5); besides, this route also offers the advantage of greater catheter stability. On the other hand, the transperitoneal route is preferred in the setting of coagulopathy and liver disease. Theoretically, the chances of procedure-related biliary peritonitis is lower with transhepatic route as compared with transperitoneal route. However, recent studies have shown similar safety profile with no significant difference in complication rates with either technique.[8]

Pancreatic Collection/Abscess

Necrotising pancreatitis includes non perfusion of both the pancreatic parenchyma and the peripancreatic tissue; the former can be diagnosed as lack of enhancement at CT scan in the first week from onset, while the latter is detected much later, usually around two weeks from the onset as a heterogeneous solid-cystic collection around the pancreas.

At CT scan, infected necrosis may show extraluminal locules of gas. Diagnosis is confirmed by demonstration of bacteria and fungi at percutaneous needle aspiration. Invasive treatment is essential in this state. Percutaneous drainage is commonly and urgently performed for such infected pancreatic collections. As these collections are usually in the retroperitoneum, a retroperitoneal course of the percutaneous drain without contaminating the peritoneal cavity should be attempted (Fig. 16.6). Sterile pancreatic necrosis can also be drained percutaneously if it is liquefied. The track of the drain insertion should be such that there is enough latitude to dilate this track (up to 20–30 Fr) in the future to permit a necrosectomy, if required.

The pseduocysts that evolve over 4–6 weeks from an acute pancreatitis are usually sterile and need not be drained. The indications for drainage of pseudocysts include recurrent pain on attempts at feeding after resolution of acute pancreatitis, an enlarging pseudocyst, secondary infection, intracystic haemorrhage, and mass effect causing biliary or bowel obstruction. Depending on the location of the pseuodcyst, it may be drained by a transgastric, transperitoneal or retroperitoneal approach. A one-time aspiration/dry tap is not adequate, with 70% recurrence rate; meanwhile, drainage with indwelling catheters have very low rate of recurrence.[9]

Pelvic Abscess

The pelvis is the most dependent portion of the abdominal cavity and hence a common site for fluid to get accumulated, infected and walled off to form an abscess. They are often seen in postoperative patients. Appendicitis, diverticulitis and pelvic inflammatory disease also commonly lead to pelvic abscess. If a

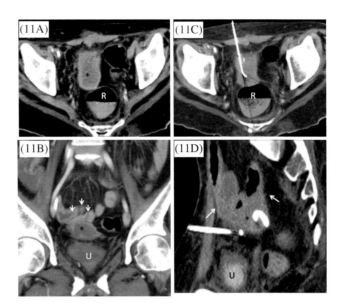

Figure 16.11.

A pelvic abscess (*) is noted in the axial (**11A**) and coronal (**11B**) images located between the rectum (R) posteriorly, bladder (U) anteromedially, and small bowel loops (*arrows*) cranially. Percutaneous guide wire localisation was done through the available narrow anterior window (**11C**) and drain inserted. The sagittal image (**11D**) shows the narrow anterior window, between the bladder and small bowel, through which the drain was inserted.

safe access through anterior abdominal wall is available, it would be the best approach for draining a pelvic abscess (Figs. 16.11 and 16.12). However, this is often unavailable and hence more tedious approaches such as the transgluteal, transrectal/vaginal, paracoccygeal–infragluteal, or perineal approach through the greater sciatic foramen may be adopted to drain a pelvic abscess.

An abscess located deep in the pelvis, adjacent to the vaginal vault or in the pouch of Douglas/rectovesical pouch may be drained with endocavitory ultrasound guidance through transrectal or transvaginal route. Transrectal drainage can also be performed under fluoroscopy guidance when the collection is anterior or lateral to the mid-to lower rectum. While using a transrectal or transvaginal approach, the operator should be aware that the technique can never be sterile. Hence, if there is any doubt that the pelvic fluid collection is only reactive and not pus, this

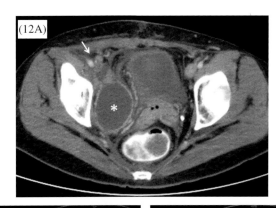

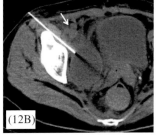
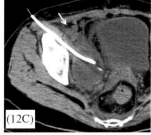

Figure 16.12.

A rim enhancing fluid collection consistent with an abscess (*) is seen along the right lateral pelvic wall in the post contrast CT scan (**12A**). There are bowel loops, iliac vessels (arrow) and urinary bladder anterior to this abscess. The transgluteal approach is not favourable here as the abscess is located more laterally in the pelvis and trying to reach it is fraught with risk of injuring the sciatic nerve and gluteal vessels. Hence, an anterolateral approach, through the iliopsoas, deep to right iliac vessels was adopted (**12B**). Note the final satisfactory position of the drain within the abscess (**12C**).

approach should be avoided as it would introduce infection into an otherwise sterile collection. The transrectal catheters, though seem awkward, are usually well tolerated by the patients.

A transgluteal approach is an effective route in draining deep pelvic abscess. Selecting a transrectal or transgluteal approach depends on the operator preference. Some studies have condemned the transgluteal approach for the pain associated with it, while some others have found it to be well tolerated by the patient. The authors generally prefer a transgluteal approach, since it provides a greater access into the deep pelvis, often allowing drainage of the more laterally and cranially placed collections that are difficult to reach transrectally. Again, transgluteal

approach is strongly favoured for pelvic collections in which infection is uncertain, because this approach allows drainage in a strictly aseptic environment. During a transgluteal approach, we keep the track as close as possible to the sacrum to avoid injury to sciatic nerve and gluteal vessels (Fig. 16.13).

Enteric Abscess

Enteric abscess is generally a complication of appendicitis, diverticulitis or Crohns' disease. This group of abscesses is best drained under CT guidance. The role of radiological drainage is often temporarising as definitive surgical procedure is frequently required at a later date. In diverticulitis, percutaneous drainage is useful in cases with limited perforation or pelvic perforation without faecal spillage. Periappendiceal abscess as a complication of acute appendicitis (Fig. 16.4) as well as post appendicectomy, benefits from percutaneous drainage. The latter often needs prolonged drainage. It is important to discriminate a periappendiceal phlegmon from an abscess before insertion of a drain. In Crohn's disease, (Fig. 16.3B) abdominal abscesses may develop spontaneosly or as a complication of surgery. These are most frequently between the leaves of the mesentery (intramesenteric), between adjacent bowel loops (interloop), between the bowel loop and the adjacent viscera or the anterior abdominal wall (enteroparietal), and less frequently in the retroperitoneoum and the pelvis. Their location often makes drainage difficult for Crohn's disease-related abscesses and they also need prolonged drainage for complete healing.[7]

Others

Splenic abscesses are rare and usually secondary to haematogenous infection. In the past, antibiotic therapy and splenectomy were the only options. However, there is a progressive trend towards splenic preservation whether in trauma or sepsis. This need has allowed percutaneous drainage to evolve as a reasonable option. Splenic abscesses have been safely treated with both percutaneous aspiration and drain insertion.[10]

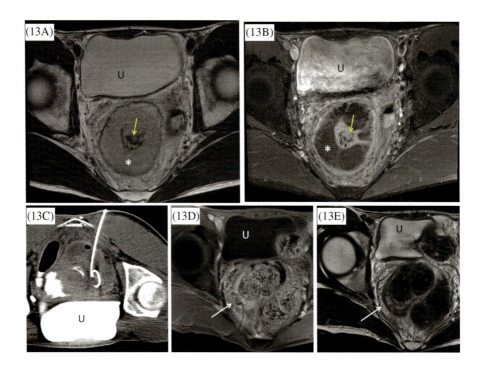

Figure 16.13.

T2 weighted (**13A**) and post contrast T1 weighted (**13B**) high resolution MRI of the pelvis shows a T2 bright, rim enhancing fluid collection surrounding the rectum (*yellow arrow*), suggestive of a pelvic abscess (*). It was drained along the trans-gluteal route (**13C**). Follow up post contrast T1W (**13D**) and T2W (**13E**) images show almost complete resolution of the abscess with the catheter within a small residual pocket of fluid (*white arrow*). Note the drain travelling close to the sacrum and hence safely away from the sciatic nerve.

Both renal and perirenal abscesses are amenable to radiologically guided percutaneous drainage. Often these are secondary to urinary obstruction and hence they also need a simultaneous percutaneous nephrostomy.

Psoas abscesses are usually seen as a complication of pyogenic or tuberculous spondylodiscitis. They can be effectively drained using CT guidance with percutaneous drain insertion (Fig. 16.2). In the past, surgery was often performed for tuberculous iliopsoas abscesses, but the failure and recurrence rate is high at 40%.[11] Therefore, percutaneous drainage has become popular as a safe and effective initial drainage option in most cases.

Conclusion

The technical feasibility and clinical efficacy of percutaneous abscess drainage have been well established. Over the years the techniques of drainage have become progressively more refined and abscesses in locations that were previously thought to be non drainable have become accessible. In experienced hands, radiological drainage of most abscesses is possible with a very low complication rate. Contraindications to percutaneous drainage are rare, with those cited in literature being often very restrictive. It is the clinical need that should determine the indication and contraindication. In our experience, the real contraindication is an unusual abdominal abscess that does not deserve a trial of percutaneous drainage; this can be determined only through a meaningful dialogue between the interventional radiologist and the clinician primarily managing the patient. Finally, active participation of the operating radiologist in monitoring the patient's progress after insertion of a drain cannot be further emphasised.

References

1. Sartelli M, Viale P, Koike K, *et al.* (2011) WSES consensus conference: Guidelines for first-line management of intra-abdominal infections. *World J Emerg Surg* **6**: 2.

2. McFadzean AJS, Chang KPS, Wong CC. (1953) Solitary pyogenic abscess of the liver treated by closed aspiration and antibiotics: a report of 4 consecutive cases with recovery. *Br J Surg* **4i**: 141–15.

3. Wallace MJ, Chin KW, Fletcher, *et al.* (2010) Quality improvement guidelines for percutaneous drainage/aspiration of abscess and fluid collections. *J Vasc Interv Radiol* **21**: 431–435.

4. Patel IJ, Davidson JC, Nikolic B. (2012) Consensus guidelines for periprocedural management of coagulation status and hemostasis risk in percutaneous image-guided interventions. *J Vasc Interv Radiol* **23**: 727–736.

5. Rothlin MA, Schob O, Klotz H, *et al.* (1998) Percutaneous drainage of abdominal abscesses: are large-bore catheters necessary? *Eur J Surg* **164**: 419–24.

6. Park JK, Kraus FC, Haaga JR. (1993) Fluid flow during percutaneous drainage procedures: an *in vitro* study of the effects of fluid viscosity, catheter size, and adjunctive urokinase. *AJR Am J Roentgenol* **160**(1): 165–9.

7. Men S, Akhan O, Köroğlu M. (2002) Percutaneous drainage of abdominal abcess. *Eur J Radiol.* **43**(3): 204–18.

8. Loberant N, Notes Y, Eitan A, *et al.* (2010) Comparison of early outcome from transperitoneal versus transhepatic percutaneous cholecystostomy. *Hepatogastro-enterology.* **57**(97): 12–7.

9. Grosso M, Gandini G, Cassinis MC, *et al.* (1989). Percutaneous treatment (including pseudocystogastrostomy) of 74 panreatic pseudocysts. *Radiology* **173**: 493–7.

10. Ferraioli G, Brunetti E, Gulizia R, *et al.* (2008) Management of splenic abscess: report on 16 cases from a single center. *Int J Infect Dis.* **13**(4): 524–30. doi: 10.1016/j.ijid.2008.08.024. Epub 2008 Dec 12.

11. Procaccino JA, Lavery JC, Fazio VW, Oakley JR. (1991) Psoas abscess: difficulties encountered. *Dis Colon Rectum* **34**: 784–9.

Chapter 17

Management of Gynaecological Emergencies

Fong Yoke Fai* and Chua Yao Dong**

Gynaecological emergencies, associated with haemorrhage, torsion or sepsis, may present as acute abdomen. They include:

I Ectopic pregnancy
II Ruptured tubo-ovarian abscess, and
III Bleeding ovarian cysts and adnexal torsion

I. Ectopic Pregnancy

Preoperative Preparation

1. Check pre-operative haemoglobin levels, Rhesus group.
2. Ensure adequate haemodynamic support with fluids and blood components.
3. The cornua are extremely vascular and profuse bleeding can occur rapidly during surgical management of cornual ectopics.

Operative procedures

Key points

1. The surgical management of ectopic pregnancy is based on several factors, including the site, size and extent of tubal damage.
2. The decision to perform a salpingostomy or salpingectomy is often made intra-operatively on the basis of the extent of damage to the affected and contralateral tubes, but it is also dependent on the patient's history of ectopic pregnancy and wish for future fertility, the availability of assisted reproductive technology, and the skill of the surgeon.
3. Whatever the surgical approach, haemostasis is essential and surgical trauma should be minimised.
4. The status of the contralateral tube is an important determinant of subsequent fertility potential.
5. Laparotomy rather than laparoscopy is performed if the patient is haemodynamically unstable, or has a cornual ectopic.
6. Other contra-indications to laparoscopy: dense pelvic adhesions, morbid obesity.
7. Consider performing bilateral salpingectomy and subsequent referral to IVF if two or more of the following risk factors are present:

— history of salpingitis
— previous ectopic pregnancy
— presence of adhesions on the contralateral tube.

1. Salpingotomy via Laparotomy

Salphingotomy preserves fertility

1. Pfannenstiel/low midline vertical incision.
2. Expose, elevate and stabilise the fallopian tube.
3. Linear incision made over distended segment of the tube at the antimesenteric wall until entry into lumen (Fig. 17.1A).

*Y.F. Fong, MBBS, MRCOG, FRANZCOG, MMed, Head of Benign Gynaecology, Department of Obstetrics and Gynaecology, National University Hospital, Singapore.
** Y.D. Chua, MBBS, Resident, Department of Obstetrics and Gynaecology, National University Hospital, Singapore.

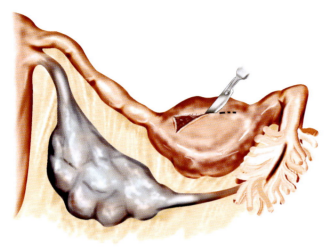

Figure 17.1A.

Linear incision made over distended segment of the tube at the anti-mesenteric wall.

4. Apply gentle pressure from opposite side of the tube to express products of conception (POC).
5. Remove any remaining fragments by profuse irrigation of the lumen, with caution to avoid trauma to the mucosa.
6. Secure complete haemostasis of the tubal mucosa.
7. Close mucosal margins with interrupted sutures.
8. Ensure no suture material is retained on mucosal surface, as this can cause adhesions.

2. Salpingotomy via Laparoscopy

1. Using a 22G injection needle, inject dilute solution of vasopressin (prepare by mixing 20U of vasopressin with 100 mL of Normal Saline) into the tubal wall at the area of maximal bulge. Inject into the mesosalpinx slightly inferior to the pregnancy and over the antimesenteric surface of the tubal segment containing the pregnancy.

   (Note: it is important not to inject the vasopressin solution into a blood vessel as this can lead to arterial hypotension, bradycardia and death.)
2. Incise along antimesenteric wall of the tube in area of maximal distension to allow for complete extrusion of products of conception (Fig. 17.1B).
3. If POC do not spontaneously extrude, use either hydrodissection or gentle tubal compression with a blunt probe/suction irrigator.
4. Tissue placed in specimen bag and removed, taking care to avoid spillage.

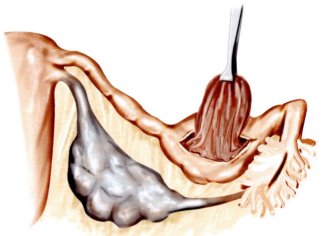

Figure 17.1B.

Complete extrusion and removal of POC.

5. After removal of tissue, irrigate carefully to dislodge trophoblasts and remove blood from peritoneal cavity. Check for haemostasis.
6. Tube can be left to heal by secondary intention or sutured.

Problems

1. Oozing from the implantation site is common and usually requires nothing more than patience. Compression using Palmer forceps can be applied.
2. In cases where the opening is too large or edges seem to be unable to come together spontaneously, a 4-0 absorbable suture can be used for reapproximation.
3. If the ectopic is located in the distal ampullary portion of the tube, occasionally the tube can be grasped with forceps and the pregnancy "milked" out of the fimbria. This can also be performed for infundibular and partially extruded tubal pregnancies.

3. Salpingectomy via Laparotomy

Salpingectomy is performed for:

1. Ruptured tubal pregnancy and uncontrolled bleeding.
2. Recurrent ectopic pregnancy in the same fallopian tube.
3. Ectopic pregnancy in a severely damaged tube.

4. Patient who has completed her family, or wants sterilisation.

1. Pfannenstiel/low midline vertical incision.
2. Elevate distended tube to reduce bleeding.
3. Mesosalpinx clamped with a succession of Kelly clamps as close to the tube as possible.
4. Tube is excised by cutting close as possible to the uterine cornu.
5. It is important to resect the tubal stump as near as possible to the tubal uterine junction to prevent tubal pregnancy from occurring in the remaining tube.
6. Figure-of-eight mattress suture of No. 0 delayed absorbable material to secure haemostasis is used to close the myometrium at the cornual end if necessary.
7. Mesosalpinx is closed with interrupted ligatures of No. 2-0 delayed-absorbable suture.

4. Salpingectomy via Laparoscopy

1. Irrigation of pelvis, evacuation of all blood clots.
2. Involved tube grasped with tooth grasper.
3. Cauterising tubal-ovarian ligament first with bipolar forceps.
4. Transect or cauterise the mesosalpinx, taking care to stay as close as possible to the fallopian tube (Fig. 17.2A).
5. Proximal tubal portion is then cauterised and transected as close to cornual as possible (Fig. 17.2B).

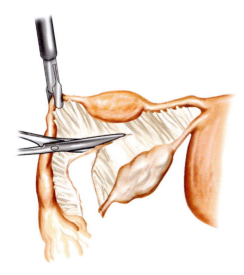

Figure 17.2A

Transect the mesosalpinx as close to the fallopian tube as possible.

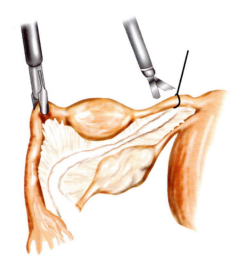

Figure 17.2B

Proximal tubal portion transected as close to the cornual as possible.

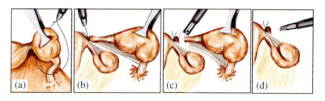

a. position of first endoloop
b. closing and securing the endoloop
c. excision of the tube
d. electrocoagulation of the tubal stump

Figure 17.2C

Salpingectomy via endo loop.

7. Care to avoid excessive cauterisation of the uterine cornu, which can lead to potential interstitial sinus tracts or diminished myometrial integrity.
8. The normal tubal portion can also be taken using the endo loop as depicted (Fig. 17.CC).
9. Retrieve specimen in an endoscopic retrieval bag and removed through port.

Postoperative care

1. Post-operative serial monitoring of BHCG values (until levels are < 5.0 IU/L).
2. No sexual intercourse.
3. Rates of recurrence

One previous ectopic pregnancy — approximately 10–15%

two or more previous ectopic pregnancies — at least 25%.

4. Rates of intrauterine pregnancy — approximately 60%.

(In patients with one remaining fallopian tube, which is patent and appears grossly normal.)

II. Ruptured Tubo-Ovarian Abscess

Of all the complications that can result from pelvic inflammatory disease, intra-abdominal rupture of a tubo-ovarian abscess has the greatest morbidity and mortality.

Complications include septic shock and generalised peritonitis.

Mortality rate can approach 10%.

Preoperative

Preoperative preparation

Combating shock is a primary concern

1. Group and match two to four units of packed red cells if necessary.
2. Close monitoring of circulation.
3. Judicious fluid resuscitation to avoid fluid overload.
4. Hourly urine output with indwelling urinary catheter to assist in fluid resuscitation.
5. Close monitoring of blood chemistry and blood gases.
6. Clinical assessment/monitoring of patient for signs of respiratory distress, shock, fluid overload.

Indications for surgical intervention

1. Failure of response to antibiotic therapy after 48–72 hr.
2. High index of suspicion for other surgical emergencies such as appendicitis.
3. Intra-abdominal rupture of a tubo-ovarian abscess.

Operative strategy

1. Primary aim is to achieve drainage and clearance of any debris.

2. In the acute inflammatory stage, more radical surgeries such as hysterectomy are not advisable
3. Speed is critical.
4. Laparoscopy only if patient is haemodynamically stable.
5. Definitive surgical treatment is usually not recommended in severely ill patients with ruptured abscess to reduce operative time and risks.
6. Surgery may be technically difficult due to high incidence of distorted anatomy.

   — Landmarks are obscured, infected tissues are edematous and friable.
   — Careful separation of densely adherent bowels is required to avoid injury.

7. Bowel serosal injury occurs frequently. Any entry into the lumen of the bowel must be repaired.

Operative procedures

1. Via laparoscopy

1. Omental and intestinal adhesions will often be present, hence the first step is usually adhesiolysis to reveal pelvic structures (Fig. 17.3).
2. The cul-de-sac is then exposed as the tubo-ovarian abscesses are often bilateral (Fig. 17.4).
3. Uterine manipulation vaginally is helpful to increase exposure of the cul-de-sac.
4. Sharp and blunt dissection is then used to expose the adnexal and pelvic side wall.

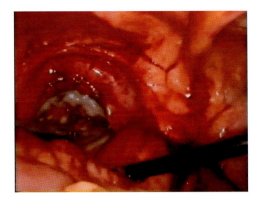

Figure 17.3.

Revealing and delineating pelvic structures using laparoscopic instruments.

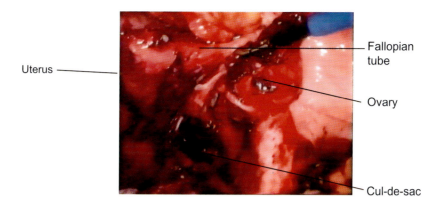

Figure 17.4.

Exposing the cul-de-sac.

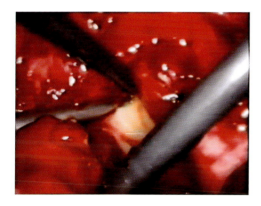

Figure 17.5.

Aspirating pus from abscess cavity.

5. The abscess cavities are often broken during this step and pus can then be washed out. Pus should also be aspirated and sent for microbiological studies (Fig. 17.5).

6. Generous peritoneal irrigation is then used and drains can be introduced via the laparoscopic ports to be placed in the cul-de-sac.

2. Via laparotomy

1. Lower transverse incision.

2. During entry into abdomen, any odour that is present should be noted.
   — An unpleasant, putrid odour is indicative of infection by anaerobic organisms.

3. Collect any pus from the abdomen using an airtight syringe
   — Gram stain, aerobic and anaerobic culture, as well as sensitivity to various antibiotics.

4. Operation of choice: removal of free pus, drainage of abscess and peritoneal washout. Adnexectomy may be possible but not necessary unless easy to perform.

5. Carefully explore the upper abdomen for collections of pus — subdiaphragmatic/subhepatic spaces.

6. Irrigate the abdominal cavity with copious quantities of warm sterile saline.

7. Consider placing a closed suction catheter to provide peritoneal drainage if haemostasis is poor or if considerable necrotic material is left behind.

8. Closure: Abdominal incision is closed with a continuous suture taking large bites of tissue. Consider delayed absorbable sutures such as PDS. Irrigate the incision with warm saline.

9. If there has been gross contamination of the incision:
   — Leave the subcutaneous fat and skin open and pack lightly with gauze soaked in an antibiotic or antiseptic solution.
   — Inspect and repack the wound on a daily basis
   — Secondary closure can be performed in four to five days if there are no further complications.

10. Once infected debris has been cleared, the patient often makes a remarkable recovery, with the right supportive treatment and choice of antibiotics.

11. Pelvic clearance (hysterectomy and bilateral adnexectomy) remains the definitive treatment but it is best to wait six weeks for the acute inflammation to settle before embarking on this.

Challenges

1. Ureter is often precariously close to the inflammatory mass.
2. Dissection of the adhesions can be bloody
   — To reduce blood loss, surgeon should aim to quickly isolate and ligate the infundibulopelvic ligament.

Precautions

1. Inflammatory tissue is friable and must be handled with extreme care.
2. If drainage is required, closed suction drains (e.g. Jackson-Pratt) should be placed in the pelvic cavity and exit from a separate abdominal stab wound.
3. The patient should not be placed in the Trendelenburg position until the abdomen has been packed.
4. The patient should also be placed no more of a dependent position than needed to avoid further dissemination of pus into the upper abdomen.
5. For laparoscopy, it is important to look at the upper abdomen at the end of the surgery to aspirate any debris and apply irrigation until the aspirate is clear.

Postoperative

1. Important considerations during post-operative care: shock, infection, ileus, fluid imbalances.
2. Septic shock: fluid resuscitation, respiratory support, inotropes/vasoactive substances.
3. Infection: Coverage with broad-spectrum antibiotics.
4. Intravenous antibiotics are continued till patient is afebrile or till the antibiotic sensitivities are available.
5. Results of antibiotic sensitivity studies on the operated specimen usually only available days after initiation of antibiotic treatment.
   — choice of antibiotics not necessarily dictated by sensitivity studies
   — change to a more effective antibiotic if patient shows evidence of continued sepsis
   — if patient is already improving clinically, not necessary to change antibiotics on the basis of sensitivity studies.

6. Look out for recurrent infection in the weeks post operatively.
   — Patients with signs of persistent intra-abdominal sepsis should have CT scans to identify collections of pus.
   — If found, CT-directed drainage may be performed.
7. Constant intestinal suction by means of a long, naso-gastric intestinal tube is very important in post-operative care.
   — Ileus can persist post-operatively for a variable period of time and is best treated with the long intestinal tube until there is evidence of peristalsis and patient is passing flatus.
8. Fluid balances and blood chemistry determination is mandatory.
   — Patients with ruptured tubo-ovarian abscess frequently have impaired renal function.
9. Patient can be discharged when well but oral antibiotics should be continued for the next 10–14 days.
10. Radiological imaging can then be used to assess resolution of the condition.

III. Haemorrhage or Leaking Ovarian Cyst and Adnexal Torsion

A. Adnexal torsion

Torsion may happen to any portion of the adnexa. It may occur in young pubescent girls or in the presence of an adnexal cyst, in neoplastic ovaries or as a consequence of hyperstimulation. Laparoscopic detorsion of adnexa is safe and reliable as primary treatment.

Operative strategy and procedure

Laparoscopy has a diagnostic and therapeutic role.

Conservative — untwisting the adnexa, followed by a procedure with no adverse effect on fertility (e.g. cystectomy).

Radical — adnexectomy of twisted adnexa is performed when there is necrotic/non-viable appearance after untwisting ischaemic adnexa.

— However, caution is needed as the surgeon's intra-operative assessment can be poor. Simple untwisting of adnexa that initially appears to be necrotic may allow ovarian function to return. Ovariopexy can be considered especially in young females with normal ovaries.

Preoperative — Benign Ovarian Cyst

Laparoscopic intervention

Laparoscopy can properly treat more than 90% of ovarian cysts.

Indications

1. No evidence suggestive of malignancy.
2. Favourable anatomy: no/minimal adhesions, no ascites/peritoneal nodules.
3. Cosmesis.

Operative strategy

1. Aim: Remove cyst intact with limited trauma to the residual ovarian tissue.
2. Complete excision is preferred over aspiration and "ablation"
   — Thermal ablation results in incomplete destruction of cyst wall, which increases recurrence risk
   — Underlying ovarian cortex may also be damaged by the heat.
3. Three ways to manage ovarian cysts
   — Intact removal
     Provides complete specimen for histological analysis
     Minimises risk of cyst recurrence
     Potentially challenging to achieve for large ovarian cysts (>18 cm in size)
   — Aspiration and excision
     Permits histological analysis of cyst wall
     More care must be taken in the scenario of potential malignancy — intraperitoneal spillage may affect disease-free survival in malignant lesions. However prognosis has not proven to be altered.

More advanced laparoscopic skills to facilitate removal have evolved, for example controlled aspiration within an endoscopic bag.
   — Aspiration with cyst wall ablation
     Ovarian cyst wall is vaporised utilising electrosurgical techniques
     Technique useful in severe pelvic adhesions that may hinder safe dissection
     Does not provide a specimen for histologic analysis and should be preceded by biopsy with frozen section evaluation

Preoperative preparation

1. Ascertain size and nature of ovarian cyst preoperatively
   Physical examination
   Ultrasound
   Serum tumour markers
2. Every patient should be prepared for cancer staging
   Consenting to an open staging procedure
   Consider bowel preparation
   Gynaeoncologist standby
3. Port placement: A port in each lower quadrant, one at umbilicus, one midway between umbilicus and symphysis pubis
   Maintain 10 cm between each port to maximise functionality
   Use 5 mm ports except for one port (10 mm or greater) to facilitate extraction

Operative procedures for benign ovarian conditions

1. Ovarian cystectomy
2. Oophorectomy
3. Salpingo-oophorectomy

1. Laparoscopic ovarian cystectomy

1. Epithelium should be incised and bluntly lifted from the cyst wall to begin (Fig. 17.6).
2. Ovarian cysts are covered by ovarian epithelium of variable thickness.
3. Select a dissection site: thin layer between the cortex and the cyst wall, anti-mesenteric border, good laparoscopic exposure.

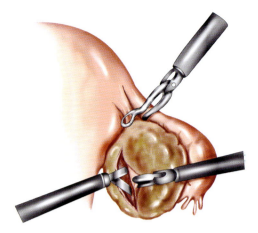

Figure 17.6.

Epithelium incised and bluntly lifted from cyst wall.

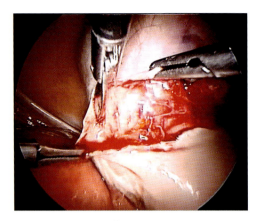

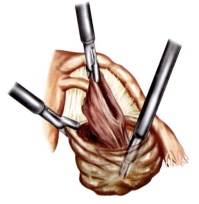

Figure 17.8.

Use grasping forceps for traction and counter traction.

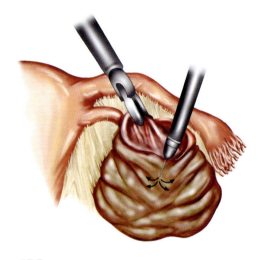

Figure 17.7.

Injecting dilute vasopressin between capsule and ovarian corfex to create a plane for dissection.

4. Inject dilute vasopressin (1:40–1:80 concentration) between the capsule and the ovarian cortex to create a plane for dissection (Fig. 17.7).
5. Incise cortex and strip the ovarian cortex away from the underlying cyst.
6. Use two to three grasping forceps and/or the suction-irrigator probe for traction and counter-traction (Fig. 17.8).
7. Tissue removal: Accomplish without spillage. Gross dimensions of the mass should be roughly known before surgery; this helps in planning regarding port sizes and sites.

Challenges

1. Ovarian endometrioma
   Do not separate readily from ovarian cortex
   Challenging in identifying a dissectible surgical plane
   Dense pelvic adhesions may increase surgical risks of bleeding and visceral organ injury
2. Intact removal of cyst larger than 8 cm laparoscopically is difficult
   Aspirate before removal.
   Large cysts may eventually require partial oophorectomy, using laser or scissors to remove the distorted portion of the ovary. Remaining cyst wall is stripped from the ovarian stroma. Consider laparotomy.
3. Difficulty identifying cyst wall
   Make a new incision with scissors.
   Resultant clean edge may reveal a different plane.

If this fails, grasp base of cyst and apply traction to the cyst with counter-traction to the ovary.

Precautions

1. Incise ovarian cortex without disrupting the cyst

   The initial incision is crucial in dissection of the right plane

   Care must be taken not to be hasty in separating the ovarian cortex

   Peeling of ovarian cortex can be facilitated with water dissection from laparoscopic suction/irrigator device

2. Do note that connections between cyst and ovary vary in strength

   In areas where connections between cortex and cyst are stronger, sharp dissection should be used. Monopolar diathermy can be used to cut these attachments while achieving haemostasis

3. Avoid spillage

   Careful aspiration of contents of ovarian cyst

   Do not attempt to pull the endoscopic retrieval bag out of the abdomen before cyst is collapsed or morcellated. This can cause rupture of the bag and contamination

   In addition, surround extraction site with absorbant material (e.g. surgical sponge, towel) to collect potential tumour spillage

   If spillage occurs, copious irrigation of the abdominal cavity should be performed, using up to 3 L of irrigation fluid

   Ensure that the abdominal incision is of adequate size; the incision may be enlarged to facilitate retrieval of the specimen if necessary

4. Potential of decreased fertility or total ovarian failure after removal of ovarian cyst

   Thought to be a result of removal of excess tissue and/or damage to surrounding stroma from electrocautery, affecting ovarian blood supply

5. Adhesion prophylaxis

   Adhesion prevention barriers promote reepithelialisation, have been shown to significantly reduce post-operative adhesions and may be considered a useful adjuvant in adhesion prophylaxis

   However they are not substitutes for established surgical techniques

2. Laparoscopic ovarian oophorectomy

Operative procedure

1. Ligation of ovarian blood supply:
2. Identify ipsilateral ureter
3. Infundibulopelvic (IP) ligament placed on tension, overlying peritoneum cut (Fig. 17.9)
4. Careful dissection to isolate IP ligament for ligature either using bipolar or surgical tie
5. After division, reflect the IP ligament medially away from the pelvic sidewall
6. Utero-ovarian ligament is divided and dissection begun at the IP ligament
7. Ovary amputated
8. Ensure haemostasis

Challenges

1. Pelvic adhesions and distorted anatomy

   Consider opening the pelvic sidewall to identify the ureter prior to transection of the IP ligament

Precautions

1. Avoidance of ureteric injuries is paramount — good knowledge of pelvic anatomy is essential

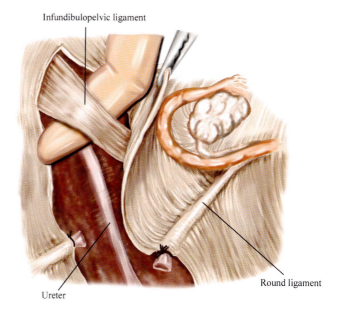

Figure 17.9.

Female pelvic anatomy.

3. Open Cystectomy

Procedure

1. Open entry (midline or Maylard)
2. Elliptic incision made through ovarian cortex (Fig. 17.10)
3. Using end of knife blade, insert and develop a plane over the cyst wall
4. Alternatively, use electrocautery to develop a plane and microsurgical scissors can be used to separate the cyst wall from the ovarian cortex
5. After separating the cyst wall from its adherent attachments with the ovarian cortex, it can be shelled out without rupture using a piece of wet gauze and applying pressure at the interface of cyst and ovarian cortex (Fig. 17.11)

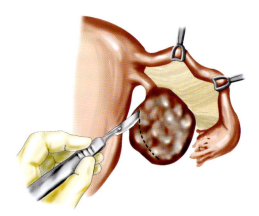

Figure 17.10.

Elliptic incision of ovary.

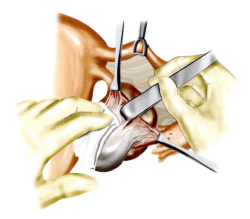

Figure 17.11.

Plane developed.

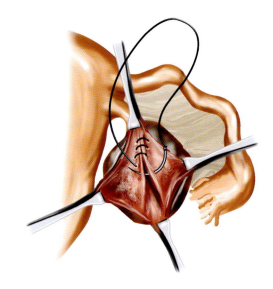

Figure 17.12.

Reconstruction.

6. Before shelling out the cyst, it is important to pack the pouch of Douglas with moist, lint-free pads to prevent any spillage from contaminating the pelvic cavity in the event of rupture
7. Ovary can be reconstructed after cystectomy using 2-0 absorbable sutures (Fig. 17.12).

Special considerations

1. Endometriotic cyst leakage.
   If severe adhesions are present, it is acceptable to perform a laparoscopic washout and leave definitive surgery for a later date if no gynaecologist is present. Under-treated endometriosis has a high recurrence rate and unfamiliarity with pelvic anatomy may increase surgical risks.
2. Special considerations in pregnancy:
   Recommended period for open or laparoscopic intervention: between 13 and 16 weeks gestation
   Tilting the table left or right to move uterus away from site of trocar insertion/abdominal incision.
   Foetal monitoring.
3. Special considerations in obese patients.
   Position the primary trocar rostral to the umbilicus (Palmer's point).
   Using peritoneal pressures of up to 20 mmHg to maximise visibility.
   Using longer trocars.

Chapter 18

Ureteric Injuries

Heng Chin Tiong*

Introduction

The ureters are structures that have over time fallen out of the realm of the general surgeon so much so that most general surgery trainees are not familiar with the principles of surgery for the ureter. In this chapter, we will discuss these general principles, as well as specific operations that deal with ureteric injuries. In any discussion of ureteric surgery, we also need to review the principles of surgery of the bladder, as some of the manoeuvres require the use of bladder wall and mucosa.

Most often, the injuries of concern will involve the middle to distal thirds of the ureter or bladder. The injury is often iatrogenic in origin, where the damage is sustained during dissection of surrounding organs such as the appendix, sigmoid colon or mesorectum.

Review of Anatomy and Exposure of the Ureter

The ureters are retroperitoneal tubular structures that run over the psoas muscles and turn in to the true pelvis around the sacroiliac joints. They then curve in the pelvis crossing the bifurcation of the common iliac artery and winding anterior to the internal iliac artery, then curve anteromedially to the base of the bladder.

For most of its journey, the ureter is closely applied to the posterior peritoneum and tends to lift off the psoas muscle with the peritoneum when mobilised. The ureter is best identified at the pelvic brim. This is achieved on the right side by lifting the caecum and retracting the small bowel mesentery medially. The bifurcation of the common iliacs can also be used as a landmark to trace the ureter. The ureter can be traced superiorly, with the colon mobilised accordingly.

On the left side, the sigmoid mesocolon will need to be retracted superomedially to expose the posterior parietal peritoneum and the ureter, similarly using the crossover at the vessels as a landmark.

When tracing both ureters distally, there will come a segment near the bladder where the vascular arcade crossing from the internal iliac artery to the bladder may obscure the path of the ureter; these may need to be divided.

The ureters are supplied by vessels from the medial side in the upper part of the ureter, and from the lateral side in the pelvic part of the ureter. This is important when considering reconstructive surgery of the ureter. The ureters are retroperitoneal organs and do not have a vascular mesentery. When mobilising the ureter, one should also take a cuff of areolar connective tissue as much as possible to maintain the vascularity of the distal segment of the ureter.

The base of the bladder is deep in the pelvis and would be familiar to pelvic surgeons. When the patient is supine, as is usually the case, the base of the bladder is often "hidden" under the curve of the pubis and surrounded by structures such as the ureters, vesical arteries

*C.T. Heng, MBBS, FRCS (Ed), FAMS (Urology), Senior Consultant, Department of Urology, National University Health System, Singapore.

and uterine arteries. In consideration of ureteric injuries and reconstruction, we should avoid this area as much as possible. What we are more interested in is the dome of the bladder, which rises out of the true pelvis as the bladder distends.

The blood vessels to the dome of the bladder ramify up from the base and cross over the midline, making the bladder dome well vascularised and not prone to ischaemia. The dome itself is largely free to move laterally, or to be pulled superiorly for such manoeuvres as the psoas hitch.

Repair of Bladder Injuries

The bladder dome is a very "forgiving" organ when it comes to its reconstruction. Even after losing a significant amount to resection (i.e. a partial cystectomy), the bladder eventually stretches and regains a significant bladder volume, thus regaining much of its original functional capacity. Injury to the bladder dome is not common if the bladder is decompressed with a urinary catheter, but may occur if there is some fibrosis pulling the bladder dome upwards, such as in a previous Caesarean section scar.

Repair of bladder dome injuries is very straightforward. The basic principle is to trim any ragged edges of the bladder, so that the apposition of the cut edges is straight. There should be a watertight mucosal repair, and structural sutures to the muscle wall. The closure can be accomplished with a single-layer running stitch. However, most urologists will perform a two-layered closure; the first being a mucosal closure, then the second closing the muscular layer (Fig. 18.1).

Basic Direct Anastomotic Repair of the Ureter

In contradistinction to the bladder, the ureters are much more "unforgiving." The bladder dome can be considered to be "free floating," allowing it to be stretched to close any defects. Ureters on the other hand are retroperitoneal, and are much more fixed. Bridging any gap of diseased or injured ureters will involve some amount of mobilisation on either end.

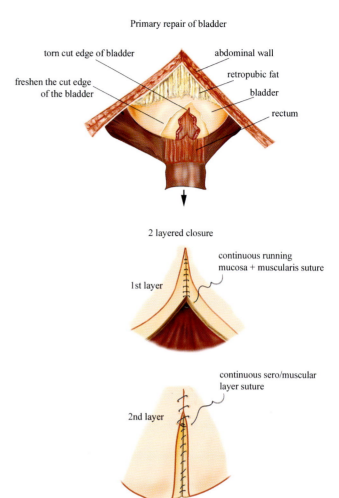

Primary repair of bladder

torn cut edge of bladder
abdominal wall
freshen the cut edge of the bladder
retropubic fat
bladder
rectum

2 layered closure

continuous running mucosa + muscularis suture
1st layer

continuous sero/muscular layer suture
2nd layer

Figure 18.1.

A simple bladder repair, freshening the edges, and closing the bladder in 2 layers.

However, the ureters do not stretch much after mobilisation, and improper technique may lead to ischaemia at the ends and subsequent strictures.

Apart from closing the gap, there needs also to be at least 1cm of overlap, as the cut ends need to be spatulated about 1–1.5 cm. The spatulation affords a wider anastomosis and reduces the risk of a stricture. To achieve this overlap without tension even without any defect to close, the ureters need to be mobilised at least 4–5 cm on either side. With an increasing defect in the ureteric segment, the amount of mobilisation will also increase. Beyond about 2 cm, this is usually impossible without tension.

As mentioned above, the mobilisation should include some of the surrounding areolar tissue so as not to devascularise the cut ends. This areolar tissue can be thinned at the ends especially at the level of the spatulations.

A single-layered closure of the spatulated ends can be made with either a running stitch or with interrupted sutures. Placement of stay sutures from the angle of one spatulation to the other ureteric edge helps to align the ureters and prevent unwanted rotation. The anastomosis is usually done over a double-j or double-pigtail catheter. The general principle is that getting the two mucosal edges to appose without tension is the key to preventing leaks and strictures. Running or locking sutures are not mandatory and reflect the surgeon's preference (Fig. 18.2).

Any defect of more than 2–3 cm will be difficult to repair directly, as it will involve too much ureteric mobilisation or put the repair under tension. Furthermore, if the injury is very distal, a direct ureteroneocystostomy will be a much more reliable repair.

Ureteroneocystostomy (Ureteric Reimplantation) and Psoas Hitch

In essence, the proximal cut end is anastomosed directly onto the dome or posterior aspect of the bladder. The bladder is distended with normal saline to bring the bladder dome up to the level of the proximal ureteric end. The proximal ureteric end is mobilised and spatulated. A small defect is created in the dome of the bladder on the ipsilateral side to match the spatulated end of the ureter.

Two stay sutures at the angles of the spatulation to the angles of the bladder dome defect bring the ureter to the bladder dome. There should be no tension or kinking of the ureter. A direct anastomosis taking the mucosa of the ureter to the mucosa of the bladder is performed with either interrupted or running stitches, over a double J-stent.

To create an antireflux mechanism at the anastomosis, a short defect can be created in the muscularis of the bladder but not incising the mucosa, in line with the initial anastomosis. The bladder wall is then closed over the anastomosis and the muscular defect, creating a submucous segment of the ureteric anastomosis. The distal ureteric segment is tied off.

This operation affords a much more reliable repair than direct ureteric reanastomosis. Furthermore, in very distal ureteric injuries, there is not enough distal ureter to be mobilised adequately.

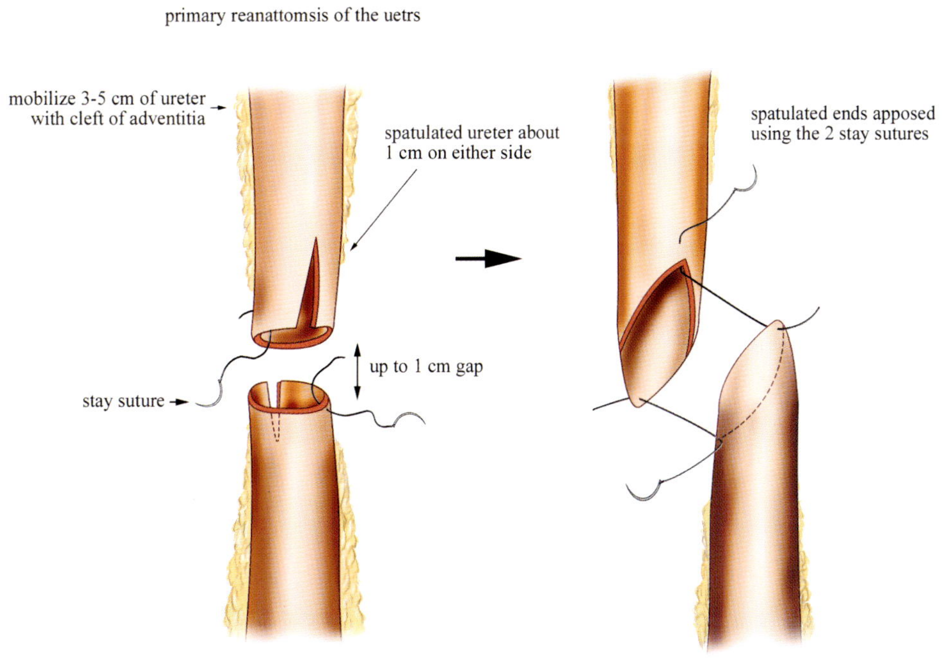

primary reanattomsis of the uetrs

mobilize 3-5 cm of ureter with cleft of adventitia

spatulated ureter about 1 cm on either side

stay suture

up to 1 cm gap

spatulated ends apposed using the 2 stay sutures

Figure 18.2.

Primary anastomosis of the ureters. The stent is omitted from the diagram for clarity.

In some situations, the ureteric end is too high and a simple ureteric reimplantation creates some tension. To reduce this tension, a modified Psoas hitch can be performed. The dome of the bladder can be stretched gently to the ipsilateral side, and several sutures used to tack the bladder to the psoas muscle. This elevates the highest portion of the bladder. The tacking sutures take much of the tension away from the anastomosis (Fig. 18.3).

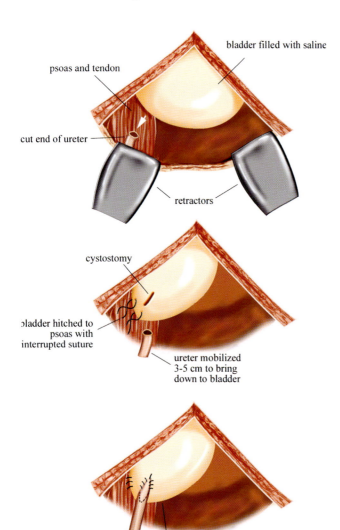

Figure 18.3.

Modified Psoas hitch. The stent is omitted from the diagram for clarity.

Boari Flap

In the event that even with a Psoas hitch, the distance to the cut end of the proximal ureter cannot be bridged, a more major reconstructive procedure will be required. This manoeuvre takes advantage of the unique properties of the bladder, in that a flap of bladder wall can be raised off the dome, and the remaining bladder closed off, while retaining much of the function of the bladder.

The flap should be based from posterolaterally on the ipsilateral side to maximise the vascular integrity of the flap. The defect is measured using a flexible ruler, and the same length off the distended bladder dome measured off. A U-shaped flap from posterolaterally with a wider base and narrower tip is raised off the bladder dome.

The defect in the bladder is then closed off. The ureteric edge can then be anastomosed directly to the tip of the flap or with a submucous tunnel, over a double-J stent. The flap is then fully tubularised. The end result should look like a smaller bladder with a horn-shaped extension which is connected to the ureter.

A Boari flap can potentially bridge very long segment defects of the distal ureter, even up to the pelvic brim or higher (Fig. 18.4).

Other Manoeuvres

Longer segment ureteric injuries in the upper ureter are particularly problematic. The Boari flap may not traverse such distances, and there may not be enough length of the ureter to mobilise to allow direct anastomosis. Reconstructive procedures such as a transureteroureterostomy or an ileal interposition graft are much more complex and are beyond the scope of this chapter. Artificial grafts are presently not a standard of care in terms ureteric surgery.

A direct cutaneous ureterostomy should not be attempted as the stoma almost inevitably will necrose and retract. If the proper facilities exist, the

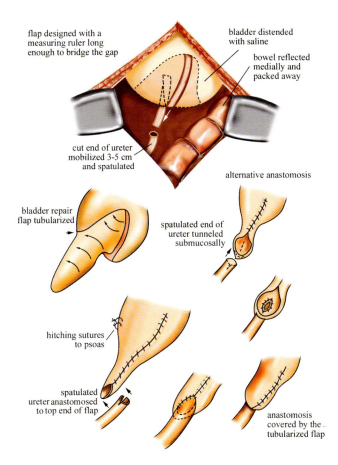

flap designed with a measuring ruler long enough to bridge the gap

bladder distended with saline

bowel reflected medially and packed away

cut end of ureter mobilized 3-5 cm and spatulated

alternative anastomosis

bladder repair flap tubularized

spatulated end of ureter tunneled submucosally

hitching sutures to psoas

spatulated ureter anastomosed to top end of flap

anastomosis covered by the tubularized flap

Figure 18.4.

Boari flap. The stent is omitted from the diagram for clarity.

proximal end should be tied off and a percutaneous nephrostomy inserted post-operatively. This preserves as much ureteric length as possible for subsequent reconstructive procedures.

Post-Operative Care

For most operations involving repair or anastomosis of the ureter, a double-pigtail urinary catheter is placed. The usual size is 6 Fr. This may be between 24 and 28 cm in length, but a multi-length catheter will fit most situations.

The bladder should be kept empty for the immediate post-operative period, to avoid reflux of urine up the stent. Additionally an abdominal drain can be considered to control the situation in the event of significant urinary extravasation.

For ureteric anastomosis, after 24–48 hours, the catheter can be removed and the patient allowed to void spontaneously. If there is any significant reflux and extravasation, it may show up in the abdominal drain at this time, which can then be removed after another 24 hours if there is no further drainage. For other operations involving the bladder, the catheter should be left for 1–2 weeks, and a check cystogram performed before it is removed.

The stent is left *in situ* for about 4–6 weeks. Some patients may develop irritation of the bladder resulting in urinary frequency and occasional haematuria. These symptoms may be managed with oral anticholinergic drugs such as tolterodine or oxybutynin. There may also be some ipsilateral loin ache during micturition, presumably from the pressure reflux during voiding. After 4–6 weeks, the stent can be easily removed with a flexible cystoscope and a rat-toothed grasper.

The healing is best demonstrated by an intravenous urogram, which gives a clear anatomical outline of the ureter or flap, as well as a qualitative depiction of urinary flow or obstruction.

Conclusion

The properties of the ureters being retroperitoneal and without any significant vascular mesentery makes repair of ureteric injuries unique as far as abdominal tubular structures are concerned. While some amount of defect can be bridged by direct mobilisation and repair, longer segments in the distal ureter or pelvic ureter are better served by utilising the bladder in the reconstruction.

Injuries to the more proximal ureters are more difficult to reconstruct and may need the bowel as an interposition. This operation should be left to the expert surgeon.

Chapter 19

Ruptured and Leaking Abdominal Aortic Aneurysms

Benjamin Chua Soo Yeng* and Peter Ashley Robless**

Ruptured or leaking abdominal aortic aneurysms are associated with a significantly high mortality rate, ranging from 50% to 80% in the preoperative period. The main determinant of survival is prompt diagnosis and emergent surgery. The classical presentation is the triad of a pulsatile abdominal mass, pallor and hypotension. These patients may give a preceding history of severe central abdominal pain with radiation to the back. In addition they have a significant history of smoking, hypertension and hyperlipidaemia. Frequently, there may not be enough time to elucidate such history from the patients.

I. General Principles of Management of Ruptured/ Leaking AAAs Include:

(1) When the patient presents with hypotension, fluid resuscitation should be aggressive but judicious. First-line fluid replacement should be with blood products (even using type O– blood if the situation requires it). Permissive hypotension should be the primary resuscitation endpoint, i.e. systolic BP of between 80 and 90 mmHg.

(2) If the suspicion is that of a frank rupture of the AAA, the patient should be rushed to the operating theatre without delay. There is no role for CT scan in a patient who is in frank hypotension or *in extremis*. However, a bedside ultrasound scan at the emergency room may be useful in aiding diagnosis. Key features of a leaking/ruptured AAA on an ultrasound include the presence of an aneurysmal aorta, free fluid in the peritoneum or a surrounding hematoma.

(3) If, however, after resuscitation, the BP is stable and the suspicion is that of a slow leaking or sealed leaking AAA, a CT scan may be useful to image the AAA and help plan the approach to management.

(4) The OT should be kept at a warm but comfortable temperature and the patient covered with warm blankets until surgery. Warmed saline for wash should be on standby at all times. Hypothermia can worsen any existing coagulopathy.

(5) In the OT, the whole surgical team must be scrubbed and the patient cleaned and draped before the patient is induced and general anaesthesia given.

*Benjamin S.Y. Chua, MBBS, MHsc (Duke), FRCS (Ed), Head and Consultant, Department of Vascular Surgery, Singapore General Hospital; Adj Asst Prof, Dept of Surgery, Yong Loo Lin School of Medicine, National University of Singapore; Adi Asst of Surgery, Duke-NUS Graduate School of Medicine.

** Peter A. Robless, MD (Lond), MBChB (Aberd), FRCS (Ed), FEBVS, Associate Professor, Department of Surgery, National University of Singapore, Singapore, and Department of Cardiac, Thoracic and Vascular Surgery, National University Health System, Singapore.

II. Perioperative Care

Several adjuncts should be considered in the perioperative period. These include the extensive use of haemodynamic monitoring devices, i.e. arterial line, central venous catheters and pulmonary arterial wedge pressure (Swan–Gantz) catheters. Expert anaesthetic help should be enlisted for the insertion and monitoring of these devices in the perioperative period. In the OT, a Level 1 rapid blood infuser should be available, as should be an auto-transfusion device. Post-surgery, all patients should be closely monitored in the ICU. We usually do not commence enteral feeding until patient is out of the critically ill period and there is at least flatus passage. In addition, in the ICU, patients should be monitored for:

(a) Severe abdominal pain — suggestive of bowel ischaemia secondary to atherosclerotic plaque/blood clot emboli.
(b) Lower limb circulation and pulses — loss of pulses and the development of dusky toes also suggest plaque/clot emboli.
(c) Cardiovascular events.
(d) Acute renal failure — signs include low urine output, rising serum creatinine levels.
(e) Acute abdominal compartment syndrome, especially if bleeding was severe and surgery prolonged — signs include decreased urine output associated with increasing abdominal girth, increasing abdominal compartment pressure (>20 mmHg when using transvesical pressure measurements) and increasing ventilatory requirements.

III. Open Repair: Surgical Technique and Principles

Open surgical repairs of ruptured AAAs are tenuous affairs that can be intimidating to the general surgeon not exposed to such events previously. However, the surgical technique of open repair is a necessary tool that every general surgeon should be familiar with and be competent at. The following principles should be applied:

(1) Insert a nasogastric tube — this will help in identification of the oesophagus during blunt

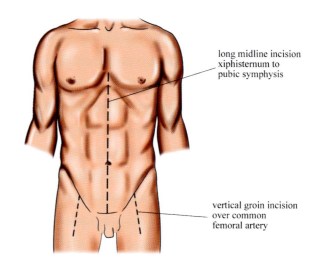

long midline incision xiphisternum to pubic symphysis

vertical groin incision over common femoral artery

Figure 19.1.

Dotted lines showing incisions to be made to gain access to aorta and common femoral arteries.

dissection to control the supraceliac aorta thus avoiding iatrogenic injury.
(2) Long midline incision from xiphisternum to symphysis pubis — use Mayo scissors to cut the Linea Alba if needed. There is no role for initial small incisions with the intent of extension when needed. The amount of blood loss can be large and control difficult. Thus, the initial abdominal wall incision should be generous (Fig. 19.1).
(3) Once abdominal cavity is entered, the overlying small bowel is lifted out of the abdomen, reflected to the right and packed into a plastic bag or with warm Penny towels. All clots are evacuated and aneurismal bleeding temporised by packing with Penny towels (Fig. 19.2).
(4) Identify the aneurysm neck by dissecting upwards from point of rupture. For juxtarenal aneurysms or aneurysms that extend beyond the celiac axis and in situations of massive uncontrollable bleeding, supraceliac clamping of the aorta should be carried out. This can be done by dividing the triangular ligament of the left lobe of the liver and reflecting the left lobe medially. Blunt finger dissection is then used to isolate the plane between the oesophagus and aorta, utilising the NG tube as a guide. If necessary, use a diathermy to divide some fibres of the left crus of diaphragm. Retract the oesophagus laterally. Once the aorta is freed

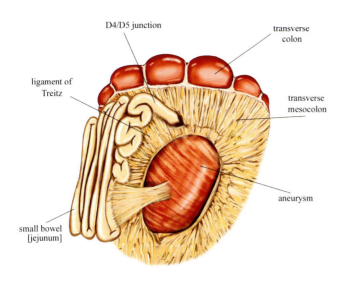

Figure 19.2.

Evisceration of the bowel to expose the retroperitoneum and infrarenal aortic aneurysm.

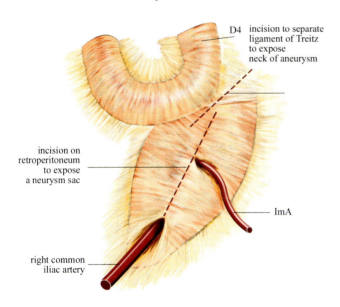

Figure 19.3.

Line of incision on the retroperitoneum to expose the aneurysm and common iliac arteries.

and felt between the fingers, an occlusive aortic clamp is applied, pressing against the vertebra. Note that if a supraceliac clamp is applied, surgery has to be expedient as irreversible ischaemia of the viscera can set in after half an hour.

(5) For infrarenal AAAs, reflect the duodenum off the aorta using sharp scissor dissection, approaching from the left paracolic gutter of the patient (Fig. 19.3). Dissection with scissors

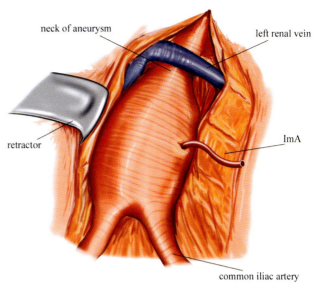

Figure 19.4.

Exposure of the aneurysm with key vessels shown.

rather than diathermy is preferred for this step to prevent cautery injury to the duodenum. Once done, the left renal vein should identified (it runs across the aorta from left to right) and retracted superiorly. If the neck is tortuous or aneurysmal beyond the left renal vein then the vein should be divided to allow better access to the neck (Fig. 19.4).

(6) Identify the inferior mesenteric artery (IMA) that travels to the left and inferiorly.

(7) Using blunt finger dissection, free all loose surrounding tissue between the left renal vein and the aneurysm neck.

(8) Free the peritoneal tissue on both sides of the aortic neck. Avoid the urge to encircle the aorta and sling it. Doing so may injure the accompanying inferior vena cava.

(9) Once the aorta can be pinched between the thumb and index fingers, using the fingers as a guide, apply an occlusive aortic clamp. If there is great difficulty in visualising the neck for clamp application, consider inserting an occlusive balloon into the aneurysm's neck for temporary control and further dissection (Fig. 19.5).

(10) Once proximal control is obtained, allow the anaesthetist to proceed with resuscitation and stabilise the patient.

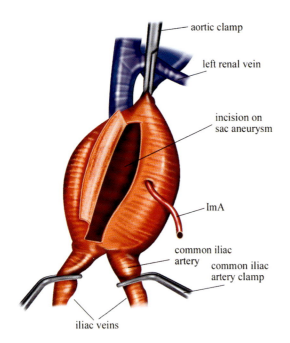

Figure 19.5.

Application of occlusive vascular clamps before opening into the aneurysmal sac.

(11) Identify the iliac bifurcation and divide the peritoneum overlying the iliac vessels. Free the peritoneum overlying the iliac arteries. Avoid injuring the ureter that lies in close proximity to the arteries at the pelvic brim. It nominally crosses the bifurcation of the common iliac artery into external and internal iliac arteries at the pelvic brim. If there is a large retroperitoneal haematoma, the position of the ureter can be distorted. A quick way to identify it is to lightly pinch it with forceps and observe for peristalsis (vermiculations). Extreme care must be taken when dissecting around the iliac artery to avoid damaging the iliac vein. Do not attempt to encircle and sling the iliac arteries as the iliac veins are closely applied and may be damaged in the process Injury to and perforation of the iliac vein can be very difficult to control and repair and can sometimes be catastrophic.

(12) Apply occlusive clamps on both iliacs and extend the opening of the aneurismal sac (Fig. 19.6).

(13) Once the contents of the aneurysm have been evacuated, identify back-bleeding lumbar artery points and oversew these with Prolene 2/0 or 1/0 sutures.

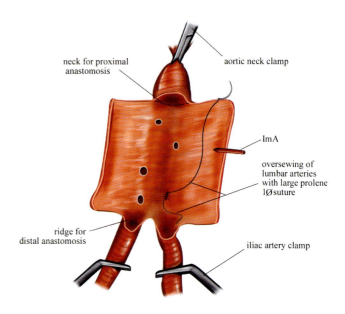

Figure 19.6.

Aneurysm sac laid open to expose the back-bleeding lumbar arteries.

(14) Identify the IMA opening from within the sac — if there is healthy back-bleeding, then this opening can be oversewn. If back-bleeding is poor, consider re-implanting the IMA.

(15) If the aneurysm extends up to the iliac bifurcation, a straight tube Dacron graft can be used — be certain to use gel-impregnated or pre-clotted grafts. If there is/are concomitant common iliac aneurysms, use a bifurcated graft.

(16) For the proximal anastomosis, incise and divided the aneurismal sac laterally in a horizontal manner to develop a circular neck for suturing the graft.

(17) Using a double-ended polypropelene 3/0 suture, begin by utilising the parachute technique. Start outside-in on the graft followed by inside-out on the native artery using one arm of the suture. Begin at the centre of the back wall and work towards yourself (Fig. 19.7).

(18) Take a series of bites on the graft first and then the aorta, making sure to take a shelf of aortic tissue.

(19) Once the anastomosis is completed, release the proximal clamp and check for leaks. Any leaking point should be sutured with polypropelene 3/0,

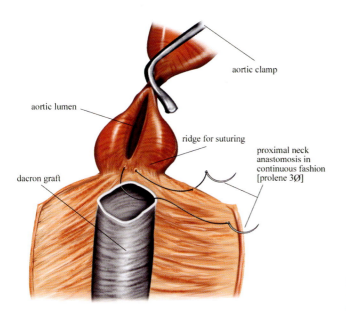

Figure 19.7.

Proximal anastomosis — suturing of the dacron graft onto the aneurysm neck using continuous prolene suture. Note occlusive clamps in position.

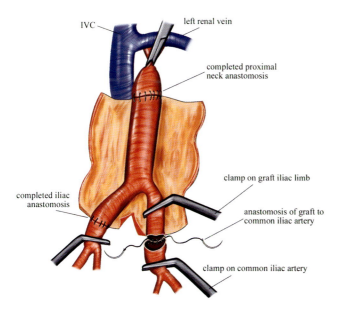

Figure 19.8.

Distal anastomosis — suturing of the dacron graft onto common iliac arteries using continuous prolene suture.

using Teflon pledgets for buttressing if needed (Fig. 19.8).

(20) If there is/are concomitant iliac anaeurysms, the bifurcated limbs of the graft should be

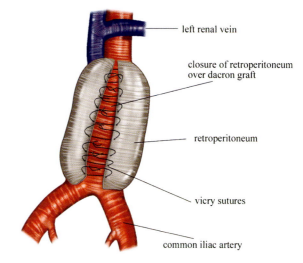

Figure 19.9.

Closure of the aneurysm sac and then the retroperitoneum over the dacron graft after haemostasis of the anastomoses.

sutured beyond the aneurysm. Either a graft to artery end-to-end or a graft end to artery side anastomosis can be used. Again, the parachute technique is useful in this context.

(21) Once the distal anastomosis is almost completed, release one of the iliac clamps and squeeze the thigh to get adequate back-bleed and flush out all distal debris. The clamp is then re-applied to the same iliac limb and the proximal aortic clamp released to allow forward flush. Then complete the anastomosis and release the iliac and then the aortic clamp. There should be a drop in the blood pressure initially following perfusion of one lower limb. Follow through with releasing the other artery iliac clamp in a similar fashion.

(22) If during back-bleeding of the iliac arteries, there is poor flow, consider passing a Fogarty Size 3 or 4 embolectomy catheters down both illiacs into the femoral arteries to evacuate emboli and debris.

(23) Close the original aneurismal sac over the inlaid graft as an extra protective layer using absorbable sutures and then the retroperitoneum over the sac (Fig. 19.9).

(24) Consider using temporary abdominal closure techniques if there is excessive bowel oedema and primary abdominal closure is under tension.

IV. Mycotic Aneurysms

Occasionally, patients can present with symptomatic AAAs with features of sepsis. In such circumstances, the presence of a mycotic aneurysm should be suspected. Emergent CT angiograms should be done. In addition, blood cultures should be collected as most of these patients will require tailored long-term antibiotic therapy post-surgery. At surgery, the presence of infected tissue precludes the insertion of prosthetic Dacron or stent grafts. As such, extra-anatomic aortic repair is the surgery of choice for mycotic aneurysms. Most surgeons will proceed to perform an axillobifemoral bypass with ligation of the aorta and debridement of the infected aneurismal sac. Even so, morbidity and mortality post-surgery is still significant.

V. Endovascular Stenting of Ruptured/Leaking AAAs

With the advent of endovascular techniques, stent grafting of ruptured/leaking AAAs is becoming a routine procedure in many units worldwide. Stent grafting has a few advantages over open repair — it can be done under local anaesthesia with IV sedation, only small groin incisions are needed, and it is suitable for patients with severe co-morbidities that may not tolerate general anesthesia. However, units planning to offer stent grafting should have a high volume of elective AAA stent graft cases have good imaging (CT scan) modalities and have a well-rehearsed and streamlined patient flow pathway from the ED to the OT. Several principles are applicable:

(1) Prompt diagnosis and imaging — the CT scan is crucial if stent graft insertion is to be done. High-resolution contrast-enhanced CT angiograms should be performed (1–3-mm thick slice cuts). There should be as minimal a delay as possible from the ED to CT scan and to OT.

(2) Judicious and aggressive fluid management with permissive hypotension. If needed, massive blood transfusion may be given, but observe for coagulopathy.

(3) The stent grafting should be performed in a fully equipped OT suite and not in a catheter lab setting as there may be a need for conversion to open repair.

(4) Consider insertion of an aortic occlusion balloon as a prelude to stent grafting, especially if the bleeding is severe.

The same inclusion criteria used for stent grafting in an elective setting is applied for emergent cases:

(1) Suitable anatomy (Table 19.1).
(2) Good renal function — should not have concurrent renal impairment as determined by a raised serum creatinine level. If, however, a decision is made for post-operative haemodialysis support, then abnormal creatinine values are not a contraindication.
(3) No contrast allergy issues.

Table 19.1.

Anatomic Requirements for EVAR

a. Neck length — at least 2 cm from the lowest renal artery
b. Aneurysmal neck angulation less than 60°
c. External iliac artery vessels — Minimal tortuosity and
d. adequate diameter (suitable for a 12 French Gauge working sheath)
e. Calcification of vessels — minimal calcification of iliac vessels

VI. Post-Surgery Follow-up

Following successful surgery, patients will require lifelong follow-up to detect early and late complications of aortic surgery. For patients who have undergone open repair, CT scans are repeated at 30 days, six months and one year. Subsequently, yearly ultrasound scans can be repeated at the discretion of the vascular surgeon. Some complications associated with open repair include anastomotic line dehiscence, graft thromobosis, graft infection with formation of graft-enteric fistulae. Patients who have had endovascular stent graft repair should have CT scans done at one month, three months, six months, one year and yearly thereafter for life. Some complications to look out for include endoleaks, graft migration and graft infection.

Chapter 20

Management of Severe Blunt Abdominal Injury

Philip Iau* and Mikael Hartman**

I. Introduction and Indications

Trauma is the leading cause of death under the age of 45 years, more common than cancer and infectious disease. This trend is likely to continue with the increase in global industrialisation and access to motor vehicles. Abdominal trauma accounts for a fifth of seriously injured patients. Recent developments have led to a decrease in preventable death rates in trauma. These include the recognition of a multidisciplinary approach, the establishment of tailored trauma care centres, improvements in resuscitation and intensive care and acceptance of the damage control concept in the treatment of the severely injured.

II. Preoperative Management

Care In EMD

A common shortcoming that emerges in trauma audits (and medico–legal discussions) is the absence of senior surgical consult at the emergency department. In our hospital, all priority one cases involve the trauma consultant attending. Our advice is to have a policy of attending the resuscitation rather than having the arrangement of being called in only when the registrar realises he (or she) is in trouble. Good trauma

surgery is all about making the correct decisions in a very truncated time interval, and maximal exposure to the patient's clinical status over time is vital for this. The subtle judgment call needed in many patients with abdominal trauma is not well-served by the phone consult. Are there other system injuries? Is the bleeding intraperitoneal, retroperitoneal or both? Does the patient have a fractured pelvis better served with external fixators and angio-embolisation rather than an opened abdomen? Do we have time for a CT or should we go straight in?

Before leaving EMD, the following should be in place: a clear surgical plan about who goes first among the different specialties in a patient with multi-system injuries; blood and plasma available; NG tube and catheter in place, and basic labs — base excess, standard coagulopathy profiles or thromboelastography and urine pregnancy test if appropriate.

III. OT Preparation

Another advantage of having a senior surgeon in the resuscitation is that decisions can be made quickly and anaesthesiologists and theatre nurses are familiar the surgeon's requirements. Among the essentials are:

- Warm theatre — in patients in shock with an open cavity this can make the difference between treatable

* Department of Surgery, National University Hospital, Singapore.
** Saw Swee Hock School of Public Health, National University of Singapore; and Department of Medical Epidemiology and Biostatistics, Karolinska Institute, Sweden.

coagulopathy and irreversible hypothermia. A 33 degree core body temperature is the equivalent of Von Willebrand disease, a condition most of us avoid doing major surgery on.

- While it may not be possible to anticipate every eventuality, certain items may be used often enough to be included in an abdominal trauma set: "liver sutures" of catgut on large blunt needles, multifire staples for finger fracture for major liver laceration, cotton tape for tying off small bowel. Get surgical towels and retractors set up, with the instrument and sutures you anticipate bowel, vascular clamps of various sizes and configurations if abdominal vascular injury is suspected.

- Have a massive transfusion protocol activated as necessary. This might save you the ordeal of having the bowel become more edematous before your eyes as the anaesthetist gives crystalloids in lieu of blood products which have not been sent fast enough.

- If the situation calls for you to "crash" theatre, tell everyone to dispense with the formal surgical scrub. Tell the nurses to gown and get trays ready and hand you the knife.

- Never leave the patient's side — be present at all times. Trauma patients are notoriously unpredictable and things can turn on a hair. As the most senior man in house, regardless of how senior you really are, you're carrying the can. Even if you are unlikely to have to perform surgery, it's on your watch until another surgeon takes him over.

IV. Operative Procedure

The standard operating position is supine with arms outstretched for vascular access. Warming blankets for the head, arms and legs are recommended (Fig. 20.1). A urinary catheter (and pregnancy test where appropriate) is done at the emergency department. Skin cleansing includes the neck to the knees in preparation for extension of surgical field as necessary.

The standard abdominal incision for the crash laparotomy is the long midline from xiphisternum to pubic symphysis. The unstable multiply injured patient who needs a crash laparotomy and then to move on to

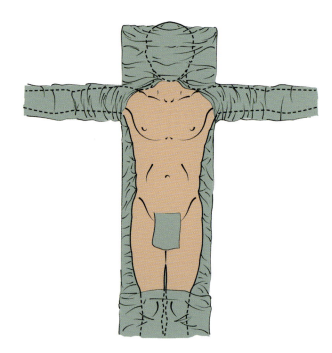

Figure 20.1.

Crash laparotomy exposure.

treatment of other associated body systems will not appreciate the diathermy entry. Use the No. 10 blade through the skin and subcutaneous tissue, the linea Alba, and then enter the abdomen with an index finger through the fairly consistent supra umbilical gap in the midline. The rest of the incision is completed with Mayo scissors up and down.

Keep in mind that by opening the abdominal cavity, whatever blood pressure is left is likely to disappear, thus have a clear plan and stick to it. In cases with severe, on-going intra peritoneal bleeding, you are now faced with the bowel floating in a bucket of blood and the blood starting to get on the drapes and onto your clogs. Hopefully this is not a surprise. How do you gain control? It is difficult to get the blood out with the bowels in place, and impossible to achieve this with suction. The fastest way to get blood out of the way and to control your mess is three simple steps:

Eviscerate. Take the bowel out of the abdominal cavity on its mesentery. If there are any obvious enterotomies, close them quickly either with Babcock forceps or cotton tape to avoid further contamination. Clamp what obvious mesenteric bleeders there are, move on.

Pack each side as the bowels are lifted out; try to pack the most obvious bleeding quadrant first. Have the nurse hand you the packs folded (the way she received them from their sterilisation wraps) — it makes packing a lot quicker and more compact

Inspect the retroperitoneal area as you take the packs out. A central expanding haematoma on the left suggests aortic injury, on the right, inferior vena cava injury. Both may need visceral rotation and sets for vascular repair. Nurses and anaesthetists like to know about these things early.

After the pooled blood has been removed, you should have some idea what you're dealing with. The next step is to see if you need to make any immediate life-saving procedures. Did his blood pressure crash to unrecordable levels in the few minutes you took to take out the blood? If so, you need to clamp the aorta. Does he continue to have no recordable vital signs despite a clamped aorta? Then you need to do a pericardial window.

Use your hands and eyes and start to prioritise what needs to be done. Is it a big liver tear that requires you to think of packing, a spleen that comes out easily, or something simple like a mesenteric tear that just needs tying off?

Damage Control Mode

Now, before you get tunnelled into your definitive surgery, stop for a minute and think tactically: Do a "surgical timeout": Are you in damage control mode? (see Table 20.1). Now that you pretty much know what's in the abdomen, does it fit his clinical picture? Is there enough blood here to account for his degree

Table 20.1.

Indications for Damage Control Surgery (DCS)

Severe metabolic acidosis pH<7.2
Core hypothermia <35°C
Coagulopathic INR >1.5
Operating time >90 min
Inaccessible venous injury
Visceral edema
Life threatening extra abdominal injuries
Need for re-look laparotomy assessment

of shock, or should you start thinking about bleeding from elsewhere? Are those chest drains that were inserted in the resuscitation room still oscillating, or are you wishing you had been there to oversee the emergency room instead of relying on secondhand information now? Where is he likely to go after your operation? How long are you likely to take, and when do you want orthopaedics or the neurosurgeons to come in? Do you need more hands in the abdomen? In other words, plan your war. Delays in transfer are fodder for the surgical audit and not good for the patient. How often have you been impressed by surgeons discussing the next step as the patient remains cold in theatre and under general anaesthesia? Cut down the dead time between interventions by planning ahead.

What happens now depends on what you have found. For ease of description, we will divide the approach into what can be removed, what can be temporised and what needs to be fixed. Fast surgeons don't have hands that move quicker, they just have to do things only once and then they move on. Mindful of this, we will describe each part of what follows in terms of key manoeuvres that are often the rate determining step to the operation and key hazards to avoid.

Splenic Injuries

The spleen is the most frequently injured organ in the abdomen. While splenorrhaphy is an accepted alternative in some cases, in our experience this is not commonly done. Patients who are stable tend to have time for a CT scan, which characterises accurately the spleens that can be conserved, and patients who are unstable deserve a splenectomy.

The key to successful splenectomy is exposure. Take the incision to the xiphisternum and have a retractor under the left subcostal. If there is a distended stomach, decompress it with the NG tube. Divide to splenic flexure between clamps and reflect the colon inferiorly. The key manoeuvre is division of the splenorenal ligament, and often this needs to be done "blind," by palpation only (Fig. 20.2). With the splenic flexure out of the way, grab the spleen in your left hand and feel the tightening of the splenorenal ligament at your fingertips. With your right hand and a pair of long Nelson scissors, divide this peritoneal reflection, and the spleen

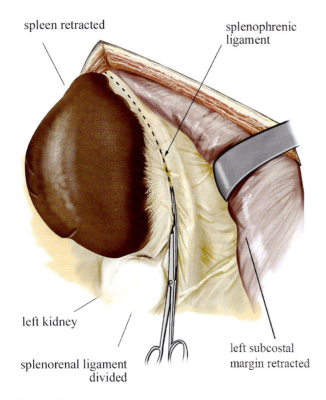

spleen retracted

splenophrenic
ligament

left kidney

splenorenal ligament
divided

left subcostal
margin retracted

Figure 20.2.

Dividing the splenorenal and splenophrenic ligament.

in your hand is now freely in the midline. The short gastric and splenic hilar vessels can now be taken between clamps. For speed and preservation of the pancreatic tail and greater curvature, we tend to use clamps on only one side as close to the spleen as possible.

Once the spleen is out, secure haemostasis and pack the splenic bed. Do your completion laparotomy (see below) and come back and check haemostasis again later. If pancreatic tail injury is suspected, leave in a drain.

Bowel Injuries

Assess bowel viability in the usual way: size of defect, peristalsis, sheen and size of contusion. When in doubt and remnant bowel length is not an issue (at least 2 m), resect. Continuity is restored with a hand-sewn anastomosis or stapling. Two special conditions should be considered in the treatment of bowel injuries. First, it may not be necessary to restore continuity: A patient in shock with splanchnic vasoconstriction from physiological and possibly even pharmacological inotropes may not be the best candidate for anastomosis of any

part of his edematous bowel. Tie off or staple off the ends, ensure a large size 18 NG tube is in its rightful place in the stomach, fashion a temporary abdominal dressing and come back in a day or two.

Second, avoid stomas. They are not necessary for the reasons given above and complicate wound management in temporary abdominal closure (see below). Much more preferable to have a dedicated re-look and join the bowel back then when warm and stable. A better appreciation of bowel viability can also be made at the time.

Kidney Injuries

A preoperative contrast CT scan is ideal for assessing the need for surgical intervention in renal injuries and has the additional benefit of demonstrating the presence of an opposite functioning remnant kidney should nephrectomy be required in unstable patients. However, time for a preoperative CT may not always be available, and the most common presentation is that of a zone 2 retroperitoneal haematoma. The key consideration then is whether the haematoma is expanding, and whether the patient has any other likely sources of exsanguination. The first assessment of this haematoma is usually carried out at the initial phase of a trauma laparotomy as intraperitoneal blood is cleared during evisceration, and a second is made a few minutes later when other life-threatening injuries have been addressed. Before deciding on exploration, a few considerations are needed.

Is exploration really necessary? In the absence of a clear tract that can be repaired in the penetrating trauma scenario, renal exploration in the setting of blunt injury almost always results in a nephrectomy. If expansion of the haematoma is not obvious or if there is only a small leak into the peritoneal cavity, packing with a planned re-look operation after stabilisation and imaging of the calyceal system is an attractive option. If the calyceal system is intact, the second operation is usually no more than a removal of packs.

However, if the expansion of the retroperitoneal haematoma is obvious even after a few minutes of entering the abdomen and especially if there are no other sites of significant surgical bleeding, you are in big trouble. The setting is that of renal injury with associated midline vascular tear, either aorta or vena cava, and now is a good time to get help. And blood products.

The initial approach depends on which of these scenarios presides. In the case of penetrating injury where repair of renal lacerations is planned, vascular control of the renal pedicles is obtained by a retroperitoneal dissection that starts just below the ligament of Treitz. Where major vascular injury is considered, access to the retroperitoneal space and its vasculature is obtained via visceral rotation (Mattox or Cattell–Brasch procedures) (see section on abdominal vascular repair); where major vascular injury is not suspected in a patient with an expanding haematoma but is otherwise clinically stable, a limited retroperitoneal exposure described here can be untaken first and extended further if necessary.

On the left side, the hazards are the spleen and tail of pancreas superiorly. Access to the retroperitoneal space is obtained by dividing the splenic flexure between clamps, and then dissecting the descending colon along its avascular plane (Fig. 20.3). On the

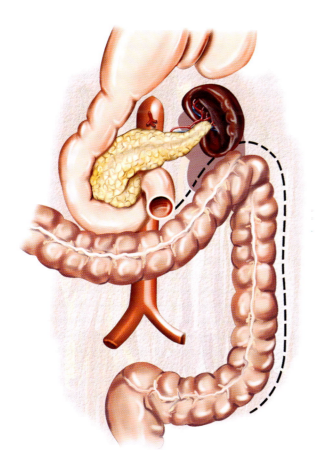

Figure 20.3.

Plane of left vicero-rotation

right, access to the kidney often requires partial Kocherisation of the duodenum followed by a similar mobilisation of the ascending colon medially. Often the required plane around the renal capsule has already been made by the retroperitoneal haematoma and dissecting the colon medially allows for blunt dissection to entirely enclose the kidney. Dissection continues to renal hilum where the renal vein is ligated and artery and ureter transfixed. A drain in the renal bed is advisable.

Pancreatic Injuries

The pancreas is more commonly injured from penetrating than blunt injuries, and blunt injuries can vary from mild contusions to life-threatening pancreaticoduodenal vascular catastrophes. Thankfully, more often than not, pancreatic injuries are detected during part of the completion laparotomy (see below), and treatment is usually straightforward.

What you need to determine (in increasing severity) is: contusion versus laceration, ductal injury or not, left or right of the superior mesenteric artery and pancreaticoduodenal complex injuries with vascular involvement. To make this decision you will need to have access to the entire pancreas.

The pancreas cannot be assessed with an intact gastrocolic ligament. As part of the standard completion laparotomy, the NG is checked in the stomach and used as an excellent splint along the greater curvature of the stomach. This allows for easy identification of an avascular approach usually found on the right side of the gastrocolic ligament. By entering the lesser sac and reflecting the stomach superiorly, the entire anterior surface of the pancreas can be assessed. Usually this is all that is required to screen for pancreatic injuries. However, if there are significant contusions, lacerations, or haematomas, complete assessment of the pancreas requires three more steps.

Kocherisation of the duodenum with reflection of the pancreatic head over the anterior surface of the IVC allows for the assessment of the head of the pancreas between left finger and thumb.

Division of the splenic flexure of the colon and mobilisation of the spleen from its peritoneal attachments allows for the spleen and tail of pancreas to be reflected medially for assessment.

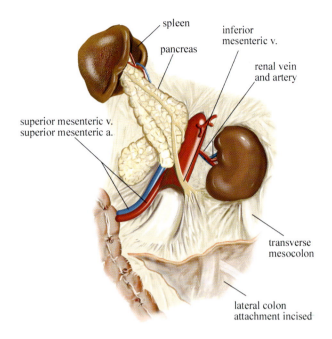

Figure 20.4.

Assessment of the pancreas after mobilisation of the splenic flexure and division of the ligament of Trietz.

Division of the ligament of Treitz at the duodenal jejunal junction and mobilisation of the third part of the duodenum left of the superior mesenteric artery allows for assessment of the posterior body and tail of the pancreas (Fig. 20.4).

Contusions which involve less than half of the width of the pancreas are unlikely to be associated with ductal injury, and these can be safely drained. Similarly superficial lacerations that are not bleeding can be left alone and the area drained. Superficial lacerations which are bleeding are best treated with some local haemostatic glue and digital pressure. The pancreatic capsule does not take sutures well.

It is the larger contusions and lacerations where the possibility of pancreatic duct involvement cannot be confidently excluded that make management difficult. Your decision should be based on the patient's condition and the site of the injury in relation to the superior mesenteric vessels. If you're at the tail end of an eventful two hours in the abdomen and everything is starting to feel cold to the touch, leave in a drain. If the patient is amenable to another 40 minutes or so of operating time, we would do a distal

pancreatectomy for injuries to the left of these vessels. While others have suggested further manoeuvres to determine the status of the pancreatic duct, we have often found them inconclusive and cumbersome, and certainly inappropriate in a multiply injured patient. Opening a perfectly normal duodenum to find the notoriously elusive ampulla of Vater for an on-table pancreatic ductogram seems like a lot of trouble for a vague, gas-filled image. Doing an on table ERCP for a trauma patient with an open abdomen is rarely helpful.

For distal pancreatectomy, while splenic preservation has been described, we have little experience with this, and splenectomy is usually carried out concurrently. Dissection for assessment of the spleen is carried out as described earlier. The splenic flexure is taken down and the colon retracted inferiorly. The spleen is freed from its peritoneal reflections and short gastric vessels divided between clamps. Dissection of the inferior border of the pancreas begins at the ligament of Treitz and extends to the right to the superior mesenteric artery. Sutures placed on the superior and inferior borders of the spleen secure the pancreatic vessels and also act as stay sutures. A 75 mm linear stapler is introduced inferiorly to superiorly and the pancreas divided and delivered with the spleen. Some bleeders in the cut pancreatic surface may need to be ligated, but there is no need to locate the pancreatic duct, or to suture the cut pancreatic surface (Fig. 20.5).

The pancreas to the right of the superior mesenteric vessels lies in the "surgical soul," as described by Hirschberg and Mattox. Injuries here are more often seen as a result of a penetrating gunshot wound than as a blunt injury. They are associated with a mortality exceeding 50%. It should be noted that this is far more often due to associated vascular injury than complications following injury to the pancreas. The treatment strategy then comprises of prioritising treatment to the vascular structures first. As far as treatment of the pancreatic injury is concerned, a few principal considerations apply.

Keep things simple. Limit resection to very obviously necrotic tissue and only when completing the job that the trauma has already nearly completed for you. Patients with pancreaticoduodenal injuries and

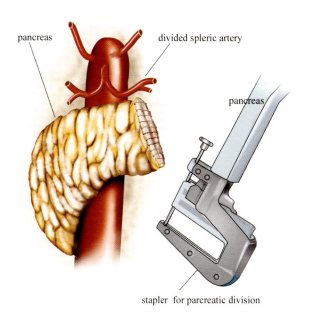

Figure 20.5.

Staple division of pancreas.

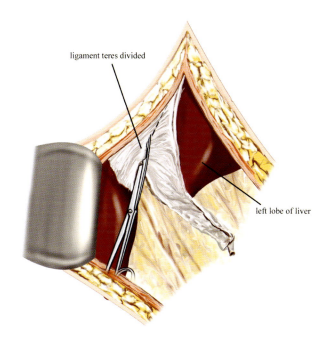

Figure 20.6.

Dividing the falciform ligament.

vascular involvement do not take well to detailed dissection in this area. Wherever possible, get haemostasis and get out.

Leave in a drain. Even in the presence of ductal injury, drainage may do just as well as resection. Accept a live patient with a controlled pancreatic fistula as a good day's work in this setting.

If resection is required, do it in stages. A high-risk anastomosis like a pancreaticojejunostomy has no place in patients in acidosis and hypothermia. Staple off the pancreas; come back another time if he makes it.

Liver Injuries

The liver is the second most often injured organ in blunt abdominal injury after the spleen. The key to successful treatment is proper assessment, and the key to successful assessment is mobilisation of the liver ligaments. These ligaments should also be divided for successful packing, so do them early in the operation. There is one notable exception (see later).

Upon entry to the abdomen, divide the umbilical ligament between clamps and follow this with a division of the falciform ligament superiorly to the

diaphragm (Fig. 20.6). Taking down this falciform ligament is the key step that will allow you access with eyes and fingers all surfaces of the liver with the exceptions of the "bare areas" which are enclosed by the coronary ligaments. A few possible scenarios now present themselves:

If there is a laceration that has already stopped bleeding, leave it alone, consider yourself lucky and move on to other things. Be very sure that there isn't a more severe liver injury elsewhere though — single liver lacerations are not all that common in blunt trauma. The posterior surface of the right lobe in Morrison's pouch immediately inferior to the right coronary ligament is a favourite hiding place.

If there is an actively bleeding laceration, don't stuff packs in the laceration. This dislodges clots, extends lacerations, and hides ongoing bleeding. Do three things: pack, Pringle and apply pressure. Packing can only be done when all the ligaments are down, so begin by applying a clamp on the hepatic ligament at the foramen of Winslow (Pringle's manoeuvre) and get to work with the ligaments. This is a two-man (er, person) job with the primary surgeon dividing the ligaments and the assistant giving proper counter-traction on the liver, at all times trying to compress the lacerated surfaces of the liver together.

The falciform ligament would have been taken down as part of your screening manoeuvre. In addition to this, take down the left coronary ligament by gentle medial traction of the left lobe, and use cautery or scissors to take the ligament off the left lobe of the diaphragm (Fig. 20.7). On the right side this is more difficult and requires an assistant to provide upwards traction on the larger right lobe with long forceps to provide counter traction downwards as the right coronary ligament is divided. It is important to divide these ligaments to the lower hepatic veins to provide adequate mobilisation (Fig. 20.8).

When properly done, the liver now hangs by its functional mesentery with the attachments to the IVC posteriorly and the clamped hepatic ligament inferiorly. It is now ready for packing. While various methods have been described, a point of agreement is that packs should be placed with the liver surface on one side and a firm surface on the other in order to achieve the necessary tamponade. The only firm surface in the vicinity is the thoracic cage. The key to successful packing is to pack the entire liver in on itself. While

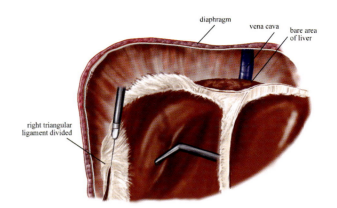

Figure 20.8.

Dividing the right coronary ligament.

there are variations, this usually means two packs in the right bare area, two each on the anterior surface right and left of the falciform and another two in the left bare area.

After packing, observe. If your packing is going to work, the effects are usually apparent in 5–10 minutes, so find something else to do (such as a completion laparotomy — see below). Remain tactical. Now that you know how things in the liver are, if there is any doubt that this is not going to work, prepare your team. Get good suction and lighting, lots of blood on standby, tissue glue, liver sutures and multifire clips. If the liver remains quiet, take off the Pringle's clamps and observe again, adjusting your packs as necessary. If things remain quiet, it is our practice to leave the packs in, devise a temporary dressing and count ourselves lucky. We have seen some surgeons remove packs and close the abdomen, but it seems counterintuitive to remove the only haemostatic measure in a patient who is almost definitely coagulopathic by now. Furthermore, bile staining on the packs at the re-look operation will mandate a search for major biliary disruption, not something to get into in the present setting.

If bleeding remains brisk, your nice options are used up and you now have to take the bull by the horns. It's not coagulopathy, it's uncontrolled surgical bleeding. Get the nurses to open liver sutures and start mixing tissue glue. If hepatic angio-embolisation is available, this is a good time to wake the radiologist up. Remove packs, re-apply Pringle's and start your finger fracture into the depths of the laceration. What

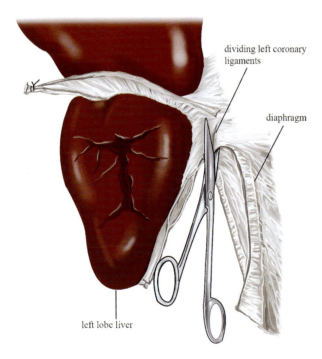

Figure 20.7.

Dividing the left coronary ligament.

we have found useful in this setting is the multifire staples we alluded to earlier. Sutures are going to be too slow. This is going to take some teamwork. Take a forceps in your left hand and with your right hand go to the heart of the laceration, pinching whatever parenchyma is in your way to the depth of the laceration. When a bleeder is identified, hold the stem of the applicator and have your assistant fire the instrument. His other hand helps you to keep the laceration edges apart. This is no time for temerity. Often we find the most significant bleeders in the deepest part of the laceration, so good lighting and suction are important. There will be some oozing from raw liver surfaces, and these respond well to tissue glue. After haemostasis is secured, apply liver sutures if possible.

The purpose of the liver sutures is to close the liver laceration on itself. This can only be done if the sutures have enough capsules to find purchase. Remember that you don't have to take the full thickness in one bite. "Coming out" in the laceration before taking the second bite is much more useful if you can get better purchase on capsule. Don't kill the knot; apposition is all you need, not an extension of the laceration by your suture. Re-pack and get out. If in any doubt of your haemostasis, go to angiography.

The one exception to taking down the liver ligaments is a haematoma that is seen in the posterior right liver, usually filling the retrohepatic space over the right diaphragm and extending downwards. This is a retrohepatic IVC tear, the beast that waits the unwary to deroof the peritoneum to get primary repair. Bleeding from this portion of the IVC is not only visible but audible. Trying to tackle it head-on results in soaked socks, a tired anaesthesiologist who will talk about it for days, an empty blood bank and oh, yes, a dead patient. The only reason the patient got into your theatre alive is because of that peritoneum and the diaphragm posteriorly giving tamponade. Deroof this and he dies. If the peritoneum is still intact, fix your other injuries, pack the liver anteriorly and get out. Even if there is a small defect in the overlying peritoneum, glue it, put a pack in and get out. If the defect is too large for glue, put in a urinary catheter blow up the balloon and get out. If you suspect a diaphragmatic rupture (rare in blunt trauma) because

of massive right hemothorax, do a right anterolateral thoracostomy and fix it from above.

V. Wound Closure

Temporary Abdominal Dressing

Staged procedures in the abdomen require dressing the laparotomy wound with a view for re-exploration. The ideal dressing should have the qualities listed in Table 20.2. We have used numerous designs in the past, including abdominal wall clips, Bogota bags and skin staples, but have now settled on either the Vac Pac (KCI) or an improvised dressing made from NG suction tubes, abdominal packs and Steri-Drapes.

Our improved dressing requires two large cardiac Steri-Drapes, four or five abdominal packs, two large NG tubes and a knife. Initially the first drape is placed with its sticky surface upwards. Depending on the size of the abdominal cavity, packs are laid out unfolded on the sticky surface, the edges of which are rolled inwards. The Steri-Drape is then turned over and cuts are made with the knife on its non-adhesive side (Figs. 20.9A and 20.9B).

The pack is then placed into the abdominal cavity with the bare surface of the packs facing away from the bowel and the Steri-Drape with its cuts in contact with the bowel. It is important in order to avoid adhesions between the bowel and the abdominal wall that this pack should be placed as far laterally and inferiorly as possible from the diaphragm to the pelvis.

With the pack in place, an NG tube is place on both sides of the shelf between the rectus fascia and muscle

Table 20.2.

Ideal Temporary Abdominal Closure

Relatively inexpensive
Easy and rapid to fashion
Preserve the abdominal fascia for definitive formal closure
Decompress the abdomen in case of abdominal compartment
    syndrome
Easy suction of abdominal fluid
Reduce bowel edema
Prevent adhesions between bowel and peritoneal walls

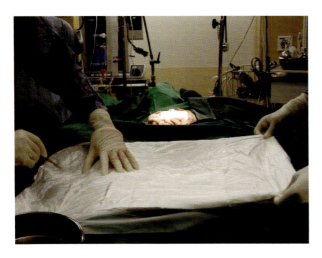

Figure 20.9A.

After towels are laid out on the steridrape, it is inverted and incisions are made on the steridrape to allow drainage of fluid.

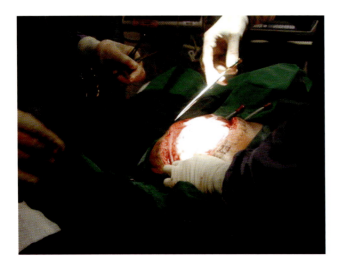

Figure 20.9B.

The dressing is placed with the plastic surface on the bowel, and nasogastric tubes placed on fascia on both sides. These are then connected to wall suction.

and sutured in place with stay sutures and brought our through the skin over the chest. A second Steri-Drape is then placed over the packs and the NG tubes placed on wall suction.

We have found this improvised device to meet most of the requirements of an ideal temporary dressing. The one major disadvantage is the leaving of packs in the peritoneal cavity can interfere with the pack

counts in an operative setting where it is usually already hard enough for the nurses to keep track. As a precaution before final closure, an on-table KUB X-ray is obtained to exclude the presence of retained packs in the peritoneum.

VI. Postoperative Care

This would depend on the anatomical and physiological disruption of each case. A simple splenectomy that was not in shock at presentation with a straightforward operation can be sent to the general ward with standard post-operative care. On the other extreme, the cold, acidotic, coagulopathic patient with a temporarily closed abdomen needs to get to the surgical intensive care (SICU).

Try to remember that the concept of damage control surgery is a package that does not just take place in the operating theatre. Before theatre, it requires strict protocols that prioritise treatment requirements, minimise missed injuries but most importantly expedite the preoperative process. The operation is done to stop bleeding, limit contamination and finish the operation. Post-operatively, the patient is warmed, coagulation restored and hypothermia addressed. The plan is to have the patient prepared for definitive operations in 24–48 hours, preferably less. There may be a difference in the location where care is being delivered, but it is a single process, and you need to keep contributing to it. While the finer points of perioperative care in the multiply injured patient are beyond the scope of this chapter, there are several areas where intensivists tend to rely on surgical opinion:

Is the continued bleeding surgical or coagulopathic? At present, this can be as much art as science. Which means that experience matters. Don't leave this to someone else; keep an eye on the patient's clinical and biochemical progress. Standard blood coagulation profiles like PT/PTT were designed for warfarin and heparin dosing in normothermic, nonacidotic patients and do not predict blood requirements in severe trauma. Thromboelastography (TEG) has shown promise in predicting the need for re-look operations in cardiac and liver transplant surgery, and its role in trauma is still being formalised. In those settings, a normal TEG in the presence of on-going bleeding is usually due to a surgical bleed that requires exploration.

The amount and appearance of blood loss can help. More than 100 mL per hour from abdominal drains is an arbitrary threshold for one of the authors. When in doubt, make sure you solve the silk deficiency (from a well-placed surgical tie) when required, as readily as his coagulation factor deficiencies.

Limit crystalloids. If your patient is bleeding from dilutional deficiencies in coagulation products, these are not found in crystalloids and need to be replaced. If he has surgical bleeding, he needs a theatre. Chances are he is already in grossly positive balance, so if no further volume replacement is needed, come off the crystalloids as much as possible. They will increase respiratory complications and bowel edema, and both those conditions can make your abdomen completely impossible to close.

Start feeding early. If bowel continuity is not a problem, this can start on the first or second post-operative day, even in the presence of an open abdomen. The benefit to infective complication rates is well accepted, and it will also simplify fluid management.

Start anticoagulation when bleeding has stopped, the exception being in cases of significant head and spinal injury. Remember that when haemostasis is secured, trauma patients shift from an anti- to a pro-coagulant state usually by the second day. Especially in the case of pelvic and lower limb fractures, start your anticoagulation by then.

Chapter 21

Abdominal Wall Reconstruction and Closure

Wei Chen Ong*, Jane Lim† and Thiam Chye Lim‡

Introduction

The abdominal wall is an important part of the body that serves many functions. It acts as a cover to protect the intra-abdominal structures, and prevents herniation of the gastrointestinal organs. It also serves to aid in movements as well as provide stability of the trunk. Other essential functions like breathing also depend on the integrity of the abdominal wall. There are several components to the abdominal wall — the most external layer being the skin and subcutaneous tissue, followed by multiple layers of muscles, fascia, and the innermost layers of extraperitoneal fat and peritoneum. Hence in reconstructing, it is important to restore structural integrity in order to maintain functional integrity of the abdominal wall.

Abdominal wall disruption and evisceration after emergency surgery is associated with considerable mortality and occurrence of ventral hernia.

Whilst immediate re-suturing may sometimes be successful, the burst abdomen in unfit patients with sepsis would best be managed as a staged operative procedure as described in this chapter.

Prior to surgical reconstruction, the negative pressure therapy system has been a valuable adjunct to patient care.

Preoperative Planning

Preoperative assessment and planning is paramount in ensuring a successful abdominal reconstruction or closure (Table 21.1).

The patient should be carefully worked up before definitive surgery. Factors such as the patient's lung function and nutritional status should be looked into. Decreased functional pulmonary capacity or a pre-existing lung problem can put the patient at increased postoperative pulmonary complications. This is especially so if abdominal wall closure increases the intra-abdominal pressure. This will further splint the diaphragm and worsen lung capacity. Suboptimal nutrition or immunosuppression can affect wound tensile strength and wound healing.

The defect to be reconstructed or repaired is assessed to determine defect size and the number of

Table 21.1.

Important Considerations in Abdominal Wall Closure or Reconstruction

- Evaluation of patient
- Aetiologic considerations
- Evaluation of structural defect
- Timing of reconstruction
- Static reconstruction vs Functional reconstruction
- Aesthetic considerations

*W.C. Ong, MBBS, MMed (Surgery), MRCS (Edin), FAMS(Plastic Surgery), Consultant, Division of Plastic, Reconstructive & Aesthetic Surgery, University Surgical Cluster, National University Health System, Singapore.
†J. Lim, MBBS, FRCS (Edin), FRS (Glasgow), FAMS (Plastic Surgery), Senior Consultant, Division of Plastic, Reconstruction & Aesthetic Surgery, University Surgical Cluster, National University Health System, Singapore.
‡T.C. Lim, MBBS (Mal), FRCS (Edin), FAMM, FAMS (Plastic Surgery), Senior Consultant & Head, Division of Plastic, Reconstructive & Aesthetic Surgery, University Surgical Cluster, National University Health System.

components (skin, soft tissue, and fascia) that need to be replaced. Infection should be controlled, and any devitalised tissue should be debrided. The presence of infection can also affect the method of reconstruction as synthetic meshes would not usually be considered. Tissue oedema can affect the mobility of tissues and the ease with which they can be advanced. It is the most significant in the first one week after initial injury. Hence reconstruction is usually delayed until inflammation and tissue oedema has settled.

The timing of closure or reconstruction is another important consideration (Table 21.2). Immediate or early closure or reconstruction is usually preferred as an open abdominal wound contributes to fluid and protein loss. It also hinders breathing and patient mobility. However, reconstruction may need to be delayed if the patient is unstable or not fit for surgery, or if the wound bed is contaminated and not ready for closure. If reconstruction poses further risks to the patient, or if the reconstruction option is limited at the time of surgery, definitive reconstruction can be performed as a delayed procedure and an interim closure or wound cover is then first performed.

The method of reconstruction is also tailored to the patient's needs and requirements. Replacing like for like tissue should be adhered to as close as possible to maintain an acceptable aesthetic outcome. Additional morbidity to the patient should be kept to a minimum whatever the method is selected for reconstruction.

Choice of Surgical Technique

There are many methods available for reconstruction, depending on the size and type of defect, the location, and the reconstruction requirements (Table 21.3). Generally, soft tissue defects of 7 cm or less can be closed primarily or with a layered closure technique[1] if there are no other factors inhibiting closure.

Approximation of the wound edges using component separation has been a popular technique since its description by Ramirez in 1990.[2] This technique is often used to close midline abdominal defects from trauma, abdominal compartment syndrome, and other midline defects.

Skin grafts can be used if the skin is the only component to be replaced. There should be sufficient support in the abdominal wall with either intact fascia or muscle layer. Generally, skin grafts are not placed on abdominal viscera as they do not provide sufficient protection, and will often break down.

Local or regional flaps from the back, lower limb and groin provide adequate skin, muscle or fascia in reconstruction. Examples include anterolateral thigh flap, tensor fascia lata, rectus femoris, and latissimus dorsi. Depending on the location of the defect, the rectus abdominis muscle can also be used. Free flaps may be required if the defect size is large, or if the regional tissue is unsuitable.

Allografts and meshes can be useful to replace fascia. There are many types of alloplastic materials currently in use. The most commonly used are synthetic meshes and dermal substitutes. However, their use is often contraindicated in infected or previously

Table 21.2.

Timing of Abdominal Wall Closure

1st week
Tissue oedema
↓
2nd week
Closure possible
↓
3rd week onwards
Retracted edges adhered down due to unopposed action of lateral muscles
↓
May need to perform temporary cover with split skin graft followed by secondary definitive surgery after 1–2 years

Table 21.3.

Factors Affecting Choice of Surgical Technique

1. Size of defect
2. Location of defect
3. Components to replace — actual tissue loss
4. Availability of tissue for reconstruction

open surgical fields. Other issues like cost, adhesions, and hernia recurrence also limit their use.

Tissue expansion is another method used in reconstruction. Expanders are first placed under the area of the skin to be expanded, usually near the planned defect. This is performed under general anaesthesia. Over a period of time, the skin can be slowly expanded by injection of saline through the port. This process is long drawn, and is not suitable in an infected field, hence limiting its use in most circumstances.

Operative Procedure

1. Component Separation Technique (Fig. 21.1)

The component separation technique was first described by Ramirez *et al.*[2] in 1990. The basis of this technique is that separation of the different component layers of the abdominal wall would allow greater mobilization than if the wall was moved as a whole unit.[3] Muscle, fascia, and skin layers are identified and

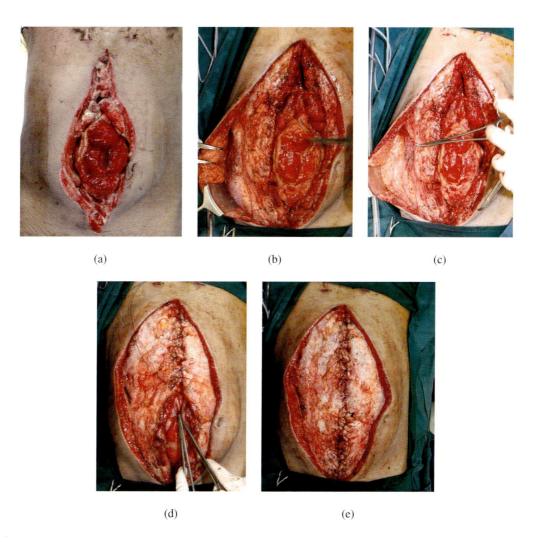

(a)   (b)   (c)

(d)   (e)

Figure 21.1.

Abdominal wound closure using component separation technique following dehisced abdominal wound from polytrauma. **(a)** Abdominal wall defect involving skin, rectus sheath and muscle. The underlying intestinal contents are exposed, **(b)** First, bilateral skin flaps are raised off the external oblique aponeurosis up to the mid axillary line, **(c)** The external oblique aponeurosis is elevated off the internal oblique muscle in the avascular plane. **(d)** The rectus sheath is then approximated in the midline using PDS suture. If the sheath cannot be approximated, the rectus muscle can be elevated off the posterior sheath to allow further mobilization to the midline. **(e)** The skin flaps are then approximated in the midline after closure of the rectus sheath.

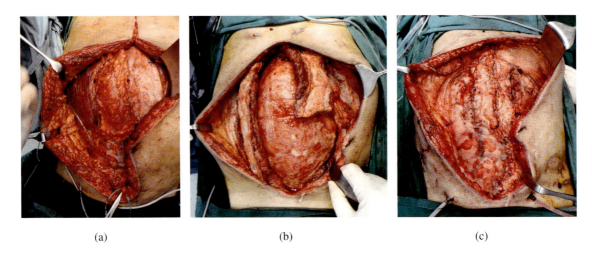

(a)   (b)   (c)

Figure 21.2.

(a) The right rectus sheath has been raised off the right rectus muscle and flipped over to cover the central defect. It is still attached to right posterior sheath, and has been sutured to the edge of the left rectus sheath. (b) One rectus muscle is raised based on the supply from the superior epigastric vessels. (c) It is then transposed to the midline, and the rest of the structures mobilised to allow closure.

individually dissected free in the different layers. Releasing incisions can be made laterally on each side, if necessary, before the layers are coapted to allow closure in the midline. This technique has been reported to be able to close defects of sizes up to 10 cm in the epigastrium, 20 cm in the mid-abdomen, and 6 cm in the lower abdomen.

As this technique involves the same surgical site, and requires no further grafts or implants, it is very versatile and can be used in an infected field.[4,5] It is now one of the most commonly employed techniques in abdominal wall closure.

2. Transposition of Rectus Sheath/Rectus Muscle (Fig. 21.2)

If the defect size is small or limited, a formal component separation may not be required. The anterior rectus sheath can be elevated off the rectus muscle and flipped over or transposed to bridge the defect.[6] Skin flaps can be raised up to the mid-axillary line to allow closure over the sheath. One limitation of this method is that movement of the rectus sheath inferior to the level of the umbilicus is limited.

Care should be taken when elevating the anterior rectus sheath off the rectus muscle to avoid inadvertent tears

in the rectus sheath, as the sheath is usually adherent to the muscle at the musculotendinous intersections.

3. Bilateral Skin Flap Advancement (Fig. 21.3)

The skin and subcutaneous layer of the abdominal wall is usually pliable and loosely adherent to the

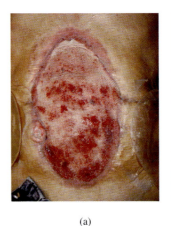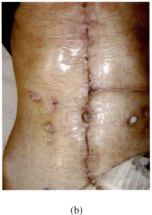

(a)   (b)

Figure 21.3.

(a) Healthy granulation over an exposed synthetic mesh over the left side of the abdomen. (b) Bilateral skin flaps are raised and advanced medially to close over the exposed mesh in the midline.

underlying sheath and aponeurosis, making it an ideal tissue layer to recruit in an abdominal wall closure. Skin flaps are easily raised in a relatively avascular plane. Perforator vessels to the skin flap should be ligated to prevent haematoma formation.

Dissection can be carried out laterally to the mid-axillary line, superiorly to the costal margin and xiphisternum, and inferiorly to the pubis to allow sufficient movement of the skin flaps to the midline. After closure is performed, a redivac drain is usually placed under the skin flaps to prevent seroma collection.

4. Use of Skin Grafts (Fig. 21.4)

Skin grafting is usually not the definitive treatment for abdominal wall closure or reconstruction. This is because the grafts are usually thin and do not offer protection nor structural support to underlying structures. They may be unstable, and may break down after the initial period of healing. Skin grafts should only be used if there is healthy underlying granulation tissue. There should not be any exposed abdominal contents or meshes. Often, when a skin graft is used as a cover over an underlying mesh, the mesh may ulcerate through, requiring further definitive reconstruction.

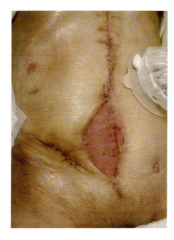

Figure 21.4.

A small area of exposed granulation tissue in the right abdominal area covered by skin graft.

A skin graft can be used as a temporizing skin cover and is a good option for temporary cover if the patient is not fit enough for a longer operation, or unsuitable for more definitive closure. Once the skin graft has taken and re-epithelialisation starts, the amount of fluid and protein loss from the wound bed is expected to decrease, reducing the caloric load to the patient, and at the same time reducing wound dressing requirements. The patient can then be rehabilitated and a more definitive closure and hernia closure performed, usually 1–2 years later.

5. Use of Alloplastic Materials (Figs. 21.5 and 21.6)

Alloplastic materials can be useful in abdominal wall reconstruction as they can provide the structural strength required. However, their use must be considered cautiously in each case. The use of mesh is limited if the wound has been left exposed for some time and potentially infected. Even when successfully used in an early setting, it can cause late problems like enterocutaneous fistula and mesh extrusion. If the intestinal contents are exposed, a mesh is usually not used to bridge the defect between the medial edges of the rectus sheath if the edges cannot be approximated in midline. This is because the mesh may cause erosions to the underlying bowel wall. If the peritoneum is intact, the rectus muscles and posterior sheath can be lifted off, and a mesh can be placed in the pre-peritoneal layer.

In addition, a mesh can be used to reinforce the closure of a sheath, especially if there is tension in the sheath closure. In this case, it is used as an onlay graft over the sheath repair. It can also be used to reinforce the oblique muscles and aponeurosis in the lateral abdominal wall, especially if they have been separated to allow central mobilisation, or if release incisions have been made to allow approximation of the sheath in midline.

A synthetic mesh is often used to strengthen the abdominal wall repair after a transverse rectus abdominis myocutaneous flap has been raised (e.g. in breast reconstruction) (Fig. 21.5). In this procedure, part of the rectus sheath underlying the skin

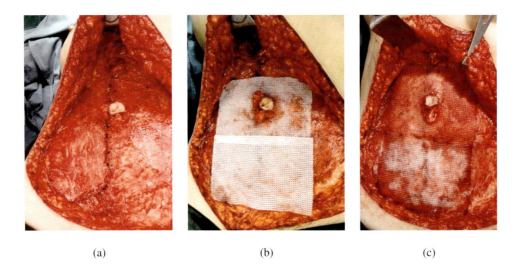

(a) (b) (c)

Figure 21.5.

(**a**) Closure of the rectus sheath after a pedicled transverse rectus abdominis myocutaneous flap where part of the rectus sheath has been excised with the flap. The sheath is closed primarily with PDS® suture. (**b** and **c**) An absorbable mesh (TIGR® matrix surgical mesh, Novus Scientific) is used as an onlay graft to strengthen the repair. It is a synthetic resorbable mesh which resorbs in about one year.

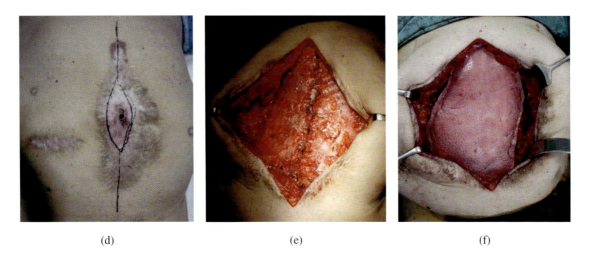

(d) (e) (f)

Figure 21.6.

(**d**) A patient with a mesh that has ulcerated through the previous midline abdominal wound. This patient also has a large midline incisional hernia and another incisional hernia of the right lower quadrant. (**e**) The mesh is removed and both hernias repaired. The sheath is approximated in the midline. (**f**) A semi-permanent dermal collagen implant (Permacol™, Covidien Surgical) is placed over both hernia repairs and to protect the closures.

island is harvested together with the rectus muscle. In most instances, the rectus sheath can still be closed but a mesh is used as an onlay graft to protect the repair. If the sheath cannot be approximated, then a permanent mesh has to be used to bridge the defect.

6. Flap Closure (Fig. 21.7)

Flap closure is often reserved for complex cases requiring reconstruction of more than one component of the abdominal wall. Usually the defect is large, and

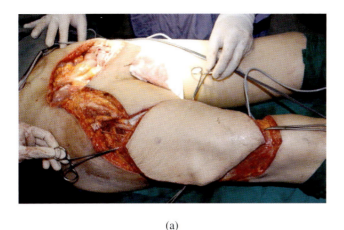
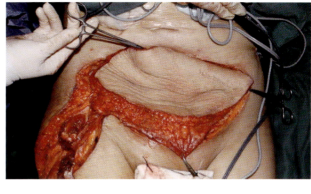

(a)   (b)

Figure 21.7.

(a) A large defect in the lower abdomen. This is a full thickness defect, exposing the intestinal contents. A pedicled anterolateral thigh flap is raised based on the supply from the descending branch of the circumflex femoral vessel. **(b)** The flap is then inset over the defect in the lower abdomen. The donor defect is closed with a skin graft.

other methods of reconstruction or closure cannot be used.

Examples of flaps that can be used for abdominal wall reconstruction include the pedicled anterolateral thigh flap,[7] pedicled tensor fascia lata flap,[8] and pedicled external oblique myocutaneous flap. If regional pedicled flaps are insufficient or not able to be used in reconstruction, then distant free flaps can be used. An example of a flap which can provide large tissue cover would be the latissimus dorsi flap.[9] This is a thin and wide muscle flap which can provide a cover for a large surface area, but a skin graft would be required to cover the muscle.

In cases where strong structural support is required, a mesh can be used under a tissue (either a muscle or skin) flap. If autologous material is preferred, fascia lata can be harvested, either separately, or together with the flap, and used as a sheath support.

7.   Adjunctions in Abdominal Wound Closure — Vacuum Assisted Closure (Fig. 21.8)

Vacuum assisted closure systems have become an important adjunct to abdominal wall closure.[10,11] This

negative pressure therapy system has been shown to reduce oedema and promote granulation if applied over a period of time.[12]

It is useful as an interim treatment for the exposed wound. This is especially so if there is too much tension and the skin or rectus cannot be brought together in the midline by component separation. With negative pressure dressing, the skin edges are pulled towards the centre of the wound, approximation with gradual of the edges and reduction of defect size. The closed drainage system helps control exudates and keeps skin edges free from maceration. Another additional benefit of this closed dressing system is that it stabilises the wound edges, thereby reducing movement of the abdominal wall when the patient is moving. The patient can then be allowed to mobilise while waiting for definitive reconstruction or closure of the abdominal wall.

Postoperative Management

Good postoperative care is necessary to ensure proper wound healing and a successful closure or reconstruction. Suction drains should be placed in the wound to minimise seroma formation. These drains are usually only removed when drainage has decreased to a

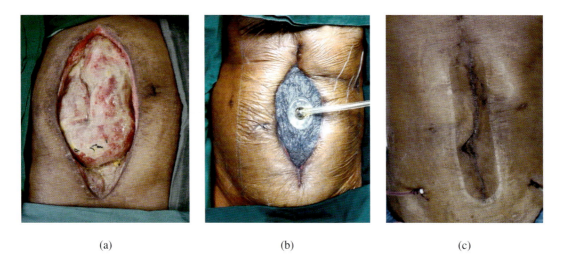

(a)   (b)   (c)

Figure 21.8.

(**a**) An exposed and infected wound in a patient who has undergone laparotomy. (**b**) Abdominal V.A.C® (KCI) dressing is applied for 2 weeks. (**c**) The wound is finally closed using component separation technique.

minimum, sometimes taking up to a few weeks. Patients are also advised to wear support garments or use abdominal binders, to protect the repair for at least one month.

References

1. Nozaki M, Sasaki K, Huang T. *Reconstruction of the Abdominal Wall*. Mathes Vol. 6, Chap. 151, pp. 1175–1195.

2. Ramirez OM, Reus E, Lee Dellon A. (1990) "Components separation" method for closure of abdominal wall defects: An anatomic and clinical study. *Plast Reconstr Surg* **86**(3): 519–526.

3. Ramirez OM. (2006) Inception and evolution of the component separation technique. *Clin Plast Surg* **33**: 241–246.

4. Kanaan Z, Hicks N, Weller C, *et al.* (2011) Abdominal wall component release is a sensible choice for patients requiring complicated closure of abdominal defects. *Langenbecks Arch Surg* **396**: 1263.

5. Yegiyants S, Tam M, Lee DJ, Abbas MA. (2012) Outcome of components separation for contaminated complex abdominal wall defects. *Hernia* **16**(1): 41–5.

6. Kushimoto S, Yamamoto Y, Aiboshi J, *et al.* (2007) Usefulness of the bilateral anterior rectus abdominis sheath turnover flap method for early fascial closure in patients requiring open abdominal management. *World J Surg* **31**(1): 2–8.

7. Kayano S, Sakuraba M, Miyamoto S, *et al.* (2012) Comparison of pedicled and free anterolateral thigh flaps for reconstruction of complex defects of the abdominal wall. Review of 20 consecutive cases. *J Plast Reconstr Aesthet Surg* **65**(11): 1525–1529.

8. Rifaat MA, Abdel Gawad WS. (2005) The use of pedicled tensor fascia lata pedicled flap in reconstructing full thickness abdominal wall defects and groin defects following tumour ablation. *J Egypt Natl Canc Inst* **17**(3): 139–48.

9. Kim SW, Han SC, Hwang KT, *et al.* (2012) Reconstruction of infected abdominal wall defects using latissimus dorsi free flap. *ANZ J Surg* Sep 26. doi: 10.1111/j.1445-2197.2012. 06286.

10. DeFranzo AJ, Argenta LC. (2006) Vacuum assisted closure for the treatment of abdominal wounds. *Clin Plast Surg* **33**(2): 213–24.

11. DeFranzo AJ, Pitzer K, Molnar JA, *et al.* (2008) Vacuum assisted closure for defects of the abdominal wall. *Plast Reconstr Surg* **121**(3): 832–9.

12. Argenta LC, Morykwas MJ. (1997) Vacuum assisted closure: A new method for wound control and treatment: Clinical experience. *Ann Plast Surg* **38**(6): 563–76.

Chapter 22

Abdominal Emergencies in Children

Vidyadhar Mali*, Dale L.S.K. Loh* and K. Prabhakaran*

There are distinct anatomic and physiologic characteristics that impact the management of a child with a surgical abdomen.

The preoperative management should emphasise:

1. The ABCs
    — Airway (apnoea is common and apnoea monitoring is routine); breathing — blood gas & biochemistry (to identify and correct metabolic acidosis); circulation — routinely administer a fluid flush 10–20 mL/kg (because although tachycardia is common, even severe hypovolemia may not manifest hypotension until late). Maintenance fluids are calculated based on body weight — 100 mL/kg for the first 10 kg weight, 50 mL/kg for the next 10 kg weight and 30 mL/kg for the subsequent weight.
    — Naso-gastric tube/Foley catheter.
    — Vit. K — neonates have a relative prothrombin deficiency.
    — Intravenous broad-spectrum antibiotics.

2. Maintenance of normothermia
    — Babies are easily prone to hypothermia because of a greater body surface area in proportion to their weight, lower amount of body fat, inability to shiver as a thermogenic mechanism and immaturity of the hypothalamic thermostat.

    — Measures to maintain normothermia include nursing in an infant warmer in the ward, heating mattress in the operation theatre, "warming" the operation theatre to 26°C, wrapping the limbs in cotton wool, using warm solutions for cleansing and prepping and for irrigation of the peritoneal cavity.

The surgical management may be discussed broadly under the headings of different treatment modalities followed by a brief description of a few typical surgical diagnoses, the aim being to highlight the differences between children and adults rather than give a full description.

We have highlighted the unique characteristics of the different treatment modalities followed by a description of different surgical conditions in neonates and older children, the aim being to emphasise the key points in their management rather than give a full account.

Laparotomy

Laparotomies in neonates and infants are performed through transverse upper abdominal incisions since it is easy to access all viscera (the abdomen is in the shape of a pot belly and the subphrenic spaces and pelvis are shallow) and these incisions heal well.

*V. Mali, MCh, FRCS (Paed), FAMS, Consultant; Dale L.S.K. Loh, FRCS (Glasg), FRCS (Paed), FAMS, Senior Consultant; K. Prabhakaran, FRCS(Glasg), FRCS(Ed), FAMS, Senior Consultant and Head, Department of Paediatric Surgery, National University Hospital, Singapore.

Midline laparotomies are employed in older children and adolescents or in case of complicated or re-do surgery in younger children. All laparotomy wounds are closed en-masse using either vicryl or polydioxanone sutures.

Since the total blood volume is about 70–80 mL/kg, even a loss of a few ml of blood in a baby weighing only a few kg may be significant. Judicious use of diathermy and gentle handling of tissues not only contribute to minimising bleeding but also hasten recovery. As such, the guiding principle for these fragile patients in an emergency laparotomy should be to "do no more than what is least required."

Intestinal anastomoses are performed using absorbable interrupted sutures (to allow future intestinal growth) in a single (to prevent narrowing of lumen) layer. Mattress sutures may be utilised for better approximation of the serosa.

Necrotising enterocolitis is an infective process that may affect any part of the gut with the potential to lead to transmural necrosis and perforation (Fig. 22.1) in neonates who are under "stress" (preterm, low birth weight, formula fed, undergone cardiac surgery). Treatment is conservative unless there is evidence of intestinal necrosis or perforation.

Meckel's diverticulectomy may be necessary for inflammation or bleeding. A narrow-based diverticulum may be safely excised by removing a wedge of the base, whereas a broad-based diverticulum may necessitate intestinal resection so as to prevent leaving

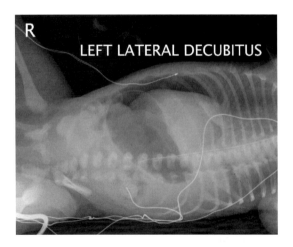

Figure 22.1.

In neonates, free air is visualised on left lateral decubitus views (in lieu of erect films) above the liver.

any ectopic mucosa behind. It is appropriate to perform an appendectomy at the same time.

Laparoscopy

Appendicectomy for acute appendicitis is often performed laparoscopically since it is possible to visualise the pelvis and subphrenic spaces for a thorough lavage and the children recover faster following laparoscopy. Nonetheless, the laparoscopy may be converted to an open approach (either McBurney's or lower midline) in cases of difficult dissections around an inflamed, friable caecum with associated phlegmon.

Laparoscopic management of torted ovarian cysts is feasible. One may have to aspirate the cyst for ease of dissection.

Laparoscopic management of neonatal abdominal emergencies is best performed by experienced hands.

Interventional Radiology

This modality is the treatment of choice for non-operative reduction of intussusceptions.

Typically, the episodes of abdominal pain are associated with curling up of legs. In between the episodes of abdominal pain, the child may look well and the diagnosis may be missed!

The classical red currant jelly stool may not be a constant feature since it occurs late due to sloughing of the ischaemic mucosa mixed with blood. Ultrasound (USG) is diagnostic and may demonstrate the oedematous walls of intussusceptum and intussuscipiens (Fig. 22.2). Doppler imaging may reveal the vascularity of the intestine within the intussusception.

Air Enema

The treatment of choice for ileocolic intussusceptions is reduction by air enema under fluoroscopic guidance. The insufflation pressures are monitored and kept below 100 mmHg.

Indications for operative reduction are failure of air enema on three consecutive attempts, suspicion of intestinal ischaemia, frank perforation and suspicion of pathological lead point (Meckel's diveticulum,

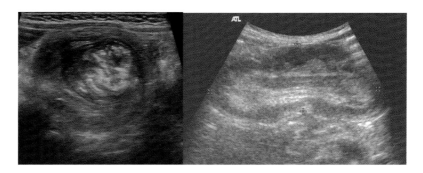

Figure 22.2.

Target sign: Transverse section; Pseudokidney sign: Longitudinal section.

polyp) on USG (especially in older children because the incidence of anatomic lead point increases in relation to age).

Manual reduction at open operation is achieved by pushing the intussuscipiens by squeezing the intestine between fingers. However, an oedematous ileocaecal valve or Peyer's patch may mimic an intraluminal mass; this does not need resection.

Laparoscopic reduction is feasible. However the technique is to gently pull the intussusceptum out of the intussuscipiens.

The common causes of bleeding from the gastro-intestinal tract (GIT) in children vary according to age:

	Upper GIT bleed	Lower GIT bleed
Neonates	Haemorrhagic disease Swallowed maternal blood Gastritis Coagulopathy	Anal fissure Necrotising enterocolitis Malrotation with volvulus
One month to one year of age	Esophagitis Gastritis	Anal fissure Intussusception Gangrenous bowel
One year to two years of age	Peptic ulcer disease	Polyps Meckel's diverticulum
Children older than two years	Esophageal and gastric varices	Polyps Inflammatory bowel disease Trauma Miscellaneous lesions (e.g. Enteric duplications)

Neonatal Intestinal Obstruction

Failure to pass meconium within the first 24–48 hrs of life, feeding intolerance, bilious vomiting, abdominal distension and erythema and oedema of the abdominal wall alert one to the diagnosis of a surgical abdomen in a neonate. The presence of green vomiting associated with abdominal distension implies a distal intestinal obstruction (Hirschsprung's disease, ileal atresia-vide infra) and without abdominal distension implies a proximal intestinal obstruction (duodenal atresia, malrotation-vide infra).

The causes of distal intestinal obstruction may be identified by performing an omnipaque enema (revealing a microcolon — Fig. 22.3) and proximal intestinal obstruction evaluated by performing an omnipaque meal. If there is suspicion of peritonitis, then one may forego the contrast studies and proceed with emergent laparotomy.

Infantile Hypertrophic Pyloric Stenosis

Hypertrophy of the circular muscle of the pylorus commonly presents as non-bilious vomiting of curd-like milky contents in a six-week-old male infant with characteristic biochemical abnormalities (hypokalemic, hypochloremic alkalosis).

Diagnosis is established by clinical palpation of the hypertrophic pylorus during a test feed and ultrasound

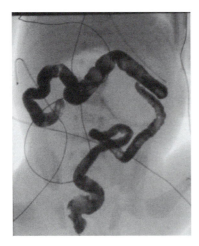

Figure 22.3.

Contrast enema showing a microcolon (unused colon).

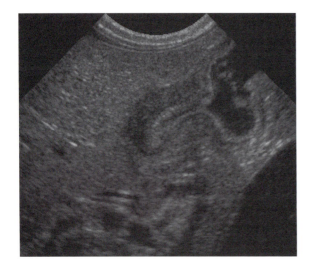

Figure 22.4.

USG view of hypertrophic pylorus.

confirmation of lengthening (15–19 mm) and thickening (3–4 mm) of the pylorus (Fig. 22.4).

The curative operation of pyloromyotomy is only performed after correction of dehydration and the abnormal biochemistry; a convenient way being to rehydrate the child to allow renal homeostasis. Preoperative gastric lavage with warm saline contributes towards prevention of post-operative gastritis.

The incision is either transverse in the right subcostal region or periumbilical.

The greater omentum is identified and delivered into the wound to identify the stomach and trace the

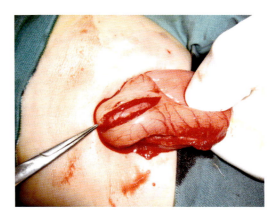

Figure 22.5.

Extent of pyloromyotomy.

greater curvature to the pylorus. Traction on greater curve to the left of the patient along with to-and-fro rocking on the antrum delivers the pylorus.

The pyloromyotomy is started by incising the serosa over an avascular area in anterior transverse plane extending from the vein of Mayo distally to the antrum proximally. Through the incision on the serosa, the muscles are split either with a knife handle or a pylorus spreader (Fig. 22.5). It is at the distal aspect of the myotomy that perforation usually occurs. However, this is managed by suture closure of the myotomy, rotating the pylorus and performing another new myotomy.

Adequacy of myotomy is confirmed by the appearance of bulging mucosa and manually moving the muscle edges in opposite directions to confirm free movement of the edges of the myotomy.

Test for perforation by instilling air into the stomach through a nasogastric tube. Any bleeding from the edges is due to venous congestion of the pylorus delivered through a narrow incision. This is stopped by depositing the pylorus back into the abdomen. Extra attention is given to the abdomen closure since it is prone to dehiscence because of sub-optimal nutrition due to vomiting.

Duodenal Atresia

Congenital atresia of the second part of duodenum (D2) (Fig. 22.6) manifests as green vomiting with

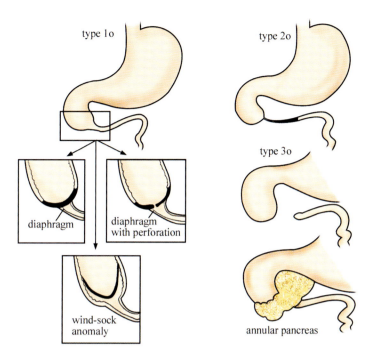

Figure 22.6.

Types of duodenal atresia encountered at laparotomy.

minimal upper abdominal fullness (if any) and the characteristic double bubble sign on abdominal radiograph.

However, a double bubble sign may also be seen in malrotation with volvulus since the obstruction occurs from D2; the distinguishing feature being that the child is more sick and there may be the presence of abdominal distension due to volvulus.

Duodenoduodenostomy

Surgical treatment is not an emergency and (having ruled out malrotation and volvulus) the child may be kept on drip and suck until specialised consult is available.

The operation involves anastomosis between the proximal distended D2 and the distal collapsed duodenum either in the form of a side-to-side or diamond shaped anastomosis (Fig. 22.7).

The essential steps involve full kocherisation of the duodenum to prevent tension and taking sutures 2 mm apart and 1 mm away from edge to prevent any injury to the ampulla of Vater in the vicinity.

Before completion of the anastomosis, it is essential to advance a feeding tube distally to rule out a wind sock deformity (Fig. 22.6). Nasogastric tubes advanced in a trans-anastomotic fashion into the jejunum may not promote anastomotic healing. Nevertheless the tubes facilitate early feeding and lesser dependence on parenteral nutrition.

Malrotation with Volvulus

Malrotation with volvulus of the entire midgut from the second part of duodenum up to the mid-transverse colon constitutes one of the most acute abdominal emergencies in paediatric surgery since potentially the entire midgut could become ischaemic, leading to either mortality or short bowel syndrome and irreversible intestinal failure.

The presentation could be either acute in the neonate/infant as GREEN vomiting and abdominal distension (90%) or subacute at a later age as malabsorption, failure to thrive or chylous ascites. One must bear in mind that in the initial stages of acute

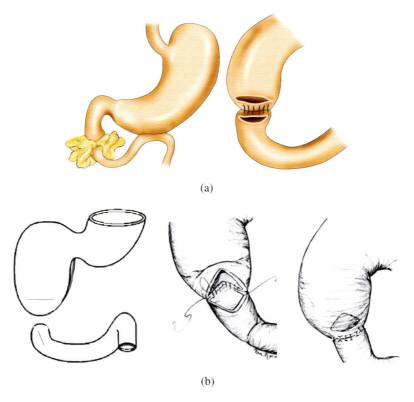

Figure 22.7.

(a) Side-to-side transverse anastomosis; (b) longitudinal and transverse enterotomies are sutured to create a diamond shaped anastomosis.

presentation, the child may LOOK WELL. However, it may be only a matter of a few hours for the situation to become irretrievable!!!!

Intestinal Atresia

Surgical management of intestinal atresia is a complex undertaking. Although resection of obviously ischaemic ends and primary anastomosis is preferable, it may be prudent to perform defunctioning stoma as a life-saving measure.

It is for this reason that paediatric surgeons will equate GREEN vomit to serious vomit and ALL instances of GREEN vomit, therefore, warrant a contrast meal to look for the normal alignment of the pylorus, duodenum and the duodenojejunal (DJ) flexure (Fig. 22.8).

An incidental finding of a high caecum on contrast enema does not equate to malrotation since the DJ

flexure may still be normally sited, in which case there is no risk for volvulus.

The normal attachment of the mesentery is broad-based extending from the DJ flexure (ligament of Treitz) in the left hypochondrium to the ileocaecal junction in the right iliac fossa (Fig. 22.8).

In malrotation (Fig. 22.9), the pathology is a narrow base of the mesentery and obstruction to duodenum because of Ladd's bands crossing the duodenum from the caecum to the abdominal wall in the right flank.

Laparotomy for malrotation and volvulus needs special mention since timely intervention may reverse a potentially morbid and, at times fatal, condition. But for the ABCs, there is simply no time to wait!

At laparotomy, the presence of blood-stained peritoneal fluid denotes intestinal ischemia. The first step is to un-twist the bowel in an anti-clockwise direction (the volvulus occurs in a clockwise manner) (Fig. 22.10).

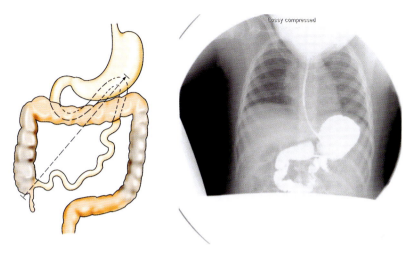

Figure 22.8.

On contrast meal, the duodenum "C" loop crosses the midline and the DJ flexure is posterior to the stomach at the same transverse level as the pylorus.

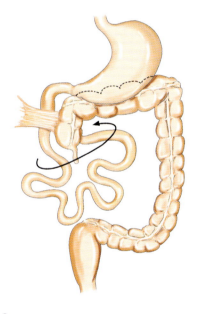

Figure 22.9.

Malrotation.

If the entire midgut is gangrenous, it may be advisable to just close the abdomen without resection and counsel the parents on the dire outlook. However, on return of colour after un-twisting or in case the bowel is not ischaemic to begin with, one should perform the Ladd's procedure (Fig. 22.11). The Ladd's bands extend from portal triad to DJ, and these should be divided near the flank.

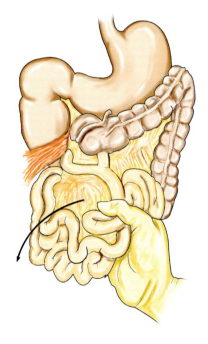

Figure 22.10.

Untwisting malrotation.

The adhesions between the small bowel and the ascending colon are released to expose the superior mesenteric vessels (SMA/SMV) near the pancreas thereby achieving widening of the mesentery. This exposure should be continued until the root of the SMA/SMV is seen. This manoeuvre broadens the mesenteric base.

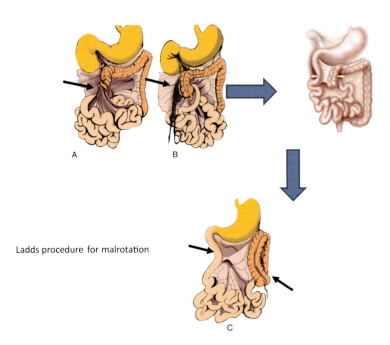

Ladds procedure for malrotation

Figure 22.11

Ladds procedure for malrotation.

At this point, the caecum comes to lie in the left hypochondrium and the entire small bowel to the right side of the abdomen. Appendicectomy is performed to avoid diagnostic confusion in the future. In the case that the bowel continues to be of doubtful viability even after un-twisting the volvulus, it is advisable to avoid any resections at this time, close the abdomen and come back for a second-look laparotomy after 24–48 hr. This period of resustitation helps to define the demarcation between viable and ischaemic bowel at the second-look laparotomy so as to resect only the frankly necrotic bowel and preserve bowel length.

Hirschsprung's Disease (HD)

Congenital aganglionosis due to absence of Meissner's and Auerbach's plexus in the rectum extending proximally for a variable distance is a functional intestinal obstruction.

Although contrast enema may show coning to indicate a transition zone between ganglionic and aganglionic bowel (Fig. 22.12), the definitive diagnosis rests on histological confirmation of absence of

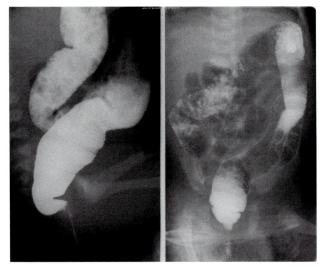

Figure 22.12.

Contrast enema in Hirschsprung's disease.

ganglion cells in rectal biopsy specimens taken at least 1.5 cm above the dentate line. Rectal biopsy does not indicate whether it is a long-segment HD which a contrast enema does.

Since there is no mechanical obstruction within the lumen, it is often possible to manage the obstruction with daily rectal washouts (the usual enemas are not good enough because invariably, they do not result in adequate evacuation and relief of obstruction).

Emergency colostomy may be indicated for failure of rectal washouts in relieving intestinal obstruction (this may be due to poor technique or long-segment HD) or enterocolitis (fever, peritonism and leucocytosis).

The principle (which is the same as that for colostomy for anorectal malformations) is to perform a divided loop, double-barrel colostomy at the ganglionic bowel well proximal to the zone of transition (coning). This level is determined by intra-operative frozen section evaluation of seromuscular biopsies of the colon at different levels.

However, one must be mindful of leaving enough bowel distally to allow a tension-free definitive pull-through at a later date.

Anorectal Malformations

Commonly known as imperforate anus, they may manifest as distal intestinal obstruction in which case they are managed by performing a colostomy at the sigmoid-descending colon junction.

Inguinal Hernia in Children

Herniation of bowel (or other viscera) through a patent processus vaginalis constitutes an urgent indication for herniotomy (even when reducible, not strangulated) at the earliest possible time because the incidence of strangulation when elective surgery is delayed approaches almost 40%. Nonetheless, the occurrence of irreducibility only occasionally necessitates an emergency operation.

The usual strategy for irreducible inguinal hernia is reduction followed by early operation after a delay of about 48 hr. This avoids having to operate when the hernia sac is likely to be oedematous and friable. Tearing of the sac during dissection may preclude complete ligation of the full circumference of the sac and cause recurrence of the hernia in the post-operative period.

Although manual "taxis" has been described for irreducibility, it may be traumatic both to the hernia contents as well as the vascular supply of the testis. Reduction is best achieved by a combination of adequate sedation (preferably morphine) and head low. Merely raising the legs of the infant under pillows is not enough; the foot end of the bed needs to be elevated using blocks from the orthopaedic ward if necessary.

Inguinal herniotomy in children differs from adults in that:

— the superficial and deep rings are almost at the same level, therefore the incision on the external oblique should be made just above the inguinal ligament, else one may end up making a high incision and encounter the conjoint tendon (roof of the inguinal canal). It is in these situations that there is a risk of injury to a distended urinary bladder.
— one must remember to pull the testis back into the scrotum before closing the wound because hooking the cord may have pulled up the testis to an inguinal position and predispose to iatrogenic undescended testis.
— for females presenting with ovary within the hernia, one could perform preoperative ultrasonography to look for the uterus or on-table per rectal examination for palpation of the cervix through the rectal wall to confirm the female gender. Karyotyping, although definitive, is not necessary.
— emergent herniotomy is indicated for irreducibility that lasts for more than a few hours and suspicion of bowel or testis ischemia. A separate abdominal incision just above the deep ring is used to aid in reduction and evaluation of the bowel. This is followed by a herniotomy through an inguinal incision.

References

1. Holcomb GW, Murphy JP. *Ashcraft's Pediatric Surgery*, 4th ed. (Pediatric Surgery (Ashcraft).
2. Spitz L, Coran AG (eds). (1994) *Pediatric Surgery (Rob & Smith's Operative Surgery* (V. 3).

Chapter 23

Instrumentation and Techniques in Emergency Laparoscopic Surgery

Davide Lomanto,* Amit Agarwal,** Vipan Kumar** and Rajat Goel**

Introduction

Acute abdomen is one of the most commonly presenting surgical emergencies and accounts for a significant part of a general surgeon's workload. Laparoscopic surgery has already been accepted as the gold standard for many emergency conditions for both diagnostic and therapeutic roles.

Diagnostic laparoscopy was first performed on humans by Jacobaeus. The widespread application and acceptance of laparoscopic surgery in 1980's revolutionised the field of abdominal surgery. For most part of the starting period, the use of laparoscopic surgery was limited to elective procedures only. However as the learning curve was overcome, the application of laparoscopy was extended to emergency setting as well. Today laparoscopy has been described as safe and feasible in a number of emergency conditions like acute appendicitis, blunt and penetrating trauma and perforated peptic ulcer, with the list expanding day by day.

Benefits of Laparoscopy in Emergency

Emergency laparoscopic surgery not only allows evaluation of the cause of acute abdominal pain but also helps in the treatment of many common abdominal disorders while avoiding a delay in diagnosis. Emergency diagnostic laparoscopy provides visual benefits without significant risks, thereby decreasing non-therapeutic laparotomies. Also, patients treated by laparoscopic surgery get all the known benefits of minimal invasive surgery like faster recovery, less pain, better cosmesis, and fewer wound complications, among others.

This chapter describes instrumentation in emergency abdominal conditions.

Indications of Emergency Laparoscopy

When considering the emergency settings, laparoscopy can be used in two ways.

Diagnostic

Disease and its severity are unknown and laparoscopy is mainly used as a diagnostic tool, like:

○ Pelvic inflammatory disease
○ Small bowel obstruction

*D. Lomanto, MD, PhD, FAMS (Surg), Department of Surgery, University Surgical Cluster, National University of Singapore; Minimally Invasive Surgery Centre, National University Hospital; and Khoo Teck Puat Advanced Surgery Training Centre, National University Hospital, Singapore.
**Department of Surgery, National University Hospital, Singapore.

○ Right lower quadrant pain and non-specific abdominal pain

The diagnostic rates of emergency diagnostic laparoscopic surgery are reported to be as high as 86–100% in unselected patients.

Therapeutic

Conditions where the diagnosis is confirmed and the role of laparoscopy is in performing the definitive therapeutic surgery, like:

○ Acute cholecystitis
○ Acute appendicitis
○ Perforated peptic ulcer
○ Acute diverticulitis

In the following sections, the role of laparoscopy will be evaluated in detail in individual emergency settings.

Instrumentation

The instruments and equipment required for emergency laparoscopic procedure can be divided into following groups:

○ Access and exposure
○ Procedure proper
○ Removal of specimen (if any)
○ Port closure

Instruments Required for Access and Exposure

1. Telescope

It is required to have 10 mm telescope of preferably 30° angles for proper exploration of whole of the abdomen. The 30° forward oblique permits far greater latitude for viewing underlying areas under difficult anatomical conditions. Today, high-definition (HD) telescope are available in the market and

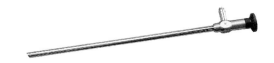

Figure 23.1.

30° telescope.

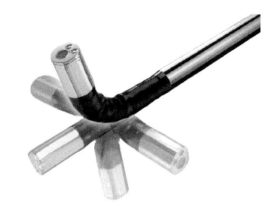

Figure 23.2.

0° Flexi-tip telescope.

utilising different technology, like full digital, where the CCD is mounted on the tip of the scope (Olympus HD EndoEYE™), or using the classical rod-lens system but with a HD camera device. The telescope comes in rigid shape (Fig. 23.1) or with a deflectable tip (Olympus LTH-VH or VP) (Fig. 23.2) to facilitate the surgical procedure. This sometimes requires additional expertise for the camera assistant for a full utilisation of the different features.

2. Light cable and light source

A high-performance halogen, xenon or newer L.E.D. light source with a fibre-optic cable to transmit the light from the light source to the telescope is required. At least a 300 watt xenon or equivalent halogen light source should be available in any O.R. with a spare system in reserve. Please note some of the commonly encountered light source problems and their simple remedies as follows:

Problem	Solution
Loose connection (source or scope)	Adjust connector
Poor vision with decreased light intensity	Go to "automatic" or increase "manual light intensity"
Bulb is burnt out	Replace bulb
Fibre optics are damaged	Replace light cable
Automatic iris adjusting to bright	Dim room lights
Reflection from instrument	Re-position instruments

3.   Endo-laparoscopic camera device or surgical imaging devices

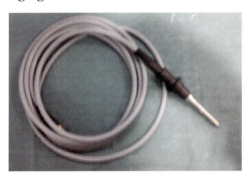

Figure 23.3.

Light Cable.

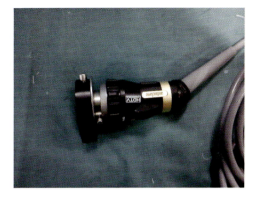

Figure 23.4.

Laparoscopic camera.

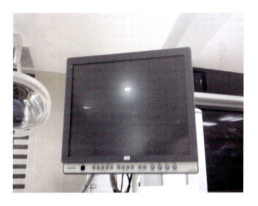

Figure 23.5.

High-definition monitor.

The endo-laparoscopic camera device is an important piece of equipment and should be of a very good quality. Cameras available today either have a single chip or three chips, both in standard or high-definition. Three-chip cameras have high horizontal image resolution of more than 750 lines. But today, we start to define these devices as imaging platforms or as surgical imaging devices since they allow different integration and usage. This system is fully integrated in a platform that allows simultaneous use of surgical endoscope and/or flexible endoscope if necessary, and is also integrated with digital recording device, additional LCDs, picture-in-picture option and other audio/video equipment in the O.R. For emergency exploration of the abdomen, it is recommended to have a high-definition imaging system that provides high-resolution imaging. Some imaging systems may have a narrow band Imaging (NBI) option and help the surgeon to differentiate benign conditions from neoplasm.

To get the best out of a laparoscopic camera, it is important to focus the camera before entering the abdomen. The scope fitted with the camera needs to be placed at a distance of approximately 5 cm away from the target. This is because during laparoscopic surgery, we keep the telescope at this distance most of the time.

It is also essential to perform white balancing before inserting camera inside the abdominal cavity. This is required for optimising the image colours.

A video management or recording system for storage of images and videos should be available. The storage of still pictures and videos is an important and powerful source of material for teaching and education. A review of the video with expert colleagues may be helpful to redeem and confirm our diagnosis in uncertain and doubtful situations. Recording devices today utilise mainly digital storage like DVD or hard disk, and the latest technology allows file-sharing within the hospital network.

4. Monitor

The image shown on the monitor depends upon the number of lines of resolution, scanning lines, pixels and dot pitch. Pixels denote the picture elements and are responsible for picture detail. The greater the number of pixels, the better the detail. High-resolution "medical" monitors (HD monitor) display colours more accurately and are a must in emergency settings. In term of size, at least a 22–26" HD monitor should be utilised to obtain sharp and good quality images.

5. Insufflator

Controlled pressure insufflation of the abdomen is required to achieve adequate working space. For this purpose, automatic insufflators are required. Carbon dioxide is the preferred gas because it does not support combustion, it is very soluble, reducing the risk of gas embolism, and it is cheap. Today, it is preferable to have a high-flow insufflator where the insufflation volume can go up to 15–20 L per minute. This allows a prompt recovery of the pneumoperitoneum in case of frequent use of suction. The device should allow an intra-abdominal pressure ranging between 0 and 30 mmHg. To ensure patient safety, there are optical and acoustic alarms as well as several mutually independent safety circuits. It is important to ensure that the CO_2 cylinder has adequate gas as may be required, tubings are connected properly and pressure and safety settings are set accordingly. Filtering or heating the CO_2 is optional and has not shown advantages in clinical practice. A preferred pressure between 12 and 14 mmHg is suggested even though in specific situations a lower (hypercarbia) or higher pressure (obese) may be needed. It is always suggested to start with low insufflations (1–2 L X min) to avoid a rapid expansion of the diaphragm with eventual vagal stimulation.

Below is a simple diagram on how to connect the different endo-laparoscopic devices with or without recording system and additional monitors.

6. Hasson trocar/Veress needle

In an emergency setting, access to the peritoneal cavity is made usually by open (Hasson's) technique to avoid any inadvertent injury. This is a very safe technique for entering the abdomen, especially in patients with multiple previous surgeries or in some emergency patients where underlying intra-abdominal disease may be hidden in dangerous situations. It is performed in an area of the abdomen distant from

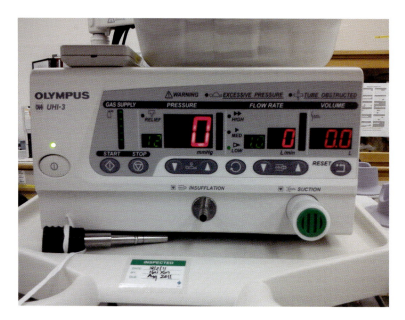

Figure 23.6.

High-flow laparoscopic insufflators.

Table 23.1.   The Diagram Shows the Most Common Way to Connect Different Surgical Devices With or Without Recording

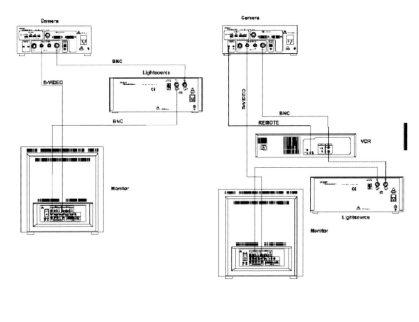

SYSTEM 1

Equipment Used: Camera, Light Source and Monitor

SYSTEM 2

Equipment Used: Camera, Light Source, Video Peripheral and Monitor. The video peripheral may be a video printer, digital capture, Hermes or VCR.

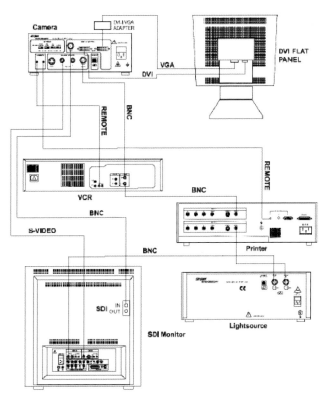

SYSTEM 3

Equipment Used: Camera, Light Source, Stryker Printer, Stryker VCR, SDI Monitor, DVI Flat Panel.

previous scars. Usually the peri-umbilical area is preferred. However the umbilicus may be used in patients who are cosmetically concerned. A 1 cm horizontal incision is made. Blunt dissection is carried out until the underlying fascia is identified. The fascia, muscle and peritoneum are incised under direct vision. Two heavy, absorbable sutures are placed on either side of the fascial incision, and these are then utilised for closure. Care must be taken when applying these sutures not to injure the underlying viscera. A 10 mm blunt trocar is advanced into the peritoneal cavity. The obturator is removed and the sleeve is secured in position with the previously placed two sutures. The Hasson trocar can be reusable or disposable, and the length can be adjusted to obtain a good access and view.

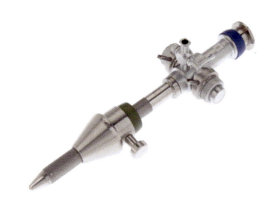

Figure 23.7.

Hasson trocar.

Figure 23.8.

Veress needle.

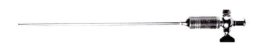

Occasionally, closed (Veress needle) technique may be used where acute bowel obstruction is not suspected to be the cause. In such cases, the Veress needle is inserted at Palmer's point (left subcostal) or the epigastric region where the least chance of intra-abdominal adhesion has been reported.

Instruments Required for Procedure Proper

1. 5 and 10–12 mm ports (3)

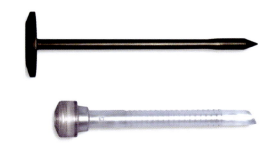

Figure 23.9.

5 mm trocar with cannula.

The use of trocars and cannulas is the first step in any laparoscopic surgery, and the surgeon should be extremely cautious. When placing the trocars and cannulas in an emergency setting where the bowel is dilated, insertion should be done under direct vision.

2. Endo-dissector

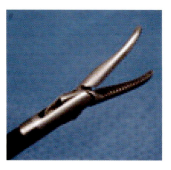

Figure 23.10.

Maryland endo dissector.

The endo dissector is a very important laparoscopic instrument both in elective and in emergency settings. It can be straight or curved, and the choice is made upon situation. It is very useful in cases of fine dissection or isolation of small structures like arteries, veins, ducts, etc. and before clipping and sectioning of them. It is very useful in cases of cholecystectomy, appendectomy, biopsies or any in other disease where fine and blunt dissection is required. The surgeons should be aware of the potential injury caused by inadvertent use.

3.   Atraumatic and traumatic grasper

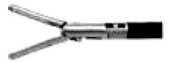

Figure 23.11.

Graspers.

Endolaparoscopic Graspers are atraumatic or traumatic. Atraumatic graspers are used to do bowel mapping during emergency surgeries with minimal trauma to minimise serosal tears and also help during bowel anastomosis. The diameter can be between 5 and 10 mm with and without a hatch. They are utilised mainly to manipulate healthy or inflamed tissue without causing serosal injuries. An atraumatic grasper is an important instrument for providing counter-traction during dissection or for retraction to explore and expose, i.e. pelvic anatomy or to "run" the small bowel.

In difficult situations as such hydrops, sclerotic or acute inflamed gallbladder or ovary, a so-called "traumatic" toothed grasper is very useful for holding or retracting the organ.

4.   Endo scissors are straight or curved (Fig. 23.12)

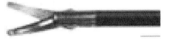

Figure 23.12.

Endo scissors.

5.   Endo-Babcock forceps

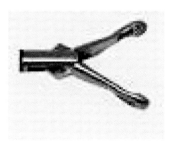

Figure 23.13.

Endo-Babcock forceps.

Endo-Babcock forceps (Fig. 23.13) are used to hold bowel and mesentery during bowel retraction and approximation for anastomosis.

6.   Laparoscopic needle holder (Fig. 23.14)

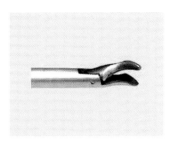

Figure 23.14.

Needle holder.

7.   Suction and irrigation cannula

Every emergency surgery should have a suction and irrigation cannula for peritoneal lavage and haemostasis (Fig. 23.15). It is a very important device in emergency surgery when there is much intra-abdominal bleeding. It is useful to have both a 5 and 10 mm cannula to exchange in case suction of large clots is necessary. This device is also useful in water-dissection in acute cholecystitis or acutely inflamed pelvic disorders where a careful dissection of adhesion is necessary.

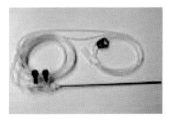

Figure 23.15.

Suction and irrigation cannula.

8.   Liver retractor (e.g. Nathanson, snake or fan retractor) (Fig. 23.16)

A liver retractor is an important instrument for emergency and bariatric emergency surgeries where liver retraction is of utmost importance. In case of duodenal perforation and right kidney injury, it is very

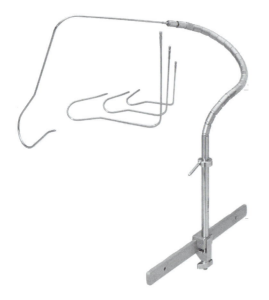

Figure 23.16.

Nathanson liver retractor.

important to retract the liver adequately for good exposure. The retractor is also useful for retracting large loops of intestine in case of exploration of the retroperitoneal area.

9. Endo-diathermy hook

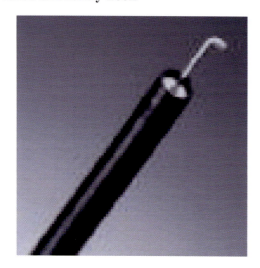

Figure 23.17.

Endo-diathermy hook.

Endo-diathermy hook (Fig. 23.17) is needed for haemostasis and for coagulation, but also for dissection of inflamed adhesion. Cholecystectomy and appendectomy are the most common procedures where the hook is utilised for dissection of the Calot's triangle or isolation of the appendicular vessel. Spreading of the thermal energy should be taken into account in case of continuous use of the hook.

10. UltraCision® harmonic scalpel

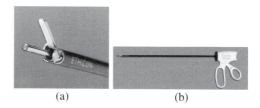

(a)   (b)

Figure 23.18.

Harmonic scalpel.

The harmonic scalpel is a cutting instrument used during emergency surgical procedures to simultaneously cut and coagulate tissue (Fig. 23.18).

11. Laparoscopic staplers with different types of cartridges (optional)

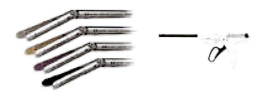

Figure 23.19.

Laparoscopic stapler with cartridges.

Linear endostaplers are sophisticated instruments for sealing and sectioning organs like bowel, liver, tube, etc. (Fig. 23.19). Reusable cartridges come in different colours and are available for the surgeons who should be aware of the different usage and familiar with the device itself before handling it. Normally a white cartridge is used for vascular sealing while a blue one is for small intestine sealing and cutting as in appendectomy or Meckel's diverticulum or small bowel resection. Green cartridges are mainly utilised for gastric tissue like antral resection for perforation or simple gastric closure. The device can be straight or articulated, allowing the surgeon to reach difficult areas. Indications for staplers in laparoscopy include necrotising appendicitis at base, where the endostapler can be used simultaneously to staple the meso-appendix and appendix, for bowel anastomosis and for revisional bariatric surgeries.

12. End loop

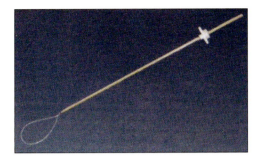

Figure 23.20.

Endo loop.

The endo loop is a premade knot of different suture material, either absorbable or non-absorbable. They are very useful in laparoscopic surgery and often utilised during an emergency. Endo loop indications include acute appendicitis to ligate the base of appendix; a large cystic duct during cholecystectomy and an irreducible inguinal hernia to seal peritoneum during total extra peritoneal or intra-abdominal repair. In some situations, it can be utilised to hold and retract an organ that is difficult to be retracted with a simple grasper.

Instruments for Removal of Specimen

Endobag

These are specially designed to isolate and remove the specimens like inflamed gall bladder, appendix and others so as to avoid spillage/contamination inside the peritoneal cavity and abdominal wall.

Instruments for Port Closure

Fascia closure needle

This is a specially designed instrument for closing ports more than 10 mm in size to avoid the risk of subsequent port site hernia formation.

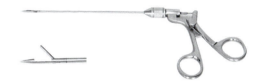

Figure 23.21.

Fascia closure needle.

Patient Position and O.T. Setup

Emergency laparoscopy requires much more expertise than elective laparoscopy, both because of undiagnosed pathology and also a less optimised patient. Surgeons need to be familiar with instruments and need to know how to make better use of each one. From a diagnostic laparoscopy to an emergency perforated ulcer in the posterior aspect of the stomach or a large bowel perforation experience, expertise and available equipment can make a big difference in the surgical outcome of the patients. All

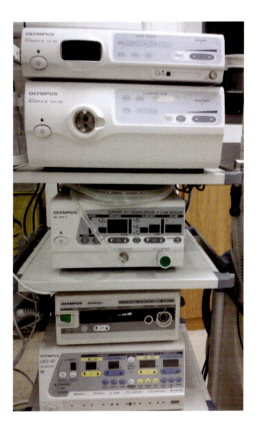

Figure 23.22.

Laparoscopic trolley.

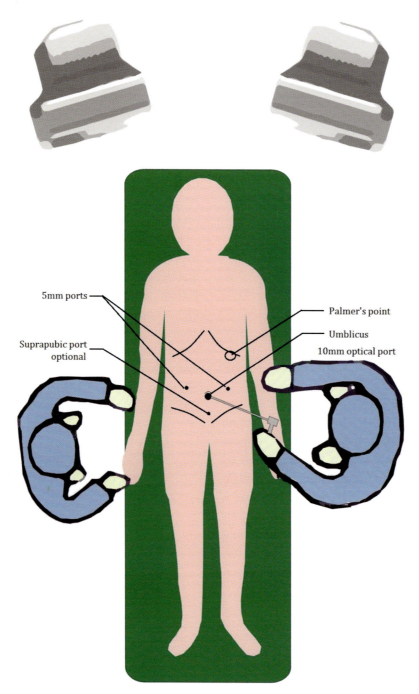

Figure 23.23.

O.T. setup.

patients should be haemodynamically optimised before surgery. It is preferable to have a hydraulic operating table which can be easily tilted in various positions as may be required during surgery. The patient is made to lie supine with legs straight in a 15° Trendlenburg position. Foley's urinary and Ryle's nasogastric tube decompression is done. The surgeon stands on the either side of the patient depending on the suspected pathology, with camera operator on the opposite side. The final position of the operating team will depend upon the nature of pathology detected.

After creating pneumoperitoneum, all the quadrants of abdomen are explored systematically beginning in the right lower quadrant. This is followed by exploration of the pelvis and the supracolic compartment, thus determining the abdominal pathology and its extent.

Dissection, Retraction and Haemostasis

Dissection may be defined as separation of tissues with meticulous haemostasis with no inadvertent damage to surrounding tissues. This usually requires a two-handed approach: one assisting and one dissecting. Part of the training of laparoscopic surgeons should be finalised to make both dominant and non-dominant hands have the same power. In laparoscopic surgery, the non-dominant hand is the best assistant, working together with the dominant in retracting and exposing tissue and organs. The assisting instrument hand provides counter-traction for the active dissecting hand. The active instrument may be non-energised (e.g. scissors and scalpel) or energised with electricity (diathermy) or ultrasonic energy.

- Blunt dissection

This is usually achieved with the help of instruments like a Maryland dissector, closed scissor tips or suction cannula. Blunt dissection is safe and is used to open planes and expose structures, especially when the anatomy is obscured by adhesions. The movement consists of forward and backward wipes accompanied by clockwise/counter-clockwise rotation of instruments. It is very important to use a combination of traumatic grasper and dissector to achieve the clearing of the desired area.

- Sharp dissection

Scissor dissection offers the benefits of giving a precise operator determined action. However, as it is a non-haemostatic approach, it needs precise usage to prevent haemorrhage and inadvertent division of blood vessels. It should be done only in safer areas where the chance to encounter hollow viscus or vessels is nil or minimal.

- Electrosurgical dissection

It is used to coagulate, fulgurate; spray coagulates or ablates tissue by using different energy sources. It can be either in the form of monopolar or bipolar diathermy or other newer alternative sources.

What is commonly used is a monopolar device attached to diathermy instrument like the "L"-shaped hook (Fig. 23.16). It is frequently utilised for dissection and ablation like cholecystectomy, oophorectomy, appendectomy, etc. However the diathermy can be attached to other dissecting hand instruments like the grasper (Fig. 23.9), dissector (Fig. 23.10) and scissors (Fig. 23.11), as mentioned above. Bipolar energy is mainly utilised for gynaecological procedure and in any surgical situation where the surgeon prefers an accurate sealing and reduced spread of the thermal energy.

When using any energy devices, we should always keep in mind the risk of complications derived by their wrong utilisation, such as: lack of insulation of the instruments, indirect contact with adjacent structure, inadvertent activation, and close proximity with other instruments, high-voltage setting, etc.

Alternative energy devices widely utilised today in surgical practice are:

- Ultrasonic dissection (e.g. Harmonic Scalpel, Johnson & Johnson USA; Sonosurg, Olympus, Japan; etc.)

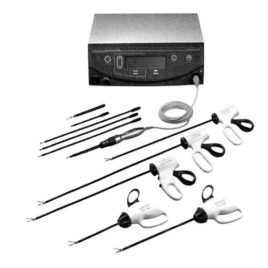

Figure 23.24.

Harmonic scalpel, Johnson & Johnson USA.

This is a unique form of energy utilising ultrasound waves (Fig. 23.24), allowing both cutting and coagulation at the precise point of impact with minimal lateral thermal spreading. This allows dissection with coagulation and cutting with less smoke and no electrical current. It is ideal for dividing and simultaneously sealing small and medium size vessels by tamponade and heat.

- Tissue response generator (Fig. 23.25) (Ligasure™, Force Triad™, Covidien , USA)

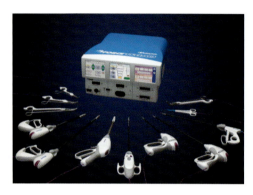

Figure 23.25.

Force Triad™, Covidien, USA.

This system has a high-current, low-voltage output generator that provides an excellent sealing of vessels up to 7 mm in diameter. It recognises changes in tissue and automatically adjusts the voltage and the current in order to achieve the adequate sealing effect. The tissue response generator has a unique tissue sealing ability with significantly reduced thermal spread as compared to a bipolar device. The seal mechanism senses the body's collagen and actually changes the nature of the vessel walls by obliterating the lumen. The collagen and elastin within the tissue melt and reform to create the seal zone.

- High-velocity and high-pressure water-jet dissection/hydrodissection

This uses the force of irrigation with clear solutions to separate tissue planes. However no haemostasis is achieved by these methods and hence their use is limited. But such methods are extremely useful in severe and dense adhesion as can be encountered in acute gallbladder, ovary torsion, endometriosis, etc. A combination of powerful hydrojet and suction can be useful to isolate structures and clear anatomy.

- Laser dissection

This is rarely used as it has no advantage over more easily available and user-friendly devices.

Suggested Reading

- MacFayden B. (2004) *Laparoscopic Sutregry of the Abdomen.* Springer-Verlag, New York.
- Neugebauer EAM, Sauerland S, Fingerhut A, *et al.* eds. (2006) *EAES Guidelines for Endoscopic Surgery.* Springer, Berlin; New York.
- Kriplani A, Bhatia P, Prasad A, *et al.* eds. (2007) *Comprehensive Laparoscopic Surgery.* IAGES.
- Oshinsky GS, Smith Ad. (1992) Laparoscopic needle and trocars: an overview of design and complications. *J Laparosc Surg* **5**:37–40.
- Zucker KA. (2001) *Surgical Laparoscopy*, USA 2nd ed. Quality Medical Pu, St Louis, MO.
- *The SAGES Manual.* (2005) Springer, New York.
- Tucker RD, Voyles CR. (1995) Laparoscopic electrosurguical complications and their prevention. *AORN J* **62**:51–3.
- Lomanto D, Cheah WK eds. (2009) Manual of Endo-laparoscopic and Single Port Surgery. 2nd ed.

Index